Psychosocial Interventions for Chronic Illness

An Avenue to Psychological Well-Being

Psychosocial Interventions for Chronic Illness

An Avenue to Psychological Well-Being

Editors

Piyanee Klainin-Yobas
National University of Singapore, Singapore

Mary Jeanette Ignacio
National University of Singapore, Singapore

Nopporn Vongsirimas
Mahidol University, Thailand

World Scientific

NEW JERSEY • LONDON • SINGAPORE • BEIJING • SHANGHAI • HONG KONG • TAIPEI • CHENNAI • TOKYO

Published by

World Scientific Publishing Co. Pte. Ltd.
5 Toh Tuck Link, Singapore 596224
USA office: 27 Warren Street, Suite 401-402, Hackensack, NJ 07601
UK office: 57 Shelton Street, Covent Garden, London WC2H 9HE

Library of Congress Control Number: 2025032524

British Library Cataloguing-in-Publication Data
A catalogue record for this book is available from the British Library.

PSYCHOSOCIAL INTERVENTIONS FOR CHRONIC ILLNESS
An Avenue to Psychological Well-Being

ISBN 978-981-98-1731-3 (hardcover)
ISBN 978-981-98-1732-0 (ebook for institutions)
ISBN 978-981-98-1733-7 (ebook for individuals)

For any available supplementary material, please visit
https://www.worldscientific.com/worldscibooks/10.1142/14420#t=suppl

Desk Editor: Shaun Tan Yi Jie

Typeset by Stallion Press
Email: enquiries@stallionpress.com

https://doi.org/10.1142/9789819817320_fmatter

About the Editors

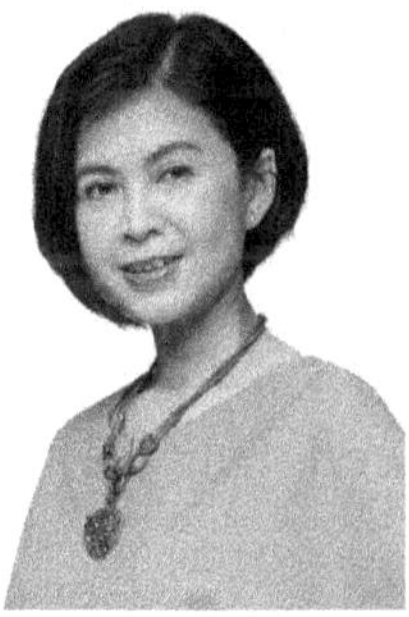

Dr Piyanee Klainin-Yobas is an Associate Professor at the Alice Lee Centre for Nursing Studies, Yong Loo Lin School of Medicine, National University of Singapore, Singapore. She holds a PhD in Nursing from Case Western Reserve University, USA. Her research interests encompass stress and health; mindfulness-based interventions for people with chronic illness and mental disorders; as well as psychosocial interventions for people with chronic illness and mental disorders. She has over 100 peer-reviewed publications, with a h-index of 46.

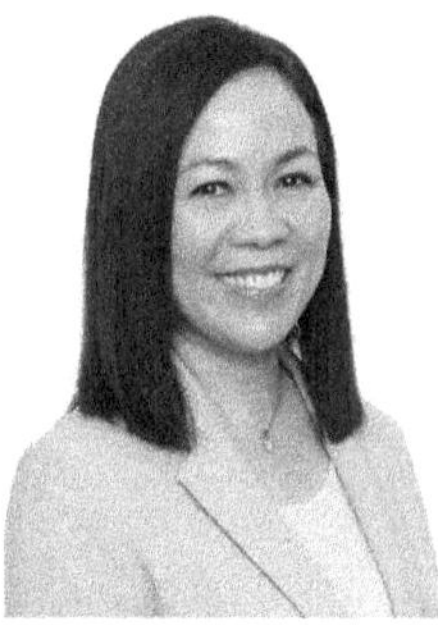

Dr Mary Jeanette Ignacio is an Associate Professor at the Alice Lee Centre for Nursing Studies, Yong Loo Lin School of Medicine, National University of Singapore, Singapore, where she is concurrently Director for the Year 1 Undergraduate Programme. She holds a PhD in Health Professions Education from Maastricht University, The Netherlands. She was one of the first few to utilize high-fidelity simulations in her pedagogy, and has been invited to conduct simulation workshops locally and internationally, such as in Hong Kong, Japan,

Thailand and the Philippines. She has also published simulation-related research in high impact peer-reviewed journals and has presented her research findings in reputable international medical, nursing and health professions education conferences in Europe and the United States. She has received the Yong Loo Lin School of Medicine's Teaching Excellence Award twice.

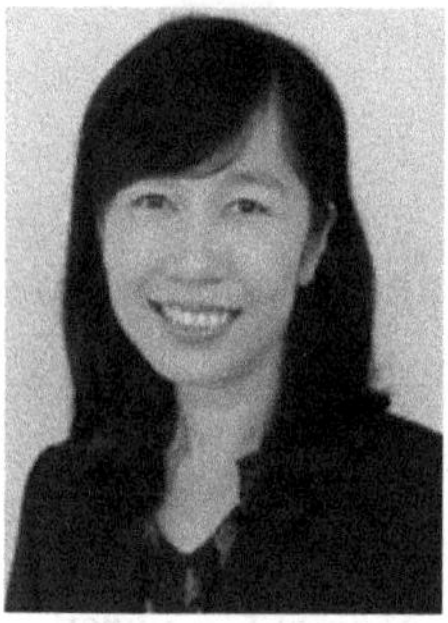

Dr Nopporn Vongsirimas is an Associate Professor at the Department of Mental Health and Psychiatric Nursing, Faculty of Nursing, Mahidol University, Thailand, where she is concurrently Head of Department. She holds a PhD in Nursing from Mahidol University, Thailand. Her clinical specialties are in depression in adolescents and women, while her research interests are in depressive symptoms in adolescents of depressed mothers and their psychosocial interventions.

https://doi.org/10.1142/9789819817320_fmatter

Preface

Chronic illness, with its lingering duration and profound impact, has emerged as one of the health challenges for global sustainable development. Regardless of its form–cardiovascular disease, diabetes, cancer, or enduring neurological problems–chronic illness extends far beyond the boundaries of biopathology. It reaches the fabric of daily living, emotions, relationships, motivation, and the sense of self. Chronic illness has created the intricate web of experiences that trigger the needs of psychosocial interventions.

The motivation for this book, *Psychosocial Interventions for Chronic Illness*, arises from the recognition that optimal healthcare requires more than physical treatments. While advances in modern technology and pharmacology continue to alleviate clinical symptoms and to prolong longevity, many individuals struggle with the psychosocial burdens of chronic disease — fear, hopelessness, stress, anxiety, and depression. The trajectory of chronic illness is not merely a physiological ordeal. Rather, individuals' emotions, coping strategies, relationships, and societal contexts all play critical roles in shaping health outcomes.

Psychosocial interventions, encompassing a diverse spectrum of therapeutic modalities (such as stress management, cognitive-behavioural therapy, and mindfulness-based interventions), have demonstrated their value in the healthcare arena. Psychosocial interventions serve as central pillars in the pursuit of psychological well-being. By offering structured guidance and the cultivation of coping skills, such interventions empower individuals to navigate the psychological complexities of chronic illness and reclaim a sense of self over their own health journeys. Ultimately, they illuminate an avenue toward comprehensive healing and psychological well-being.

Empirical evidence has provided solid support on the efficacy of psychosocial interventions in improving mental health, reducing stress, and enhancing well-being among people with chronic conditions. Mindfulness-based intervention appears to cultivate self-awareness, emotion regulation, and thought management skills amidst the adversity. Cognitive-behavioural strategies empower individuals to reframe unhelpful thoughts and behaviours, mitigating the impact of depression and anxiety. Positive psychology approach helps illuminate individuals' strength and intrinsic capability to thrive. The ripple effect of these interventions extends to families and caregivers, whose well-being is inextricably linked to people's experiences.

This book offers an exploration of theoretical frameworks and empirical evidence concerning psychosocial interventions. The first section introduces theoretical foundations and the psychological well-being promotion model that we created to guide our own research and clinical practice. The second section emphasises how psychosocial interventions can be implemented to promote health outcomes among healthy and at-risk individuals. The third section illuminates evidence-based psychosocial interventions for clinicians, researchers, and policymakers, while centring the experiences of people affected by chronic illness. We explore the nuances of delivering attuned care, leveraging technology for remote interventions, and addressing the unique needs of diverse populations.

It is our hope that this book will serve as a catalyst for incorporating psychosocial programs into routine chronic illness management. We hope to inspire healthcare professionals to envision the person behind the patient, and to offer interventions that fit the full complexity of clients' experience. In doing so, we can help foster a healthcare culture where every individual's psychological well-being is valued and upheld.

Piyanee Klainin-Yobas, PhD, RN
Alice Lee Centre for Nursing Studies,
Yong Loo Lin School of Medicine
National University of Singapore

https://doi.org/10.1142/9789819817320_fmatter

Contents

Section Three: Evidence-Based Psychosocial Interventions for Chronic Conditions

https://doi.org/10.1142/9789819817320_0001

Chapter 1

Psychosocial Interventions in Healthcare

Piyanee Klainin-Yobas[1,*] and Dhananja Kaushalya[2]

[1]*Alice Lee Centre for Nursing Studies, Yong Loo Lin School of Medicine, National University of Singapore, Level 5, Centre of Translational Medicine, Block MD6, 14 Medical Drive, Singapore 117599*

[2]*Illangasinghe Estate and Urban Health Unit, Ministry of Health and Mass Media, Sri Lanka*

**Corresponding author: nurpk@nus.edu.sg*

Psychosocial interventions have been implemented by healthcare professionals to help individuals achieve optimal physical health and psychological well-being. This chapter begins with defining and describing psychosocial interventions, providing a list of psychosocial interventions, and elaborating common ones, including cognitive-behavioural interventions, stress management, motivational interviewing and positive psychology. Psychosocial interventions can be integrated into healthcare in three levels: primary, secondary and tertiary interventions. The applications of psychosocial interventions on chronic illness are also provided with the focus on cardiovascular diseases, diabetes mellitus and cancer.

1.1 Definition of Psychosocial Interventions

According to the World Health Organization (WHO), health is a state of complete physical, mental and social well-being, not merely the absence of disease or infirmity [1]. Furthermore, there is a link between physical and mental health. Evidence suggests that people with chronic illnesses (such as cardiovascular diseases, metabolic disorders, cancer, and chronic kidney diseases) experience different psychological symptoms including stress, depression and anxiety [2].

Psychosocial interventions refer to evidence-based treatments with psychological and social elements to enhance individuals' psychological well-being, resilience, coping mechanisms, and social interconnections [3]. They take into consideration biological, behavioural, cognitive, emotional, interpersonal, social and environmental factors for improving health and well-being [3]. Psychosocial interventions entail different elements, such as psychosocial support, social support, skill training and empowerment [3]. Unlike biomedical treatments, psychosocial interventions address mental, emotional, and social aspects comprehensively.

WHO [4] recommended different psychosocial interventions for different mental health disorders. Specifically, cognitive behavioural therapy (CBT) is recommended for people with epilepsy, depression, bipolar disorders, anxiety, acute traumatic symptoms, attention deficit hyperactive disorder, dementia, and substance abuse, among others. Other recommended psychological treatments encompass behavioural activation/intervention, social skills training, cognitive stimulation therapy, cognitive training, contingency management therapy, eye movement desensitisation and reprocessing, motivational enhancement therapy, and stress management, among others. Additionally, the third wave of therapies have been well-known. These therapies entail mindfulness-based interventions, acceptance and commitment therapy, metacognitive therapy, and dialectical behavioural therapy.

Psychosocial interventions can be delivered in individual, group and self-help formats [4]. The individual interventions allow the opportunity to build rapport between a client and healthcare provider, to share personal and sensitive information, and to ascertain confidentiality [4]. However, this intervention format requires more manpower and other resources. Group interventions involve one or two healthcare providers hosting multiple clients at the same time, which is considered less resource-intensive [4]. The group format permits group members to share experiences, validate feelings and support each other during the sessions. However, the arrangement of multiple members can be challenging and ensuring confidentiality can be harder, in comparison to individual intervention. For self-help interventions, clients access the interventions by themselves or with the assistance of healthcare providers. The former is called "unguided self-help" and the latter "guided self-help" [4]. Additionally, psychosocial interventions can be delivered face-to-face or via technology platforms such as websites, virtual reality, augmented reality, mixed reality, mobile applications and artificial intelligence.

1.2 Major Theories Adapted in Psychosocial Interventions

This section describes psychosocial interventions that are frequently used in healthcare, encompassing CBT, stress management interventions, motivational interviewing and positive psychology.

1.2.1 *Cognitive Behavioural Therapy*

CBT has been effective for various psychosocial problems including depression, anxiety, alcohol and drug addiction, marital problems, and eating disorders [5, 6]. A systematic review [7], involving 45 randomised controlled trials (RCTs), suggested that CBT was effective in improving physical conditions (such as chronic fatigue syndrome, fibromyalgia, irritable bowel syndrome, and cancer), mental health problems (such as depression, anxiety, eating disorders, and attention deficit disorder) and behavioural problems (such as substance abuse, gambling, smoking, overweight, and antisocial behaviours). Short-term effects of CBT were reported in most RCTs. Long-term effects of CBT were positive, yet with limited evidence [7].

CBT was derived from Aaron Beck's model of cognitive therapy [8]. CBT postulates that individuals' cognition influences their emotional reactions and behaviours. Within CBT, irrational thoughts commonly contribute to various psychological disturbances, including depression. However, when people learn to reconstruct their thoughts, they will experience less negative emotions and less maladaptive behaviours [8]. CBT's main therapeutic goals are in identifying and rectifying irrational thoughts, thus achieving better psychological outcomes. CBT therapists utilise different techniques, encompassing Socratic questioning, cognitive restructuring, behavioural activation, skill building, exposure therapy, among others [8]. *Socratic questioning* involves the use of probing questions to explore and challenge irrational thoughts and beliefs. *Cognitive restructuring* helps identify irrational thoughts and replace them with positive ones. *Behavioural activation* refers to encouraging individuals to engage in positive activities to improve emotions and normal functions.

CBT treatment requires a sound therapeutic relationship. A collaborative effort between a therapist and client is required to develop an understanding of a problem and to establish a treatment strategy [9]. CBT is educational and clients learn through exercises during therapeutic sessions, and "homework" exercises outside of the sessions. The clients are to develop coping skills, where they can learn to change their own thinking, problematic emotions, and behaviour [9]. CBT therapists point out what is going on in the person's current life, rather than past difficulties [9]. Though this method needs a certain amount of information about one's history, the focus is primarily on moving forward in time to develop more effective ways of coping with life.

1.2.2 *Stress Management*

Stress is a fact of life, especially in the modern world of ongoing demands and dramatic changes. The stress management theory envisions stress as the body's response to undesirable situations [10]. With this theory, stress can be a positive motivator if it is well-managed. Otherwise, excessive and/or unmanaged stress can trigger physical conditions, psychological problems, job dissatisfaction and decreased projectivity [10]. Stress management refers to strategies for managing stress so as to prevent negative consequences on health and to achieve optimal well-being [10].

Stress management is relevant to healthy individuals and people with chronic illnesses. A systematic review involving 46 studies was conducted to test the effects of different stress management programs on college students. Results indicated that stress management reduced stress, psychological distress, depression and anxiety [11]. Furthermore, *CBT-based interventions* (stress inoculation and cognitive restructuring), *third-wave intervention* (mindfulness-based stress reduction) and *mind-body interventions* (meditation, muscle relaxation, breathing exercise, guided imaginary, and biofeedback) show greater effects than skill training programs [11]. Stress management can be delivered face-to-face and/or via technology platforms. Another systematic review [12] examined 150 studies that utilised stress management applications. Results indicated that most studies (n = 121) utilised a "*personalisation strategy*", interventions that were tailored to participants' personal profiles (such as demographic and clinical data). Some studies (n = 77) used "*self-monitoring*" that encouraged users to record their health condition and activities. Other stress management apps used *simulation* (n = 43), *tailoring* (n = 32), *rehearsal* (n = 14), *reduction* (n = 12) and *tunnelling* (n = 11) [12].

1.2.3 *Motivational Interview*

People with chronic conditions and mental disorders are required to modify their behaviours and lifestyle to achieve positive health outcomes. Motivational interviewing (MI) is based on the assumption that individuals have the motivation to change. However, such motivation may ebb and flow during their journey to recovery [13]. MI is a patient-centred method for promoting behavioural changes among clients, especially those with chronic illnesses. MI can be implemented in many healthcare settings and other environments to foster improved health practices in challenging situations. By using principles of therapeutic communication, a health professional can act as a coach for patients to help them make better health choices. MI is a collaborative process that edifies patients and encourages them to make responsible decisions with regard to behavioural choices. A systematic review and meta-analysis revealed that MI significantly improved willingness to change, treatment adherence, physical activity, dental hygiene, alcohol consumption and weight reduction [14].

There are four basic principles of MI: Express empathy, develop discrepancy, roll with resistance, and support self-efficacy [15]. During the healing process, the therapist needs to *express empathy* and understand the world of the clients with a non-judgemental attitude and without harsh criticisms [15]. The therapist uses active listening, validates the clients' experiences, refrains from confrontation and blame, and encourages open communication. *Develop discrepancy* reflects the therapist's ability to help the clients see the gap between their goals and current behaviours [15]. As an example, a client wishes to be a healthy person but he smokes two packs of cigarettes per day. The therapist helps the client enhance his intrinsic motivation and find the reasons to change his behaviour (such as quit smoking). Sustainable changes usually come from intrinsic motivation, rather than external forces. Furthermore, resistance and ambivalence are considered normal and expected during the change process. The therapist *rolls with resistance* and uses it as a tool to further explore the client's internal experiences. Finally, self-efficacy reflects individuals' belief that they can modify and sustain a behavioural change. The therapist *supports self-efficacy* by using empowering statements, affirming the client's strengths, pointing out past successes, and encouraging hope [15].

1.2.4 *Positive Psychology*

Traditional psychosocial interventions generally focus on the "disease model", addressing psychopathology such as stress, depression, anxiety, aggression, violence and addiction. On the contrary, positive psychology emphasises human flourishing and a path to well-being. The positive psychology model (PERMA) postulates that humans innately avoid danger, loss and injustice; nevertheless, they have the potential to grow and to achieve well-being [16]. Within the PERMA model, well-being comprises five major elements: positive emotions, engagement, relationships, meaning and accomplishment [17]. *Positive emotions* encompass various positive experiences such as contentment, happiness and satisfaction. *Engagement* reflects how individuals are in the flow and being consumed in various activities in their surroundings. *Relationships* refer to both quantity and quality of social connections within family and community. *Meaning* reflects a sense of purpose in individuals' lives. Lastly, *accomplishment* is linked with successful progression toward individuals' goals. A systematic review [18] was conducted using 347 studies with more than 72,000 participants from clinical and non-clinical settings in 41 countries. Results suggested that positive psychology interventions had significant small to medium effects on quality of life ($g = 0.48$), well-being ($g = 0.39$), strengths ($g = 0.46$), stress ($g = -0.58$), depression ($g = -0.39$) and anxiety ($g = -0.62$).

1.3 Integration of Psychosocial Interventions in Healthcare

Psychosocial interventions can be applied to many occasions in healthcare, including primary, secondary and tertiary care. Firstly, they can be used to promote healthy behaviours and to mitigate risk factors related to chronic diseases, such as hypertension, hyperglycaemia, and hyperlipidaemia. Secondly, psychosocial interventions can be offered to people with chronic diseases, such as cardiovascular disease, diabetes, cancers, chronic kidney diseases and mental disorders. Psychosocial interventions can be complementary with medications and other biological treatments.

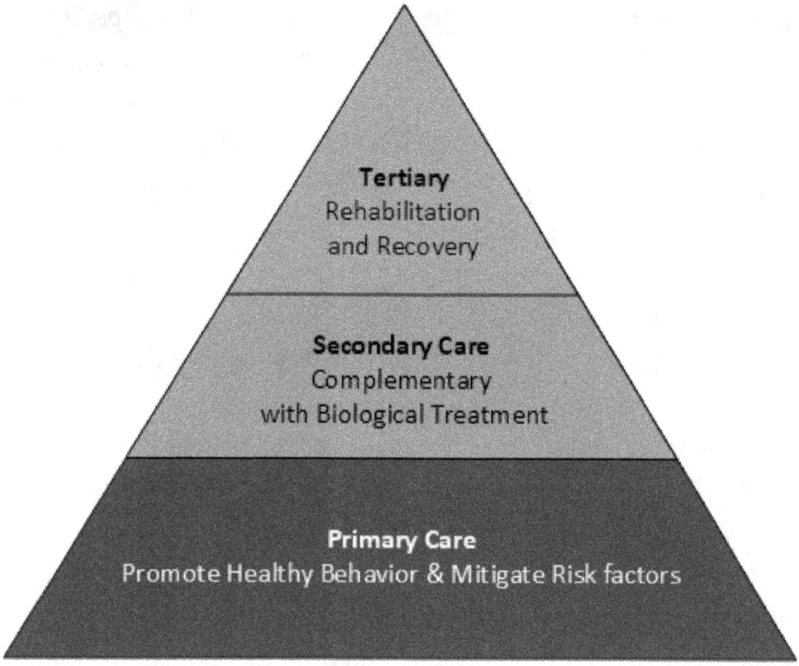

Figure 1.1 Levels of psychosocial interventions in the journey of chronic illness in healthcare.

The integrated model of biological and psychosocial care can be implemented by healthcare professionals in hospital settings. Thirdly, the psychosocial interventions come into action at a tertiary level of prevention. They can be integrated into rehabilitation and recovery care for people with chronic illnesses.

All these levels of psychosocial interventions can be integrated together to achieve a common goal at an individual or community level. The integrations also cater to different levels of the chronic illness (Figure 1.1).

1.4 Psychosocial Interventions for Chronic Illness

Chronic illnesses (or non-communicable diseases) refer to long-term medical conditions resulting from biological, behavioural and environmental factors [19]. Chronic illnesses are commonly associated with individuals' sociological status. Specifically, people with lower sociological classes tend to have poorer health. They are more likely to use harmful products (such as tobacco), consume unhealthy diets, and have limited access to health services [19]. In low-resource settings, healthcare costs for chronic illnesses quickly drain household resources. Direct and indirect costs of illnesses, including expensive treatments in combination with the loss of income, force millions of people into poverty annually. Ultimately, poverty may lead to psychological pain, frustration and hopelessness among people with chronic illnesses [19].

1.4.1 *Psychosocial Interventions for Cardiovascular Diseases*

Psychosocial interventions play an essential role in the recovery and management of individuals with different cardiovascular diseases. Among patients with chronic heart failure, a systematic review of 16 RCTs indicated that psychosocial interventions improved quality of life with a small effect size (SMD = 0.46) [20]. Traditional face-to-face interventions had larger intervention effects than telephone interventions [20]. Furthermore, interventions delivered by multidisciplinary teams tended to be more effective than those by non-multidisciplinary approaches [20]. A systematic review involving 1,358 participants examined the effects of psychosocial interventions for patients with coronary heart diseases with depression [21]. The interventions encompassed CBT, interpersonal therapy, and counselling delivered via face-to-face or telephone. Results suggested that the intervention significantly decreased depressive symptoms (SMD = −0.15), social support (SMD = 0.17), and quality of life [21].

For people with different cardiovascular diseases, another systematic review (involving 30 studies) examined the effectiveness of psychosocial interventions on health outcomes [22]. Specifically, psychoeducation programs and stress management reduced participants' stress and anxiety. Psychotherapy, mindfulness-based interventions and stress management diminished depression and anxiety [22]. Additionally, a recent review involving three RCTs examined the effect of psychosocial interventions on depression and anxiety among people with congenital heart diseases [23]. The interventions included rational emotive behaviour therapy, mindfulness-based stress reduction, and CBT. Findings indicated that the interventions did not reduce anxiety; however, they improved depression with a large effect size (SMD = −1.04) [23].

1.4.2 *Psychosocial Interventions for Diabetes Mellitus*

Diabetes mellitus (DM) is considered a 'non-infectious epidemic', affecting more than 500 million people globally [24]. Patients with DM are required to perform self-management activities, including adherence to prescribed treatments, self-adjustment to dietary plans, regular physical activities, self-monitoring of blood glucose, and doctor visits [25]. To accomplish optimum self-management tasks in adults with DM, health education and psychosocial interventions, such as CBT and motivational interviews, generated positive results [25, 26]. For adolescents with DM, family-based interventions, group interventions, social skills training, and effective coping strategies are essential to achieve optimal glycaemic control [25]. Several studies examined the effectiveness of psychosocial interventions on people with DM. A systematic review of 96 studies suggested that CBT and counselling appears to be clinically effective and CBT was found to be cost-effective among adults with type 2 DM [27]. Furthermore, psychosocial interventions were found to reduce glycated haemoglobin levels while improving dietary behaviour and quality of life [27].

In addition to a face-to-face traditional approach, psychosocial interventions were delivered using digital technology. A systematic review of 10 studies reported that eHealth psychosocial interventions reduced depressive symptomatology among patients with types 1 and 2 DM at post-intervention, short-term (3 months), and long-term follow-up (6 and 12 months) [28]. In this review, CBT, behavioural activation treatment, systematic behavioural activation with problem solving, and healthy outcomes through patient empowerment were delivered using different formats, encompassing telephone, website, and video call [28]. Another systematic review involving 20 RCTs reported that technology-based psychosocial interventions improved health outcomes, including diabetes distress, self-efficacy, and HbA1c levels with small effect sizes [29]. Telephone-delivered problem-solving therapy, online behavioural program with telephone consultations, and telephone coaching were effective in reducing diabetes distress [29]. Computer-assisted self-management programmes, motivational interviews, and telephone health coaching on self-management improved self-efficacy among people with type 2 DM [29].

1.4.3 *Psychosocial Interventions for Cancer*

Cancer is a devastating illness, contributing to poorer quality of life and mortality. New cases of cancer were estimated to be 20 million in 2022, and will increase 77% by 2050 [30]. Recent advances in cancer care encompass both pharmacological and psychosocial interventions. Such interventions can be offered in different formats: group, individual, and family therapy. A systematic review (involving 68 RCTs) reported the applications of psychosocial care on people with advanced cancer [31]. Such interventions encompassed CBT, meaning-enhancing therapy, dignity therapy, life review, counselling, education, music therapy, and expressive writing, among others. These psychosocial interventions were delivered in person, and/or mobile applications, videos, or online platforms. The number of sessions ranged from 1–15 with most studies (90%) conducted within five sessions.

Results suggested that education interventions could be delivered earlier in the advanced cancer trajectory. Time-limited CBT-based interventions could be offered to improve quality of life, mitigate distress, and manage symptoms for patients with reasonable conditions and prognosis (six months or more) [31]. Meaning-centred psychotherapy appears to increase participants' spiritual well-being, sense of meaning and quality of life [31]. Narrative-based interventions aim to elevate the meaning of life and dignity, and they can be offered to patients at terminal stage. Music therapy can be more suitable for palliative care settings and for patients closer to the end of life [31].

Accumulated evidence suggests that mindfulness-based interventions are promising for cancer patients and survivors. A systematic review was conducted involving 29 studies with 3,476 participants [32]. Those who received mindfulness-based interventions showed significant improvement on anxiety, depression, fatigue, stress, quality of life, post-traumatic growth, and mindfulness levels [32]. Mindfulness-based art therapy produced the strongest intervention effect on anxiety (SMD = −2.48) and depression (SMD = −2.21), followed by mindfulness-based stress reduction program and mindfulness-based care recovery. The interventions were effective across different cancer types [32]. In another systematic review, 18 studies were included [33]. The eHealth-mindfulness interventions reduced anxiety (SMD = −0.28) and depression (SMD = −0.24) among cancer patients/survivors with small effect sizes. Effects on quality of life (SMD = 0.25) and mindfulness (SMD = 0.29) were also observed [33].

Psychosocial interventions can be delivered by a multidisciplinary healthcare team (Figure 1.2). Specifically, the interventions are applicable to different levels, encompassing: a) family and caregivers, b) hospitals, c) non-healthcare sectors, and d) governmental levels.

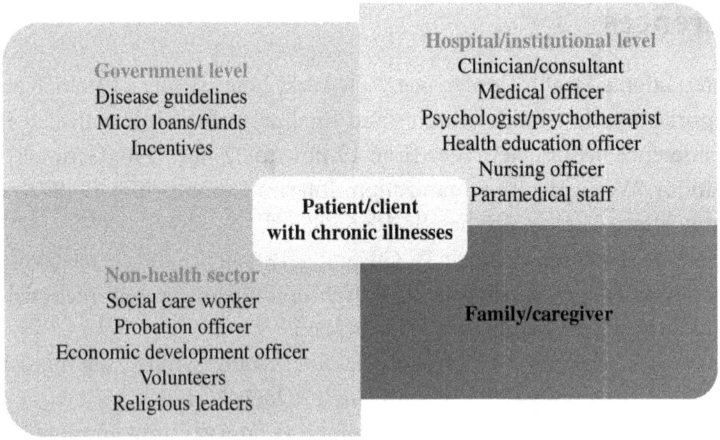

Figure 1.2 Tips for multidisciplinary psychosocial interventions for chronic diseases.

1.5 Conclusion

Psychosocial interventions encompass evidence-based treatments that target individuals' physical and psychological well-being. WHO has recommended various psychosocial interventions such as CBT, behavioural activation, social skills training, cognitive stimulation therapy, cognitive training, contingency management therapy, eye movement desensitisation and reprocessing, motivational enhancement therapy, and stress management, among others. This chapter elaborates on common psychosocial interventions, including cognitive-behavioural interventions, stress management, motivational interviewing and positive psychology. Furthermore, psychosocial interventions can be integrated into healthcare at three levels: primary, secondary and tertiary interventions. The applications of psychosocial interventions on chronic illness are also provided, with the focus on cardiovascular diseases, diabetes mellitus and cancer.

References

1. International Health Conference, New York, June 19–July 22 1946. Summary report on proceedings, minutes and final acts of the International Health Conference held in New York from 19 June to 22 July 1946. Geneva: United Nations, World Health Organization, Interim Commission; 1948. Available from: https://iris.who.int/handle/10665/85573
2. Swathi M, Manjusha S, Isatrin JV, Gururaj A. Prevalence and correlates of stress, anxiety, and depression in patients with chronic diseases: a cross-sectional study. Middle East Curr Psychiatry. 2023;30(1):66.
3. Edwards L. The power of psychosocial interventions: nurturing mental well-being. J Community Public Health Nurs. 2023;9:427:1–6.
4. World Health Organization. Psychological interventions implementation manual: integrating evidence-based psychological interventions into existing services. Geneva: World Health Organization; 2024.
5. American Psychological Association. What is Cognitive Behavioral Therapy? PTSD clinical practice guideline. [Internet]. 2024. Available from: https://www.apa.org/ptsd-guideline/patients-and-families/cognitive-behavioral
6. Beck A. The Instructor's Manual accompanies the DVD Aaron Beck on Cognitive Therapy with Aaron T Beck, M.D. (Institutional/Instructor's Version) [Video]. 2012. Available from: psychotherapy.net
7. Henrich D, Glombiewski JA, Scholten S. Systematic review of training in cognitive-behavioral therapy: summarizing effects, costs and techniques. Clin Psychol Rev. 2023;101:102266.
8. Beck AT, Rush AJ, Shaw BF, Emery G. Cognitive therapy of depression. New York: Guilford Press; 1979.
9. Beck JS. Cognitive behavior therapy: basics and beyond. New York: Guilford Publications; 2020.
10. Rachmad YE. Stress management theory. Saarbrücken: Saar Buch Internationaler Verlag; 2022. Available from: https://doi.org/10.17605/osf.io/5ut3k
11. Amanvermez Y, Rahmadiana M, Karyotaki E, de Wit L, Ebert DD, Kessler RC, Cuijpers P. Stress management interventions for college students: a systematic review and meta-analysis. Clin Psychol Sci Pract. 2023;30(4):423–444.
12. Alhasani M, Mulchandani D, Oyebode O, Baghaei N, Orji R. A systematic and comparative review of behavior change strategies in stress management apps: opportunities for improvement. Front Public Health. 2022;10:777567.
13. Burke BL, Lundahl B, Arkowitz HA. Motivational Interviewing in the Treatment of Psychological Problems. 3rd ed. New York: Guilford Press; 2025.

14. Bischof G, Bischof A, Rumpf HJ. Motivational interviewing: an evidence-based approach for use in medical practice. Dtsch Arztebl Int. 2021;118(7):109–115.
15. Miller WR, Rollnick S. Motivational Interviewing: Helping People Change. 3rd ed. New York: Guilford Press; 2013.
16. Seligman M. Flourish: a new understanding of happiness and well-being and how to achieve them. London: Nicholas Brealey Publishing; 2011.
17. Seligman ME. The Hope Circuit: a psychologist's journey from helplessness to optimism. London: Nicholas Brealey Publishing; 2019.
18. Carr A, Cullen K, Keeney C, Canning C, Mooney O, Chinseallaigh E, O'Dowd A. Effectiveness of positive psychology interventions: a systematic review and meta-analysis. J Positive Psychol. 2021;16(6):749–769.
19. World Health Organization. Noncommunicable diseases [Internet]. 2023. Available from: https://www.who.int/news-room/fact-sheets/detail/noncommunicable-diseases
20. Samartzis L, Dimopoulos S, Tziongourou M, Nanas S. Effect of psychosocial interventions on quality of life in patients with chronic heart failure: a meta-analysis of randomized controlled trials. J Card Fail. 2013;19(2):125–134.
21. Ski CF, Jelinek M, Jackson AC, Murphy BM, Thompson DR. Psychosocial interventions for patients with coronary heart disease and depression: a systematic review and meta-analysis. Eur J Cardiovasc Nurs. 2016;15(5):305–316.
22. Klainin-Yobas P, Ng SH, Stephen PDM, Lau Y. Efficacy of psychosocial interventions on psychological outcomes among people with cardiovascular diseases: a systematic review and meta-analysis. Patient Educ Couns. 2016;99(4):512–521.
23. Magon AM, Invernizzi SI, Arrigoni CA, Flocco S, Devecchi SDV, Nedesca RB, Caruso R; *et al.* The effect of psychosocial interventions on anxiety and depression in congenital heart disease population: a systematic review and explorative meta-analysis. Eur J Cardiovasc Nurs. 2024;23(suppl_1):zvae098.012.
24. International Diabetes Federation. IDF Diabetes Atlas. 10th ed. Brussels: International Diabetes Federation; 2021.
25. Harvey N. Psychosocial interventions for the diabetic patient. Diabetes Metab Syndr Obes. 2015;9:29–43.
26. Bilgin A, Muz G, Yuce GE. The effect of motivational interviewing on metabolic control and psychosocial variables in individuals diagnosed with diabetes: systematic review and meta-analysis. Patient Educ Couns. 2022;105(9):2806–2823.
27. Winkley K, Upsher R, Stahl D, Pollard D, Kasera A, Brennan A, Heller S, Ismail K. Psychological interventions to improve self-management of type 1 and type 2 diabetes: a systematic review. Health Technol Assess. 2020;24(28):1–232.

28. Varela-Moreno E, Carreira Soler M, Guzmán-Parra J, Jódar-Sánchez F, Mayoral-Cleries F, Anarte-Ortíz MT. Effectiveness of eHealth-based psychological interventions for depression treatment in patients with type 1 or type 2 Diabetes mellitus: a systematic review. Front Psychol. 2021;12:746217.
29. Yap JM, Tantono N, Wu VX, Klainin-Yobas P. Effectiveness of technology-based psychosocial interventions on diabetes distress and health-relevant outcomes among type 2 diabetes mellitus: a systematic review and meta-analysis. J Telemed Telecare. 2024;30(2):262–284.
30. World Health Organization. World Cancer Day [Internet]. 2025. Available from: https://www.emro.who.int/media/news/world-cancer-day-2024.htm
31. Teo I, Krishnan A, Lee GL. Psychosocial interventions for advanced cancer patients: a systematic review. Psycho-Oncology. 2019;28(7):1394–1407.
32. Xunlin N, Lau Y, Klainin-Yobas P. The effectiveness of mindfulness-based interventions among cancer patients and survivors: a systematic review and meta-analysis. Support Care Cancer. 2020;28:1563–1578.
33. Fung JYT, Lim H, Vongsirimas N, Klainin-Yobas P. Effectiveness of eHealth mindfulness-based interventions on cancer-related symptoms among cancer patients and survivors: a systematic review and meta-analysis. J Telemed Telecare. 2022;30(3):451–465.

https://doi.org/10.1142/9789819817320_0002

Chapter 2

Mindfulness-Based Interventions

Piyanee Klainin-Yobas[1,*], Wareerat Thanoi[2], Nopporn Vongsirimas[2], Lian Kwang Tang[3], Debbie Ramirez[4], Zenaida Fernandez[4], and Jenneth Sarmiento[4]

[1]*Alice Lee Centre for Nursing Studies, Yong Loo Lin School of Medicine, National University of Singapore, Level 5, Centre of Translational Medicine, Block MD6, 14 Medical Drive, Singapore 117599*

[2]*Department of Mental Health and Psychiatric Nursing, Faculty of Nursing, Mahidol University, 2 Prannok Road, Bangkoknoi, Bangkok, Thailand 10700*

[3]*Raffles Hospital, 585 North Bridge Road, Singapore 188770*

[4]*College of Nursing, Angeles University Foundation, 2009 Angeles City, Philippines*

**Corresponding author: nurpk@nus.edu.sg*

Mindfulness-based interventions are regarded as third wave psychotherapies given their effectiveness and popularity in healthcare research. This chapter will begin with definitions and description of mindfulness from the perspectives of well-known researchers. Examples of mindfulness-based interventions will also be provided and elaborated. Furthermore, measurements of mindfulness are listed with an emphasis on the Mindfulness Awareness Attention Scale (MAAS). Additionally, our research testing psychometric properties of the MAAS on five large samples will be presented.

2.1 Mindfulness

The concept of "mindfulness" has received considerable attention from researchers, educators and healthcare professionals worldwide. Mindfulness, derived from "Sati" in Pali language, has its origin and historical root in Buddhist traditions. According to Kabat-Zinn [1,2], mindfulness is defined as paying attention in a particular way, on purpose, to the

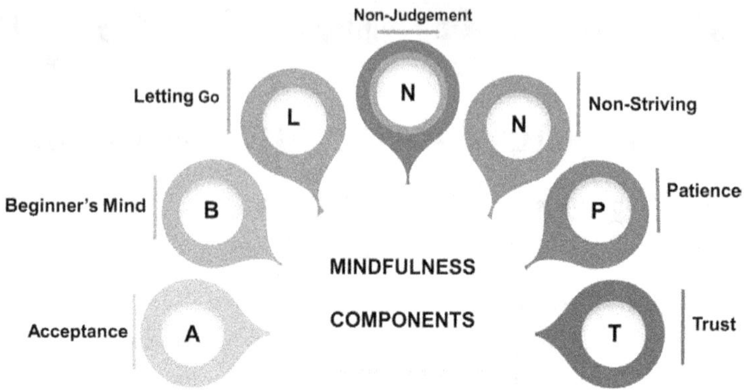

Figure 2.1 Elements supporting core mechanisms of mindfulness.

current moment with a non-judgemental attitude. Mindfulness can be cultivated by various practices such as mindful breathing, body scan and yoga (mindful movements). Mindfulness practices are based on seven attitudinal foundations: non-judging, patience, beginner's mind, trust, non-striving, acceptance, and letting go (Figure 2.1) [2, 3].

The *non-judging* attitude requires individuals to observe their own thoughts, emotions and other experiences without judging them or labelling them as right, wrong, good or bad. *Patience* is considered a form of wisdom, whereby individuals allow things or matters to unfold in their own time. There is no need to be judgemental, agitated, or frightened. *Beginner's mind* refers to the mind with the willingness to see everything as if it is seen for the first time. This attitude is important because it will enable individuals to practice mindfulness and to obtain the richness of current-moment experiences [3]. *Trust* emphasises confidence in individuals' self, feelings and wisdom. The *non-striving* attitude highlights that mindfulness practice is not necessarily linked with any outcome or expectation. Being in the moment is more important. *Acceptance* is regarded as part of the healing process and positive changes. Acceptance reflects how individuals see things as they actually are in the process. Finally, *letting go* refers to letting things be or letting go of unpleasant thoughts/emotions [3].

Shapiro and her colleague proposed a model of mindfulness with three axioms originating from Kabit-Zinn's definition of mindfulness. Specifically, the three axioms encompass intention (on purpose), attention (paying attention), and attitude (in a particular way). Intention plays a crucial role in mindfulness practice. During mindfulness practice, individuals' *intention* shifts to self-regulation, leading to self-exploration and finally to self-liberation. Attention is a critical element of a healing process. *Attention* enables individuals to observe their moment-to-moment experiences, contributing to cognitive inhibition (an ability to inhibit secondary elaborative processing of thoughts, emotion and body sensations) and self-regulation. Attitude is also essential to the healing process. *Attitude* reflects the seven attitudinal foundations of mindfulness [2]. Shapiro *et al.* postulated a potential mechanism of mindfulness, whereby paying intention and attention with non-judgement will contribute to *reperceiving* (a significant shift in perspective). Reperceiving allows individuals to dis-identify themselves from unpleasant thoughts, emotions and body sensation, leading to positive health outcomes.

Brown and Ryan provided a definition of mindfulness with a slightly different focus: "A receptive attention to and awareness of present events and experiences" [4]. *Awareness* refers to the conscious registration of various stimuli, entailing five physical senses (vision, audition, olfaction, gustation, and tactition), kinaesthetic senses (awareness of body's positions and movements) and mind activities [5]. Mindful individuals have a clear awareness of their internal and external worlds, encompassing five physical senses, thoughts, actions, emotions and surroundings [5]. Awareness reflects reality, without any bias from individuals' judgement, concepts, labels, beliefs and ideas. With such a definition, mindfulness interventions are directed towards a non-judgemental attitude to experiences and acceptance. The mindfulness interventions are perceived to ameliorate impulsive reactions to unpleasant experiences and to enhance individuals' insight to self and others [5].

2.2 Mindfulness-based interventions

The promise of mindfulness interventions in enhancing psychological well-being and other positive outcomes has been recognised worldwide. The mindfulness-based stress reduction program (MBSR) was the first, developed at University of Massachusetts Medical School [2]. MBSR was offered as an outpatient program in behavioural medicine to help patients manage stress-related symptoms and chronic pain. This group-based programme was conducted in eight weeks, lasting 2–2.5 hours each session, with a full-day retreat between the sixth and seventh week. All participants were instructed to practice mindfulness at least 45 minutes per day. Mindfulness practices encompass mindful breathing, body scan, raisin exercise, yoga, walking meditation, sitting meditation, among others [2, 3]. Group discussion and exploration are crucial components to help participants comprehend mindfulness practice and the integration of practice in daily living.

Mindfulness-based cognitive therapy is an extension of MBSR, with the integration of cognitive therapy that aims at preventing the relapse of depression [6]. It is a manualised, group-based, eight-week program which involves weekly group discussion, different mindfulness practice, one day retreat, and home-based mindfulness practice. Each week participants learn and discuss different topics, entailing: 1) awareness and automatic pilot, 2) living in our heads, 3) gathering the scattered mind, 4) recognising aversion, 5) allowing/letting be, 6) thoughts are not facts and relapse prevention, 7) take care of self, and 8) maintaining and extending new learning. Mindfulness practices include raisin exercise, body scan, mindfulness of the breath, mindful movements, and mindful walking [6].

Other programs were subsequently developed, such as Acceptance and Commitment Therapy [7], Dialectical Behavior Therapy [8], and Mindfulness-based Cancer Recovery [9].

Mindfulness-based interventions have been delivered through a face-to-face approach and technology-based platforms such as websites, virtual reality, mobile applications, among others. The digital mindfulness-based psychoeducation for cancer survivors (Digital-MindCAN program) was developed to help cancer survivors manage their stress, unpleasant thoughts, and problematic emotions [10]. The Digital-MindCAN program is delivered in real time via a videotelephony platform using an interactive group format. The program has two major components (discussion and mindfulness practices) and home-based practice. The weekly topics entail: 1) The mindfulness world, 2) Mindful management of stress, 3) Mindful body sensations, 4) Mindful emotions: Calmness and composure, 5) Mindfulness: The powerful mind, 6) Mindful communications, 7) Loving kindness and compassion, and 8) Mindful living [10].

2.3 Measurement of Mindfulness

It is essential to use well-validated and reliable measurements to capture the concept of mindfulness in research studies to ensure credible findings. Thus far, at least eight self-reported questionnaires have been developed. The 14-item Frieburg Mindfulness Inventory [11] was originally devised in Germany and later translated into English [12]. The 15-item MAAS, rooted in the self-regulatory theory, captures the presence or absence of attention and awareness [4]. The Kentucky Inventory of Mindfulness [13] contains 39 items and was developed under the Dialectical Behaviour Therapy's concept of mindfulness [14]. The 12-item Cognitive and Affective Mindfulness Scale Revised covers four factors of mindfulness, including attention, awareness, non-judgement, and present focus [15]. The 13-item Toronto Mindfulness Scale was developed according to Bishop's concept of mindfulness [16]. The 39-item Five Facet Mindfulness Questionnaire covers five factors: act with awareness, describing, observing, non-judging, and non-reactivity [17]. The 16-item Southampton Mindfulness Questionnaire captures four dimensions: decentred awareness of cognitions, letting cognitions pass, allowing one's attention to remain with difficulty cognition, and accepting difficult thoughts and images [18]. Lastly, the 20-item Philadelphia Mindfulness Scale measures two components: acceptance and awareness [19].

All aforementioned scales have shown sound psychometric properties in previous studies. However, only the MAAS is the focus of this chapter given that the questionnaire's contents have its roots in the mindfulness conceptualisation and self-regulatory theory. The scale contains only 15 items, which are simple, short, and easy to administer to people in hospital and community settings. Brown and Ryan defined mindfulness as "enhanced attention to and awareness of current experiences or present reality" [4]. With this definition, they developed the 15-item MAAS to cover the degree to which individuals pay attention to their activities (such as walking, doing jobs/tasks, listening to conversations, driving to places, and eating), notice their emotions and physical tensions, stay focused on present events, forget names, are preoccupied with the past and the future, and run on autopilot mode [4].

A series of validation studies of the MAAS were conducted across different samples in America [4]. Firstly, factor analyses suggested a one-factor solution with strong factor loadings. Secondly, convergent and discriminant validity were supported through its correlations with measures of well-being. Thirdly, the MAAS appeared to distinguish mindfulness levels between two groups of adults: meditators and non-meditators. Fourthly, the MAAS was found to predict autonomy and affect among adults and students. Finally, the MAAS was a significant predictor of psychological outcomes in clinical settings across time. Apparently, the aforementioned evidence suggested that the MAAS is a valid and reliable measure of mindfulness for American participants [4].

According to the principle of cross-cultural psychology, culture plays a crucial role in a person's development, behaviour, and socialisation [20]. Therefore, the concept of mindfulness may not be universal across different countries, contexts, and cultures. To avoid culturally blind issues [21], it is imperative to ensure that the measures of mindfulness are valid and reliable in different cultures and populations. Thus far, the MAAS has been translated and extended in its use to other languages, including Chinese, French, Norwegian, Spanish, and Thai [22]. A comparative study examined the MAAS on configural (baseline model), metric (equality of factor loadings), and scalar (equality of intercepts) invariances across American and Thai university students [22]. The results supported the equivalence of all factor loadings and some intercepts across the two subgroups. Other studies documented that the Chinese, French, Spanish, and Swedish versions of the MAAS had adequate psychometric properties with a unidimensional structure [23-26].

Mindfulness interventions have been implemented in some Asian countries, including Thailand and the Philippines. There is a need to further conduct validation studies of the MAAS on Asian samples given the limited research in the literature. Furthermore, most previous studies examined the scale on cross-sectional samples; thus, it is unclear if the results are maintained across time. Therefore, we conducted a study aiming to (a) initially examine a factorial structure of the MAAS among Thai secondary school students and (b) test whether the psychometric properties (construct validity, concurrent validity, and reliability) remain stable across two repeated cross-sectional samples among youths in Thailand and in the Philippines.

2.3.1 *Method*

Research Design and Participants

A descriptive correlational research was conducted in two countries (Thailand and the Philippines), and five datasets were collected (Sample A, B1, B2, C1, and C2). Conventionally, the sample size estimation for confirmatory factor analyses (CFA) was based on the observations-estimated parameter ratio whereby a 5:1 ratio would be acceptable [27]. Given the 30 parameters (15 factor loadings and 15 variances) (Figure 2.2), the minimal adequate sample size would be 150 students for each data set.

Sample A was a convenient sample of students who were recruited from three different secondary schools in Thailand. One school contained only male students, one had only female students, and one contained both male and female students (mixed sample). This data collection commenced after receiving ethics approval from the university. The researchers liaised with school principals to arrange out-of-class meetings with the students to explain the study, distribute participant information sheets, and request their involvement. The students were then advised to discuss with their parents. Interested students and their parents were asked to sign consent and assent forms respectively and to complete self-reported paper-and-pencil questionnaires.

Samples B1 and B2 were two repeated cross-sectional samples. They involved undergraduate university students from a public university in Thailand. Upon approval from the university's institutional review board (IRB), the researchers sought permission from deans of all faculties to recruit participants. Then, we began recruiting participants by organising meetings with students and distributing personal information sheets. Interested participants each signed a consent form and completed a self-reported paper-and-pencil questionnaire (Sample B1). One year later, we recruited another sample (Sample B2) using the same data collection process.

Samples C1 and C2 were two repeated cross-sectional samples. They encompassed undergraduate students at a university in the Philippines. Following ethics approval, the researchers sought permission from university administrative personnel to conduct the study. Following permission, we emailed a letter of invitation to all students during their academic year (Sample C1). Each interested participant was asked to visit the study website, sign an online consent form, and complete an online questionnaire. One year later, we recruited another sample (Sample C2) using the same data collection process.

Measurements

Data were collected using paper-and-pencil questionnaires (Samples A, B1, and B2) and online questionnaires (Samples C1 and C2).

Demographic variables were collected, including each student's age, gender, religion, and satisfaction with his/her family income. The 15-item MAAS was devised to measure trait mindfulness. Students were asked to identify their experiences on a six-point scale, ranging from one (almost always) to six (almost never). Scores for all items were reverse-coded, in that the highest score signified the highest level of mindfulness. The Thai version of the MAAS was administered on Samples A, B1, and B2 whereas the English version was used in Samples C1 and C2.

Psychological well-being was measured with the 18-item Psychological Well-Being Scale (PWBS) [28]. Researchers translated and back-translated the Thai version of the PWBS using Brisline's method [29]. Three nurse educators with research experience reviewed the Thai and English versions of the PWBS to ascertain the meanings of the questionnaire items. Factor analyses in a previous study revealed two distinct factors of the PWBS: the autonomy and growth factor and the negative triad factor [30]. The Cronbach's alpha values of the former were 0.81 to 0.85 and the latter were 0.56 to 0.74, respectively [30]. The PWBS served as an external measure for testing the concurrent validity of the MAAS.

Data analyses

Univariate analyses were performed to describe samples and study variables. A severe non-normal distribution would be observed if its skewness was larger than two and its kurtosis was larger than seven for samples larger than 300 [31]. To explore a factor structure of the MAAS on Sample A, exploratory factor analyses (EFA) were performed using principal axis factoring as an extraction method and different rotation methods, including Varimax and Oblimin. To determine the number of factors to extract, we used the following criteria: parsimony, interpretability of the extracted factor, content validity, and previous evidence [32]. We also examined statistical parameters including eigenvalue and scree plots. A factor loading of 0.30 or higher was used to determine a sufficient relationship between each item and its underlying factor [33].

The results from the EFA were then submitted to CFA using IBM SPSS AMOS version 25.0. Model fit was examined via (a) chi-square per degree of freedom (χ^2/df) < 5 [34], (b) confirmatory fit index (CFI), Tucker-Luwis Index (TLI) > 0.90 as acceptable fit and > 0.95 as well-fit, and (c) root mean square of error of approximation (RMSEA) < 0.05 as well-fit and < 0.08 as reasonable fit [35-37]. Regarding the measurement invariance across samples, we first determined the baseline model of each sample separately. Then, we performed multiple-group CFA using the available features in AMOS [35]. For Model 1, we ran the analyses and allowed all parameters to be freely estimated without any equality constraints (baseline model). For Model 2, we imposed quality constraints on all factor loadings across two samples. For Model 3, all covariances were imposed to be equal, while Model 4 imposed equality constraints on measurement residuals. The measurement invariance (equivalence) would be assumed if there was no significant decrease in model fit (in comparison with Model 1), evidenced by insignificant $\Delta\chi^2$ ($p > 0.05$) and ΔCFI < 0.01 [35, 38].

Concurrent validity was estimated using IBM SPSS. Pearson product moment correlations were used to determine relationships between the MAAS and the two-factor PWBS. If the MAAS items really captured the construct of mindfulness, they would exhibit positive correlations with the autonomy and growth factor and negative correlations with the negative triad factor of the PWBS. Correlation coefficients of 0.10, 0.30, and 0.50 would be regarded as weak, moderate, and strong, respectively [39]. The internal consistency reliability of the MAAS was then estimated using a reliability analysis. Cronbach's alpha values (α) greater than 0.70 would signify an acceptable reliability [40].

Ethical considerations

This research was reviewed and received approval from two IRBs. The IRB in Thailand approved the study conducted in secondary schools and universities in Thailand. The IRB in the Philippines approved the study conducted in a university in the Philippines. All participants received written information concerning the research project and signed the informed consent form prior to completing the self-reported questionnaires. The researchers also emphasised voluntary participation and confidentiality.

2.3.2 *Results*

Characteristics of Participants

Table 2.1 displays characteristics of the study participants in Samples A (n = 624), B1 (n = 966), B2 (n = 695), C1 (n = 221), and C2 (n = 409). Most students were female across the five samples. Average

Table 2.1 Characteristics of the study participants.

	Sample A (n = 624)		**Sample B1 (n = 966)**		**Sample B2 (n = 695)**		**Sample C1 (n = 221)**		**Sample C2 (n = 409)**	
	n	**%**	**n**	**%**	**n**	**%**	**n**	**%**	**n**	**%**
Gender										
- Male	265	42.50	307	31.80	217	31.20	55	24.90	78	19.10
- Female	359	57.50	650	67.30	473	68.10	158	71.50	244	59.70
- Missing	—	—	9	0.90	5	0.70	8	3.60	87	21.30
Religion										
- Buddhism	574	92.00	913	94.50	649	93.40	147	66.50	211	51.60
- Christian	26	4.20	20	2.10	18	2.60	—	—		
- Islam	9	1.40	13	1.30	12	1.70	—	—		
- Others	—	2.40	—	—	16	2.30	65	29.40	110	26.90
- Missing	15		20	2.1	—	—	9	4.10	88	21.50
	Mean	**SD**	**Mean**	**SD**	**Mean**	**SD**	**Mean**	**SD**	**Mean**	**SD**
Age	16.14	0.97	20.21	1.51	20.34	1.43	19.56	1.74	19.56	1.76

Note: Sample A = secondary school students, Thailand; Sample B1 = university students, Thailand (sample 1); Sample B2 = university students, Thailand (sample 2); Sample C1 = university students, the Philippines (sample 1); Sample C2 = university students, the Philippines (sample 2).

age was 16.14 years (standard deviation (SD) = 0.97) for Sample A, and in the range of 19.56 to 20.34 years for the other samples (SD ranging from 1.43 to 1.76).

Exploratory factor analyses: Sample A

We conducted EFA on Sample A (n = 624) to initially explore the factorial structure of the Thai-version MAAS. To compare findings across schools, we subsequently examined the factorial structure on the three subsamples, including Subsample A1 (male school, n = 194), Subsample A2 (female school, n = 231), and Subsample A3 (mixed-gender school, n = 199). The results suggested that the MAAS had one factor for the total sample and three schools (Table 2.2). This accounted for 28.16% of the variance on questionnaire items and all items had sufficient factor loadings ($\lambda > 0.30$). For the total sample and three schools, items 7–10 and 14 had the strongest factor loadings. Internal consistency reliability was good for the total sample and the three schools (Cronbach's alphas were in the range of 0.84 to 0.86). All evidence in this section supported the single dimension of the Thai version of the MAAS.

Measurement invariance across samples: Samples B1 and B2

Given the results of EFA on Sample A, we performed CFA on Thai university students (Samples B1 and B2) separately and simultaneously. We submitted the one-factor structure of the MAAS into AMOS and tested for measurement invariance across samples. The results of the modification indices suggested that three pairs of error variances (Mind 2-Mind 3, Mind 9-Mind 10, and Mind 13-Mind 14) were correlated. We carefully examined the contents of each pair and found that the contents overlapped to some degree. Hence, we allowed correlations among the variances. As an example, Mind 2 (Break or spill things because of carelessness, not paying attention, or mind wandering) and Mind 3 (Difficult to stay focused on situations in the present moment) contained similar information (Figure 2.2).

Table 2.2 Factor loading (λ) of the MAAS items among secondary school students (n = 624).

	Total Sample A (n = 624)	**School A1 (n = 194)**	**School A2 (n = 231)**	**School A3 (n = 199)**
Mind1 Experience emotions and not be conscious until later	0.55	0.55	0.56	0.56
Mind2 Break or spill things because of carelessness, not paying attention, or mind wandering	0.38	0.52	0.41	0.41
Mind3 Difficult to stay focused on situations in the present moment	0.54	0.53	0.58	0.58
Mind4 I walk quickly without paying attention to the present	0.45	0.44	0.37	0.37
Mind5 Not notice feelings of physical tension or discomfort until later	0.51	0.48	0.57	0.57
Mind6 Forget a person's name almost immediately	0.47	0.48	0.48	0.48
Mind7 Run on automatic without much awareness of the current actions	**0.65**	**0.67**	**0.60**	**0.60**
Mind8 Rush through activities without really paying attention	**0.68**	**0.73**	**0.61**	**0.61**
Mind9 Focused on the goals but lose touch with current actions	**0.58**	**0.63**	**0.49**	**0.49**
Mind10 Do jobs/tasks automatically without being aware of them	**0.63**	**0.67**	**0.60**	**0.60**
Mind11 Listen to someone with one ear and do another thing simultaneously	0.42	0.42	0.43	0.43
Mind12 Travel to places on automatic pilot	0.45	0.47	0.43	0.43
Mind13 Preoccupied with the future or the past	0.53	0.44	0.53	0.53
Mind14 Do things without paying attention	**0.64**	**0.64**	**0.68**	**0.68**
Mind15 Snack without being aware of it	0.39	0.31	0.49	0.49
Cronbach's alpha (α)	0.85	0.86	0.85	0.84

Note: School A1 = male-only students; School A2 = female-only students; School A3 = both male and female students.

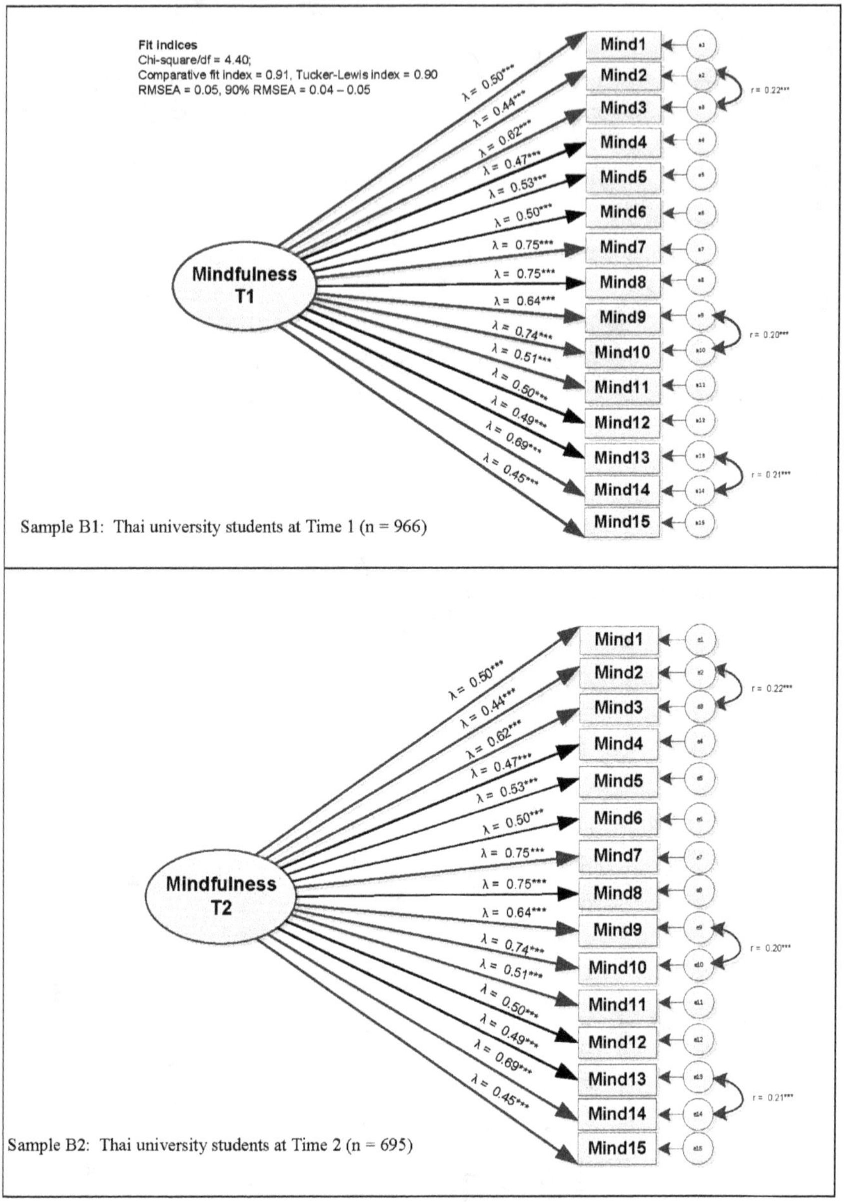

Figure 2.2 (*Continued*)

←

Figure 2.2 The factorial structure of the MAAS in university students in Thailand. Mind1 = Experience emotions and not be conscious until later; Mind2 = Break or spill things because of carelessness, not paying attention, or mind wandering; Mind3 = Difficult to stay focused on situations in the present moment; Mind4 = I walk quickly without paying attention to the present; Mind5 = Not notice feelings of physical tension or discomfort until later; Mind6 = Forget a person's name almost immediately; Mind7 = Run on automatic without much awareness of the current actions; Mind8 = Rush through activities without really paying attention, Mind9 = Focused on the goals but lose touch with current actions; Mind10 = Do jobs/tasks automatically without being aware of them; Mind11 = Listen to someone with one ear and do another thing simultaneously; Mind12 = Travel to places on automatic pilot; Mind13 = Preoccupied with the future or the past; Mind14 = Do things without paying attention; Mind15 = Snack without being aware of it.

The findings (Table 2.3) indicated that Model 1 (with no equality constraints between Samples B1 and B2) had an adequate fit with the sample data (χ^2/df = 5.03, CFI = 0.91, TLI = 0.91, RMSEA = 0.05, 90% RMSEA = 0.46, 0.53). However, after imposing quality constraints, Models 2, 3, and 4 did not have significant reductions in fit indices. Therefore, we can conclude that: (a) the MAAS has a one-factor structure and (b) all parameters (factor loadings, covariances, and residuals) were invariant across the two samples. Furthermore, Figure 2.2 showed that all factor loadings achieved statistical significance and items 7–10 and 14 had the strongest factor loadings.

Measurement invariance across samples: Samples C1 and C2

For these analyses, we submitted a single-factor structure of the English version of the MAAS into AMOS to test measurement invariance across samples on university students in the Philippines.

Table 2.3 Fit indices for confirmatory factor analyses on four samples.

	χ^2/df	CFI	TLI	RMSEA	90% Confidence Interval	$\Delta\chi^2$ (p-value)	ΔCFI
Sample B1 (n = 966) and Sample B2 (n = 695)							
Model 1: No equality constraints between Sample B1 and Sample B2	5.03	0.91	0.89	0.05	0.05, 0.05	Reference group	Reference group
Model 2: Equality constraints on factor loads between two groups	4.73	0.91	0.90	0.05	0.04, 0.05	15.69 (0.33)	0.00
Model 3: Equality constraints on factor loadings and covariance	4.73	0.91	0.90	0.05	0.04, 0.05	19.55 (0.19)	0.00
Model 3: Equality constraints on factor loadings, covariance and residuals	4.40	0.91	0.90	0.05	0.04, 0.05	35.58 (0.34)	0.00
Sample C1 (n = 221) and Sample C2 (n = 409)							
Model 1: No equality constraints between Sample C1 and Sample C2	2.17	0.95	0.94	0.04	0.04, 0.05	Reference group	Reference group
Model 2: Equality constraints on factor loads between two groups	2.04	0.95	0.95	0.04	0.04, 0.05	4.75 (0.99)	0.00
Model 3: Equality constraints on factor loadings and covariance	2.03	0.95	0.95	0.04	0.04, 0.05	6.55 (0.97)	0.00
Model 3: Equality constraints on factor loadings, covariance and residuals	1.96	0.95	0.95	0.04	0.03, 0.05	28.56 (0.69)	0.00

Note:
(a) Sample B1 = university students, Thailand, Time 1; Sample B2 = university students, Thailand, Time 2.
(b) Sample C1 = uiversnity students, the Philippines, Time 1; Sample C2 = university students, the Philippines, Time 2.
(c) CFI = confirmatory fit index; TLI = Tucker-Lewis Index; RMSEA = root mean square of error of approximation.

After viewing the modification indices output, three pairs of variances were suggested to be correlated. This included Mind 2-Mind 3 (pair 1), Mind 4-Mind 5 (pair 2), and Mind 14-Mind 15 (pair 3). Given that the contents of each pair were similar, we allowed the variance correlations (Figure 2.3). Additional results suggested that Model 1 (with no equality constraints between Samples C1 and C2) fit reasonably well with the sample data ($\chi^2/df = 2.17$, CFI = 0.95, TLI = 0.94, RMSEA = 0.04, 90% RMSEA = 0.04, 0.05) (Table 2.2). Nevertheless, Models 2, 3, and 4 did not have significant reductions in fit indices. Therefore, we can conclude that (a) the MAAS has a one-factor structure and (b) all parameters (factor loadings, covariance, and residuals) were invariant across sample C1 and C2. In addition, all factor loadings achieved statistical significance and items 7–10 had the strongest factor loadings (Figure 2.3).

Concurrent validity

Table 2.4 illustrates the correlation between the MAAS and the PWBS across samples. All correlation coefficients achieved statistical significance ($p < 0.01$). As anticipated, the English version of the MAAS was positively correlated with the autonomy and growth factor (Sample C1, $r = 0.38$, $p < 0.01$; Sample C2, $r = 0.34$, $p < 0.01$) and negatively correlated with the negative triad factor (Sample C1, $r = -0.48$ $p < 0.01$; Sample C2, $r = -0.40$, $p < 0.01$).

Similarly, the Thai version of the MAAS was positively associated with the autonomy and growth factor (Sample B1, $r = 0.43$, $p < 0.01$; Sample B2, $r = 0.41$, $p < 0.01$) and negatively associated with the negative triad factor (Sample B1, $r = -0.41$, $p < 0.01$; Sample B2, $r = -0.50$, $p < 0.01$). This information supported the concurrent validity of the English and Thai versions of the MAAS across the two repeated cross-sectional samples.

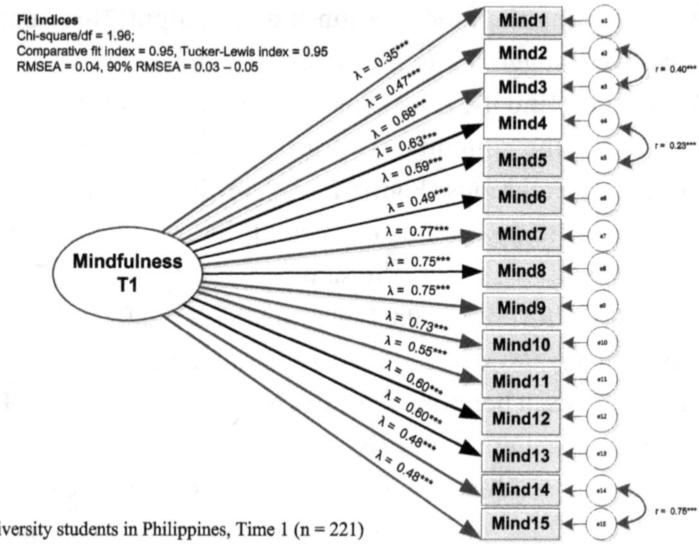

Sample C1: University students in Philippines, Time 1 (n = 221)

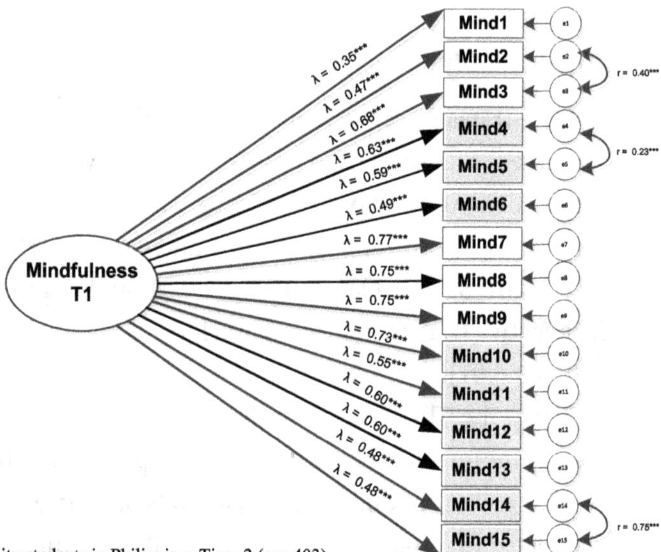

Sample C2: University students in Philippines Time 2 (n = 403)

Figure 2.3 (*Continued*)

Figure 2.3 The factorial structure of the MAAS in university students in the Philippines. Mind1 = Experience emotions and not be conscious until later; Mind2 = Break or spill things because of carelessness, not paying attention, or mind wandering; Mind3 = Difficult to stay focused on situations in the present moment; Mind4 = I walk quickly without paying attention to the present; Mind5 = Not notice feelings of physical tension or discomfort until later; Mind6 = Forget a person's name almost immediately; Mind7 = Run on automatic without much awareness of the current actions; Mind8 = Rush through activities without really paying attention, Mind9 = Focused on the goals but lose touch with current actions; Mind10 = Do jobs/tasks automatically without being aware of them; Mind11 = Listen to someone with one ear and do another thing simultaneously; Mind12 = Travel to places on automatic pilot; Mind13 = Preoccupied with the future or the past; Mind14 = Do things without paying attention; Mind15 = Snack without being aware of it.

Table 2.4 Correlations between the MAAS and PWBS.

Variables (Psychological Well-Being)	**Correlation coefficient (r): Thailand**		**Correlation coefficient (r): the Philippines**	
	Sample B1 (n = 966)	**Sample B2 (n = 685)**	**Sample C1 (n = 221)**	**Sample C2 (n = 409)**
Autonomy and growth factor	0.43**	0.41**	0.38**	0.34**
Negative triad factor	−0.41**	−0.50**	−0.48**	−0.40**
Cronbach's alpha of the MAAS	0.88	0.86	0.90	0.89

Note:
(a) **Correlation is significant at the 0.01 level.
(b) Samples B1 and B2 used the Thai version of the MAAS; samples C1 and C2 utilised the English version of the MAAS.

Internal Consistency Reliability

The MAAS had acceptable internal consistency reliability for all samples. Specifically, Samples B1 and B2 had Cronbach's alpha values of 0.88 and 0.86, respectively (Table 2.4), while Samples C1 and C2 had Cronbach's alpha values of 0.90 and 0.89, respectively (Table 2.4).

2.3.3 *Discussion*

This study aimed to test the psychometric properties of the 15-item MAAS on five data sets of Thai and Filipino youths. Three samples (A, B1, and B2) used the Thai version of the MAAS whereas two samples (C1 and C2) utilised the English version of the MAAS. For all five samples, the findings consistently supported the unidimensional structure of MAAS and all questionnaire items had sufficient factor loadings. This information suggested that all items were suitable to capture the underlying concept of mindfulness. Moreover, statistical parameters demonstrated invariant characteristics (equality) across two repeated cross-sectional samples for both Thai and Filipino participants. The evidence in this study provided strong support for the construct validity of the Thai and English versions of the MAAS. Previous studies also reported the unidimensional structure of the MAAS among American, Thai, Colombian, and Spanish undergraduate students [4, 21, 25, 40] and French high school students and community participants [24]. Another study conducted a cross-cultural validation and found configural, metric, and scalar invariances between Thai and American samples [21].

For all five samples, items 7–10 showed the strongest factor loadings, suggesting that they were the best items to capture the concept of mindfulness. Item 14 was one of the strongest items for only three samples (A, B1, and B2). The factor loadings of the five items ranged from 0.60 to 0.77 across all samples. Item 7 states how a person runs on autopilot without awareness of his/her current actions, item 8 addresses rushing through activities without paying attention, item 9 mentions focusing on the goals but losing touch with current actions, and item 10 indicates how an individual does a job automatically without awareness. Additionally, item 14 states doing things without paying attention. The abovementioned items reflect the conceptual definition of mindfulness provided by Kabat-Zin [41] and Brown and Ryan [4]. Specifically, Kabat-Zin originally defined mindfulness as paying cautious attention to the present moment non-judgementally, while Brown and Ryan viewed mindfulness as enhanced attention and awareness to the present reality. Our findings concurred with those in a previous investigation whereby items 7–10 and 14 had the strongest factor loadings among undergraduate students in America that ranged from 0.71 to 0.78 for the total sample and male/female subgroups [40]. A study in Norway tested the short version of the MAAS, which contained only items 7–10 and 14, and reported that the five-item MAAS was an adequate instrument of mindfulness in Norwegian adolescent samples [42].

The concept of mindfulness appears to be associated with psychological well-being. Brown and Ryan [4] proposed four mechanisms underlying the link between mindfulness and an individual's well-being. First of all, the vividness of one's current experience minimises autonomic thoughts, habits, and unhealthy behaviours. Secondly, attention engages people in gathering factual information associated with healthy behaviours. Thirdly, attention is a key role in a healthy regulatory process. Finally, mindfulness enhances the quality, enjoyment, and flowing activities of the current experiences. In line with the conceptualisation and mechanisms, our findings suggested that the Thai and English versions of the MAAS had significant moderate relationships with measures of psychological well-being (the autonomy and growth factor and the negative triad factor) across two assessment points. This evidence then supported the concurrent validity of the scale. Our results were comparable with other studies. Using the English version of the MAAS, Brown *et al.* [43] documented significant correlations between the scale and several measures of well-being, including negative affect, positive affect, life satisfaction, substance use coping, and healthy self-regulation. The French version of the MAAS appeared to link depression and cognitive emotion regulations. The Spanish version of the MAAS was found to be negatively associated with measures of stress, depression, and anxiety and positively correlated with life satisfaction [25].

This study has strengths concerning the use of five data sets with a large sample size. Five datasets were collected, and the findings confirmed the psychometric properties of the MAAS. Two languages (Thai and English) and two data collection methods (paper-and-pencil and online questionnaires) were used, which might have increased the generalisability of the findings. Moreover, correlations between the scale and other measures were tested. Nevertheless, there were a few limitations, in that we tested the psychometric properties on convenient healthy samples; thus, the findings might not be applicable to people with clinical conditions. Furthermore, we used only self-reported questionnaires, which hampered the possibility to perform a multitrait-multimethod matrix to test the convergent and divergent validity of the MAAS.

2.4 Conclusion

This chapter summarises definitions and descriptions of mindfulness. Mindfulness interventions have been implemented for diverse populations around the world to minimise stress and maximise psychological outcomes (such as psychological well-being). There is a need to measure changes in mindfulness before and after the mindfulness interventions to confirm the effectiveness of the interventions. Nevertheless, the evidence to support psychometric properties of the MAAS among Asian populations is lacking. This study provides solid evidence to support construct validity, concurrent validity and reliability of the MAAS across two languages (English and Thai), two formats (paper-and-pencil versus online questionnaires) and five samples (The Philippines and Thailand).

References

1. Kabat-Zinn J. An outpatient program in behavioral medicine for chronic pain patients based on the practice of mindfulness meditation: theoretical considerations and preliminary results. Gen Hosp Psychiatry. 1982;4(1):33–47.

2. Segal ZV, Williams JMG, Teasdale JD. Mindfulness-based cognitive therapy for depression. 2nd ed. New York: Guilford Press; 2013.
3. Kabat-Zinn J. Full catastrophe living: using the wisdom of your body and mind to face stress, pain and illness. New York: Delacorte; 1990.
4. Buchheld N, Grossman P, Walach H. Measuring mindfulness in insight meditation (vipassana) and meditation-based psychotherapy: the development of the Freiburg Mindfulness Inventory (FMI). J Meditation Meditation Res. 2001;1:11–34.
5. Kabat-Zinn J. Full catastrophe living: using the wisdom of your body and mind to face stress, pain and illness. New York: Bantam Books; 2013.
6. Brown KW, Ryan RM. The benefits of being present: mindfulness and its role in psychological well-being. J Pers Soc Psychol. 2003;84:822–848.
7. Brown KW, Ryan RM, Creswell JD. Mindfulness: theoretical foundations for its salutary effects. Psychol Inq. 2007;18(4):211–237.
8. Hayes SC, Strosahl KD, Wilson KG. Acceptance and commitment therapy: the process and practice of mindful change. New York: Guilford Press; 2011.
9. Linehan MM, Wilks CR. The course and evolution of dialectical behavior therapy. Am J Psychother. 2015;69(2):97–110.
10. Carlson LE, Beattie TL, Giese-Davis J, Faris P, Tamagawa R, Fick LJ, *et al.* Mindfulness-based cancer recovery and supportive-expressive therapy maintain telomere length relative to controls in distressed breast cancer survivors. Cancer. 2015;121(3):476–484.
11. Klainin-Yobas P, Hounsri K, Chng WJ, Ang NKE, Goh YSS. Preventing psychological symptoms among cancer survivors through a digital mindfulness psychoeducation program: protocol of a randomized controlled trial. Preprint. 2023. doi:10.1101/2023.01.05.23284230.
12. Walach H, Buchheld N, Buttenmüller V, Kleinknecht N, Schmidt S. Measuring mindfulness: the Freiburg Mindfulness Inventory (FMI). Pers Individ Dif. 2006;40:1543–1555.
13. Baer RA, Smith GT, Allen KB. Assessment of mindfulness by self-report: the Kentucky Inventory of Mindfulness Skills. Assessment. 2004;11:191–206.
14. Linehan MM. Cognitive-behavioural treatment of borderline personality disorder. New York: Guilford Press; 1993.
15. Feldman G, Hayes A, Kumar S, Greeson J, Laurenceau JP. Mindfulness and emotion regulation: development and initial validation of the Cognitive and Affective Mindfulness Scale-Revised (CAMS-R). J Psychopathol Behav Assess. 2007;29:177–190.
16. Lau MA, Bishop SR, Segal ZV, Buis T, Anderson ND, Carlson L, *et al.* The Toronto Mindfulness Scale: development and validation. J Clin Psychol. 2006;62:1445–1467.

17. Baer RA, Smith GT, Hopkins J, Krietemeyer J, Toney L. Using self-report assessment methods to explore facets of mindfulness. Assessment. 2006;13:27–45.
18. Chadwick P, Hember M, Mead S, Lilley B, Dagnan D. Responding mindfully to unpleasant thoughts and images: reliability and validity of the Southampton Mindfulness Questionnaire (SMQ). Br J Clin Psychol. 2008;47:451–455.
19. Cardaciotto L, Herbert JD, Forman EM, Moitra E, Farrow V. The assessment of present-moment awareness and acceptance: the Philadelphia Mindfulness Scale. Assessment. 2008;15:204–223.
20. Berry JW, Poortinga YH, Segall MH, Dasen PR. Cross-cultural psychology. 2nd ed. Cambridge: Cambridge University Press; 2002.
21. Scholten S, Velten J, Bieda A, Zhang XC, Margraf J. Testing measurement invariance of the Depression, Anxiety, and Stress Scale (DASS-21) across four countries. Psychol Assess. 2017;29:1376–1390.
22. Christopher MS, Charoensuk S, Gibert BD, Neary TJ, Pearc KL. Mindfulness in Thailand and the United States: a case of apples and oranges? J Clin Psychol. 2009;65:590–612.
23. Black DS, Sussman S, Johnson A, Milam J. Psychometric assessment of the Mindful Attention Awareness Scale (MAAS) among Chinese adolescents. Assessment. 2012;19:42–52.
24. Hansen E, Lundh L, Homman A, Wanby-Lundh M. Measuring mindfulness: pilot studies with Swedish versions of the MAAS and Kentucky Inventory of Mindfulness Skills. Cogn Behav Ther. 2009;38:2–15.
25. Jermann F, Billieux J, Larøi F, Argembeau A, Bondolfi G, Zermatten A, Linden MV. MAAS: psychometric properties of the French translation and relations with emotion regulation strategies. Psychol Assess. 2009;21:506–514.
26. Ruiz FJ, Suarez-Falcon JC, Riano-Hernandez D. Psychometric properties of the MAAS in Colombian undergraduates. Suma Psicol. 2016;23:18–24.
27. Bentler PM, Chou C. Practical issues in structural modeling. Sociol Methods Res. 1987;16:78–117.
28. Ryff CD. In the eye of the beholder: views of psychological well-being among middle-aged and older adults. Psychol Aging. 1989;4:195–210.
29. Brislin RW. The wording and translation of research instruments. In: Lonner WJ, Berry JW, editors. Field methods in cross-cultural research. Thousand Oaks: Sage Publications; 1986. p. 137–164.
30. Klainin-Yobas P, Thanoi W, Vongsirimas N, Lau Y. Evaluating the factor structure of the psychological well-being scale among students across Thai and Singaporean samples. Psychol (Tokyo). 2020;11:71–86.
31. Kim HY. Statistical notes for clinical researchers: assessing normal distribution (2) using skewness and kurtosis. Restor Dent Endod. 2013;38:52.

32. Fabrigar LR, MacCallum RC, Wegener DT, Strahan EJ. Evaluating the use of exploratory factor analysis in psychological research. Psychol Methods. 1999;4:272–299.
33. Tabachnick BG, Fidell LS. Using multivariate statistics. 4th ed. Boston (MA): Allyn & Bacon; 2001.
34. Schumacker RE, Lomax RG. A beginner's guide to structural equation modeling. 3rd ed. New York: Routledge; 2010.
35. Byrne BM. Structural equation modeling with AMOS: basic concepts, applications, and programming. 2nd ed. New York: Routledge; 2009.
36. Hu LT, Bentler PM. Cutoff criteria for fit indexes in covariance structure analysis: conventional criteria versus new alternatives. Struct Equ Modeling. 1999;6:1–55.
37. Marsh HW, Hau KT, Wen Z. In search of golden rules: comment on hypothesis testing approaches to setting cutoff values for fit indexes and dangers in overgeneralizing Hu and Bentler's findings. Struct Equ Modeling. 1999;11:320–341.
38. Chen FF. Sensitivity of goodness of fit indexes to lack of measurement invariance. Struct Equ Modeling. 2007;14:464–504.
39. Meyers LS, Gamst G, Guarino AJ. Applied multivariate research: design and interpretation. 2nd ed. Thousand Oaks: Sage; 2013.
40. Cronbach LJ. Coefficient alpha and the internal structure of tests. Psychometrika. 1951;16:297–334.
41. Mackillop J, Anderson EJ. Further psychometric validation of the MAAS. J Psychopathol Behav Assess. 2007;29:289–293.
42. Kabat-Zinn J. Wherever you go, there you are: mindfulness meditation in everyday life. New York: Hyperion; 1994.
43. Smith ORF, Melkevik O, Samdal O, Larsen TM, Haug E. Psychometric properties of the five-item MAAS in Norwegian adolescents. Scand J Public Health. 2017;45:373–380.
44. Brown KW, West AM, Loverich TM, Biegel GM. Assessing adolescent mindfulness: validation of an adapted MAAS in adolescent normative and psychiatric populations. Psychol Assess. 2011;23:1023–1033.
45. MacCallum RC, Widaman KF, Zhang S, Hong S. Sample size in factor analysis. Psychol Methods. 1999;4:84–89.

https://doi.org/10.1142/9789819817320_0003

Chapter 3

The Psychological Well-Being Promotion Model

Piyanee Klainin-Yobas[1,*] and Nopporn Vongsirimas[2]

[1]*Alice Lee Centre for Nursing Studies, Yong Loo Lin School of Medicine, National University of Singapore, Level 5, Centre of Translational Medicine, Block MD6, 14 Medical Drive, Singapore 117599*

[2]*Department of Mental Health and Psychiatric Nursing, Faculty of Nursing, Mahidol University, 2 Prannok Road, Bangkoknoi, Bangkok, Thailand 10700*

**Corresponding author: nurpk@nus.edu.sg*

Healthcare professionals play a crucial role in assisting individuals to achieve happiness and psychological well-being. This chapter highlights the concept of "psychological well-being" and its link with positive health outcomes. Moreover, we propose a theoretical model to guide our clinical practices and research.

3.1 Psychological Well-being

Psychological well-being represents a crucial construct within positive psychology and mental health. Rather than simply addressing the absence of mental illness, psychological well-being reflects the presence of positive psychological attributes. These encompass ***subjective well-being*** (positive effect, happiness and life satisfaction) [1] and ***eudaimonic well-being*** (autonomy, environmental mastery, purpose in life, personal growth, positive relations and self-acceptance) [2]. In recent years, there has been a paradigm shift towards promoting both physical and psychological health, supported by several empirical evidence.

Psychological well-being is closely linked with favourable biological outcomes. A systematic review, involving 29 studies, indicated that positive psychological well-being had a significant correlation with lower inflammatory biomarkers (interleukin–6, and C-reactive protein) [3]. Psychological well-being is associated with lower incidence and slower progression of cardiovascular diseases [4, 5]. Such positive association may result from a healthier lifestyle, better stress management strategies, and reduced inflammation [4]. Furthermore, psychological well-being is perceived to be a vital indicator of positive affective states, optimal functioning and social life [6-8]. Decreased psychological well-being was associated with increased depression and anxiety among people with diabetes [9]. Given the importance of the psychological well-being in predicting other health outcomes, it is essential to promote psychological well-being among people with various sociocultural backgrounds such as adolescents and young adults.

3.2 Psychological Well-being Promotion Model

We proposed the Psychological Well-being Promotion Model, developed based on Neuman's system theory [10] and eudaimonic psychological well-being [11] (Figure 3.1). Within the model, there are four major constructs: stress, resource protection factors, psychological well-being, and prevention intervention.

Stress is defined as a state of biopsychological changes occurring when individuals encounter undesirable circumstances. Such changes may include increased heart rate, hypertension, hyperventilation, elevated blood sugar, suppressed immunity, feelings of nervousness, anxiety and irritability. A systematic review (involving 19 studies) was conducted on various clinics and hospital settings (such as emergency departments, burn units, and intensive care units) [12]. Stress was linked with physical health (such as pain and healthcare utilisation), mental health (such as

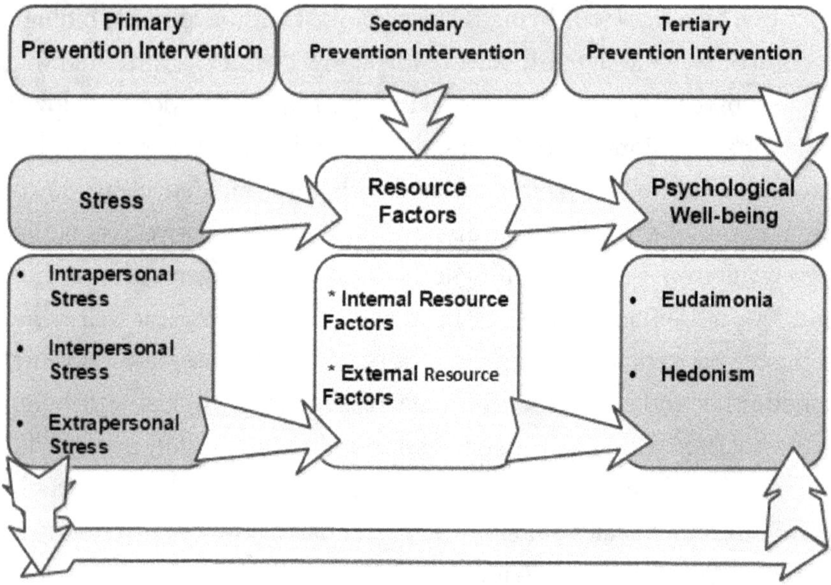

Figure 3.1 The psychological well-being promotion model.

depression, anxiety, and phobia) and behavioural outcomes (alcohol consumption). Within the model, it is postulated that stress has both direct and indirect effects (through resource protection factors) on psychological well-being.

Health refers to the state of wellness or equilibrium where individuals' components (physiological, psychological, sociocultural, spiritual, and developmental) interact with one another in harmony [10]. With this conceptualisation, psychological well-being reflects individuals' best possible psychological state at any given time. Health is in line with eudaimonic psychological well-being, which emphasises living well to the fullest potential [11].

Resource protection factors refer to factors which are activated to protect the individuals from negative effects of stress or unpleasant situations [10]. Resource protection factors comprise internal factors (such as resilience, self-efficacy, and mindfulness) and external factors (such as social support). Existing studies revealed that psychological well-being is linked to resilience [13, 14], self-efficacy [15, 16], mindfulness [17–19], and social support [20, 21].

Prevention intervention helps individuals achieve the state of psychological well-being. The intervention encompasses three levels: primary (promoting health and preventing stress among healthy individuals); secondary (restoring health among people who suffer from stress-related symptoms); and tertiary (regaining and maintaining normal functioning). Prevention intervention may aim to strengthen individuals' resource protection factors, including resilience, self-efficacy, mindfulness, social support, among others.

3.3 Conclusion

The psychological well-being promotion model comprises four main constructs: stress, resource protection factors, psychological well-being and prevention intervention (primary, secondary, and tertiary levels). This model may inform clinical practice in hospital and community settings. Healthcare professionals may provide different levels of prevention in response to clients' needs and their health conditions. The model can be used to guide different research, such as one that tests effectiveness of psychosocial interventions on people with chronic illnesses and/or healthy individuals. The model can guide different research methodologies, including qualitative, descriptive, and randomised control trials.

References

1. Diener E. Subjective well-being. Psychol Bull. 1984;95:542–575.
2. Ryan RM, Deci EL. On happiness and human potentials: a review of research on hedonic and eudaimonic well-being. Annu Rev Psychol. 2001;52:141–166.
3. Zuccarella-Hackl C, Princip M, Auschra B, Meister-Langraf RE, Barth J, von Känel R. Association of positive psychological well-being with circulating

inflammatory markers: a systematic review and meta-analysis. Neurosci Biobehav Rev. 2023;150:105186.

4. Hernandez R, Bassett SM, Boughton SW, Schuette SA, Shiu EW, Moskowitz JT. Psychological well-being and physical health: associations, mechanisms, and future directions. Emotion Rev. 2018;10(1):18–29.
5. Ryff CD. Psychological well-being revisited: advances in the science and practice of eudaimonia. Psychother Psychosom. 2014;83:10–28.
6. Ryff CD. Psychological well-being in adult life. Curr Dir Psychol Sci. 1995;4: 99–104.
7. Ryff CD, Singer B. Psychological well-being: meaning, measurement, and implications for psychotherapy research. Psychother Psychosom. 1996;65:14–23.
8. Kumari A, Thapa K. A Systematic literature review on psychological well-being. Int J Futur Manag Res. 2025;7(2):1–10. Available from: https://www.ijfmr.com/papers/2025/2/43237.pdf
9. Ramkisson S, Pillay BJ, Sartorius B. Anxiety, depression and psychological well-being in a cohort of South African adults with type 2 diabetes. S Afr J Psychiatry. 2016;22:a359.
10. Neuman B, Fawcett J. The Neuman systems model. 4th ed. Upper Saddle River, NJ: Prentice Hall; 2002.
11. Ryff CD, Keyes CLM. The structure of psychological well-being revisited. J Pers Soc Psychol. 1995;69:719–727.
12. Garfin DR, Thompson RR, Holman EA. Acute stress and subsequent health outcomes: a systematic review. J Psychosom Res. 2018;112:107–113.
13. Li ZS, Hasson F. Resilience, stress, and psychological well-being in nursing students: a systematic review. Nurse Educ Today. 2020;90:104440.
14. Tay PKC, Lim KK. Psychological resilience as an emergent characteristic for well-being: a pragmatic view. Gerontology. 2020;66(5):476–483.
15. Priesack A, Alcock J. Well-being and self-efficacy in a sample of undergraduate nurse students: a small survey study. Nurse Educ Today. 2015;35:e16–e20.
16. Tamannaeifar MR, Motaghedifard M. Subjective well-being and its sub-scales among students: the study of role of creativity and self-efficacy. Iran J Psychiatry Behav Sci. 2014;8(1):19–25.
17. Sulosaari V, Unal E, Cinar FI. The effectiveness of mindfulness-based interventions on the psychological well-being of nurses: a systematic review. Appl Nurs Res. 2022;64:151565.
18. Widha WL, Rahmat HK, Basri ASH. A review of mindfulness therapy to improve psychological well-being during the COVID-19 pandemic. Rev Mindfulness Ther COVID-19 Pandemic. 2021;4(1):383–390.

19. Chua JYX, Shorey S. The effect of mindfulness-based and acceptance commitment therapy-based interventions to improve the mental well-being among parents of children with developmental disabilities: a systematic review and meta-analysis. J Autism Dev Disord. 2022;52(6):2770–2783.
20. Cnen TW, Chiu YC, Hsu Y. Perception of social support provided by coaches, optimism/pessimism, and psychological well-being: gender differences and mediating effect models. Int J Sports Sci Coach. 2021;16(2):272–280.
21. Brunsting NC, Zachry C, Liu J, Bryant R, Fang X, Wu S, Luo Z. Sources of perceived social support, social-emotional experiences, and psychological well-being of international students. J Exp Educ. 2021;89(1):95–111.

https://doi.org/10.1142/9789819817320_0004

Chapter 4

Emotional Training in Healthcare: Addressing Stress and Anxiety for Better Clinical Outcomes

Jeanette Ignacio

Alice Lee Centre for Nursing Studies, Yong Loo Lin School of Medicine, National University of Singapore, 10 Medical Drive, Singapore 117597

nurimjj@nus.edu.sg

4.1 Introduction

In the dynamic landscape of the healthcare setting, critical thinking and efficiency are of utmost value. Healthcare professionals are continually faced with challenges that impact on their critical thinking and efficiency, hence affecting their work performance and outcomes. High stress levels resulting from managing high-acuity patient conditions, dealing with distraught patient relatives or a non-collaborative interprofessional team, and adjusting and adhering to strict hospital policies and protocols, among others, affect patient care and outcomes. Additionally, the high-stress nature of the clinical environment also influences the healthcare providers themselves such that they become preoccupied with anxious thoughts and impending burnout that threaten their overall well-being. Burnout impacts the effectiveness of treatment [1]. Studies have shown that burnout in healthcare professionals has a detrimental effect on practitioners, on the effectiveness of treatment for their clients, and on the health of organisations [2, 3]. Workplace-related sustained stress is considered an occupational hazard [4] and can influence individual well-being. Its twofold effects underscore the potential development of physical and mental conditions as sustained stress can lead to cardiovascular conditions while concurrently increasing anxiety and even depression. It is thus imperative for healthcare professionals to be able to manage stress and anxiety by utilising effective stress management techniques. These techniques facilitate the optimisation of the healthcare professional's clinical performance, bringing about the delivery of safe quality care to patients.

Stress is a response to highly charged clinical events that is closely associated with emotions [5]. In the healthcare setting, the patient's responsiveness to treatment has been found to be closely associated with the health professional's connection with the patient [2]. It is vital, therefore, that stress management strategies be underpinned by emotional training principles. By doing so, an individual is equipped to better recognise triggers of stress, respond to them appropriately by regulating emotions associated with stress, and manage stressful events effectively. Emotional training, as the foundation of stress management, improves one's skills to understand and manage emotions more successfully. However, achieving the goals of emotional training to better manage and cope with stress requires time and consistency. Hence, an early initiation of intervention, i.e., prior to clinical practice in the workplace, is recommended. In fact, in a group of medical and nursing students who underwent an emotional training intervention focusing on improving emotional intelligence, positive results were observed in several areas which included stress coping [6]. The findings also suggest that time has the potential to augment the benefits of the intervention [6], hence providing emotional training early and more frequently better equips healthcare professionals to deal with the potential work-related challenges in the course of their clinical careers.

As one of the main goals of emotional training is to help individuals adjust their emotions in response to certain triggers, emotional regulation is intrinsic to this training. Emotional regulation has been defined as "the processes by which individuals influence which emotions they have, when they have them, and how they experience and express these emotions" [7, p. 275]. Successful emotion regulation is important for maintaining wellness and mental health. This is especially crucial for healthcare professionals as they have been entrusted with patient care and safety. The significant role of emotion regulation in improving emotional wellness, job performance, clinical safety, and healthcare effectiveness has been highlighted by research. It has been noted that better emotion regulation leads to a reduction in the perceived stress in professional settings [8]. Various levels of stress occur in different clinical environments. A study by Pálfi *et al.* [9], conducted at the emergency department and participated in by emergency healthcare professionals, emphasised the need for stress management and mental wellness strategies to counter burnout and mental distress resulting from work-related stress. Thus, a reduced use of adaptive emotion regulation strategies was found to be associated with higher burnout levels in staff [9]. The implementation of emotional training that highlights the ability to regulate emotions can enhance the mental wellness of healthcare professionals, thus successfully mitigating burnout and ultimately improving quality of care and patient outcomes. In another study by Martín-Brufau *et al.* [10], it has been suggested that developing targeted emotion regulation strategies can help healthcare professionals manage stress more effectively and decrease the risk of burnout.

Clinical decision-making and response to high-acuity clinical events are also influenced by emotions, consequently affecting patient safety [11]. Healthcare professionals are embedded in emotionally charged environments that oftentimes cause stress leading to negative consequences such as burnout, absenteeism and a high staff turnover rate; unregulated emotions of healthcare professionals thus potentially compromise patient safety and the efficient delivery of healthcare to patients [12]. The importance of patient safety and efficient healthcare delivery cannot be overemphasised, hence critical steps to assist healthcare professionals in regulating their emotions should be taken. This is to offset the deleterious effects of stress and anxiety pervasive within clinical settings. Emotion regulation, an integral component of emotional training, therefore plays an essential part in stress and anxiety management in healthcare professionals. Exploring existing stress and anxiety management strategies, and how they help in reducing the ill effects of stress and anxiety in clinical staff, are key in implementing the appropriate strategies for a targeted group of healthcare professionals. Carrying out such an intervention has wide-ranging outcomes that impact individual well-being and promote work performance, ensuring patient safety and quality of care.

4.2 Understanding Stress and Anxiety in Healthcare

Stress is the body's natural response to any external demand or challenge, whether physical, mental, or emotional [13]. Acute stress is a normal part of life whereas chronic stress can have dire consequences physically, mentally and emotionally. Often, anxiety and stress are used interchangeably. However, these two concepts, although closely linked, are not technically the same. Whereas stress is a bodily response, anxiety is an emotion. According to the American Psychological Association [14], anxiety is "an emotion characterised by feelings of tension, worried thoughts, and physical changes such as increased blood pressure". Stress and anxiety are interrelated, each having an influence on the other.

In the healthcare setting's context, there are variable factors that lead to stress and anxiety among staff. Consequently, these levels of high stress lead to burnout and reduced well-being. Psychological and physical exhaustion as well as potential compromise of quality patient care and safety often result. In fact, high workload and long shift hours in the healthcare professions have been linked to emotional exhaustion, particularly in nurses [15]. According to Dall'Ora *et al.* [16], healthcare professionals working 12 hours or more report significantly higher levels of stress as compared to those who work in standard 8-hour shifts. In a classic paper by Maslach and Jackson [17], it was noted that chronic stress can be emotionally draining, leading to emotional exhaustion and subsequently to burnout. Burnout has been found to be more prevalent in frontline specialties which are more work intensive and have greater emotional demands on the healthcare professional, such as in emergency medicine and family medicine [18]. The significant emotional burden of patient care experienced by healthcare professionals impacts their ability to provide effective patient care and develop empathy to the patients. For instance, emotional exhaustion leading to compassion fatigue often stems from longstanding exposure to patient suffering [19]. Compassion fatigue, if not prevented, can permanently negatively affect compassion ability [20], an essential in healthcare service.

Decision-making, a competency that can potentially be impacted by stress, is vital for healthcare professionals as this requires a careful analysis of complex clinical scenarios under time pressure. Stress increases cognitive load by impairing the brain's capacity to understand and synthesise information from various sources. Attention, necessary for sound decision-making, can be affected [21]. Additionally, emotional distress associated with a highly stressful clinical environment redirects cognitive resources from analytical thinking [22], hence affecting decision-making. Some evidence further suggests that stress weakens reward valuation, a key process in decision-making [23]. The studies highlighted are only a few of those that underscore the significant consequences of stress on the healthcare professionals' decision-making competency. However, aside from the effect of stress on clinical decision-making, interprofessional incivility and conflicts are associated with increased stress in healthcare [24]. Poor team dynamics can compromise patient safety and reduce the quality of care provided. In a study by Ramsay [25], it was highlighted that poor communication is a considerable trigger for conflicts in the clinical setting, noting that from the healthcare professional's perspective, communication, whether the lack of it or being unclear, is a primary cause of discord among healthcare staff. Addressing and managing these conflicts proactively can thus reduce the healthcare professionals' stress and improve quality of care provided to the patients.

Overall, the effects of stress and anxiety in healthcare professionals profoundly impact the individual and the healthcare institution. Individually, psychological effects of stress such as burnout and emotional exhaustion have been well documented in literature [17, 26]. Cognitive effects also lead to decreased decision-making ability that translates to suboptimal clinical performance, patient care and management [5, 21, 27]. Additionally, like in any other occupation, work stress can lead to increased risk for negative physiological effects like cardiovascular conditions [28, 29]. Fatigue can also result from the prevalence of emotionally charged situations in the clinical setting and this considerably impacts patient safety [30]. It is therefore imperative that strategies mitigating stress and anxiety within the confines of the healthcare environment be implemented. Such a move will consequently translate to more efficient clinical management and better patient outcomes resulting from healthcare professionals' enhanced well-being and increased job satisfaction.

4.3 Stress and Anxiety Management Strategies

4.3.1 *Personal Coping Strategies*

Emotional training is crucial for healthcare professionals as the clinical setting is a high-stress environment. To facilitate well-being among healthcare professionals, a multifaceted approach is essential. Utilising various methods and interventions from different angles to tackle a complex issue such as stress and anxiety in the clinical setting has the potential to provide more innovative solutions that result in more valuable and comprehensive outcomes.

Personal coping strategies are at the forefront of emotional training. An individual's ability to cope is a manifestation of emotional stress regulation that leads to adaptation [5]. In healthcare, multiple strategies are currently being utilised to facilitate the health professionals' coping and adaptation for better stress and anxiety management. These strategies are essential for them to be able to function optimally in the clinical setting, ensuring competency in analysing clinical situations, soundness in clinical decision-making and efficiency in delivering care to patients.

Mindfulness is a concept that espouses present moment awareness and a non-judgemental attitude on everything occurring at that moment [31]. It has gained popularity as an effective technique for stress and anxiety management because of its evidence-backed benefits, adaptability across different fields, and its accessibility. A meta-analysis of 29 studies by Khoury *et al.* [32] noted that mindfulness-based stress reduction is moderately effective in decreasing stress and anxiety in healthy individuals. There is also evidence that mindfulness practice can increase grey matter in brain areas responsible for regulating emotion [33], hence mitigating the stress response. As a versatile stress management approach, mindfulness-based strategies are adaptable in various fields and in multiple settings. For instance, it has been used to moderate stress in clinical settings and in institutions of higher learning for healthcare professionals [34].

Meditation is considered a type of mental training to enhance one's psychological abilities, resulting in improved well-being [35] and often serves as a technique to nurture the mental state of mindfulness. Meditation and mindfulness are intricately linked. According to Hölzel *et al.* [36], mindfulness meditation works through mechanisms such as attention regulation, body awareness, and emotional regulation. Thus, mindful meditation is an essential component of any mindfulness-based stress management strategy.

Aside from mindfulness and meditation, other effective stress and anxiety management strategies work on changing how individuals think and react to less than ideal situations, such as when faced with challenges or acute critical events. These strategies utilise the cognitive-behavioural approach. One construct involved in this approach is self-reflection. In self-reflection, one takes time to learn about and be aware of oneself — one's thoughts, emotions and values, among others. This generally leads to enhanced mental well-being [37]. Another cognitive-behavioural approach to managing stress and anxiety is called positive reappraisal which involves viewing a stressful event in an optimistic light, that is, it is not harmful but rather beneficial to oneself, thus improving mental health [38].

Physical activity can also reduce stress because activities stimulate immune, physiological and psychological mechanisms resulting in the mitigation of anxiety, stress and depression [39]. According to Anderson and Shivakumar [40], a multifaceted relationship between exercise and anxiety exists and this involves both physiological and psychological mechanisms. Physiologically, regular exercise regulates the hypothalamic-pituitary-adrenal axis, resulting in lessened stress hormone levels and enhanced response to stress, and neurogenesis and neurotransmitter function are also contributors to better emotional regulation [40]. Psychologically, exercise serves as a distraction from stressors, boosts self-efficacy, and provides a sense of accomplishment, all of which can reduce anxiety levels. Anderson and Shivakumar [40] further note that while the exact mechanisms are complex and not fully understood, the cumulative evidence supports the role of physical activity as a beneficial intervention for anxiety management. They advocate for incorporating exercise into treatment plans for individuals with anxiety disorders, emphasising its potential as a complementary strategy alongside traditional therapies. Furthermore, consistent exercise has been shown to reduce symptoms of anxiety and depression, making it a vital component of stress management programs. By incorporating physical activity into daily routines, individuals can experience both immediate relief and long-term protection against the negative effects of stress.

4.3.2 *Institutional Support Strategies*

Individuals in high-pressure environments, such as in healthcare and education, benefit from peer support and mentorship programmes that contribute to stress management. In the healthcare context, peer support involves the "provision of emotional, appraisal, and informational assistance by a created social network member who possesses experiential knowledge of a specific behaviour or stressor" [41, p. 329]. This principle can apply to both patients and healthcare professionals. Thus, peer support can provide structured opportunities that allow individuals to receive emotional, informational, and appraisal support from others within the organisation. Such a provision gives encouragement and assists in coping with challenges in the working environment.

Mentorship is another safety net that not only promotes professional development, but also has the potential to contribute to emotional wellness. As a result of having a mentorship programme, mentees reported reduced anxiety and an enhanced psychological autonomy [42]. Additionally, mentors contribute to mentees' success by offering emotional and moral support, nurturing their development in both personal and professional domains, and serving as advocates and protectors within their institutions [43]. Mentorship, therefore, is associated with job and career satisfaction, with the potential effect of increasing retention [42].

Other strategies that are increasingly gaining attention as important strategies for stress and anxiety management in healthcare settings are resilience and emotional intelligence training. These strategies aid healthcare professionals face workplace challenges such as high workloads, emotional fatigue, and stressful decision-making situations. Skills to regulate emotions, cope with stressors, and maintain psychological wellness are harnessed through these training programmes. Resilience training focuses on an individual's ability to persevere and cope despite challenges and setbacks. In essence, resilience training helps an individual cultivate traits that are protective against the ill effects of potential stressors and may include strategies such as mindfulness and cognitive-behavioural therapy, among others [44]. Emotional intelligence training, meanwhile, facilitates emotional regulation that enhances one's ability to respond to emotions appropriately, thus minimising the negative effects of stress and anxiety. It has been shown that emotional training programmes can improve work performance, raise organisational commitment, and increase job retention [45].

4.3.3 *Simulation-Based Training for Emotional Preparedness*

Simulation-based training for emotional preparedness is an essential element of emotional training strategies in healthcare. It facilitates an engaging, practical and realistic approach to developing not only clinical competence, but also emotional resilience to withstand the challenges in high-acuity clinical settings. The use of role-playing, virtual reality and standardised patients are usually involved in simulation-based training. The utilisation of standardised patient interactions to create realistic clinical scenarios elicit authentic psychological responses similar to those encountered in actual practice [46]. As realistic emotions are evoked during the simulations, healthcare professionals become more prepared to manage stress and anxiety in similar clinical settings in the future. In addition, experiential learning, which underpins simulation-based training, allows for reflective practice that is of benefit when engaged in emotionally charged clinical events. Simulation-based training therefore supports individual wellness and, at the same time, adds value to patient care by enabling the healthcare professional to deliver more emotionally attuned care to patients.

4.4 Challenges in Implementing Emotional Training in Healthcare

The overall stigma around mental health issues and the fear of being judged as psychologically weak or emotionally vulnerable remain as major barriers that prevent individuals from actively seeking emotional support. Expectations of being discriminated against promote a non-help-seeking behaviour which discourages participation in mental wellness interventions and programmes [47]. Furthermore, the heavy workloads and prolonged working hours, among others, are factors that result in chronic stress — a contributor to burnout [48]. These factors intensify time pressures within clinical settings, thereby limiting healthcare professionals' capacity to engage in emotional training initiatives.

As have been highlighted, there are various approaches to emotional training that involve an array of content, duration and delivery methods. This variety makes evaluation of emotional training difficult in terms of outcomes and effectiveness. Standardised curricula and validated outcome measures are needed to ensure robustness and usefulness of any implemented emotional training programme. In addition, the disparity of mental wellness resources among institutions needs to be addressed to guarantee all health professionals and healthcare students equal access to mental health resources.

4.5 Future Directions and Recommendations

Clinical environments are inherently high-pressure settings, marked by frequent exposure to emotionally intense situations that can precipitate considerable stress and anxiety among healthcare professionals. Such stress not only affects the well-being of healthcare professionals but may also impair clinical decision-making and communication, thereby adversely influencing patient care and outcomes. It is crucial, therefore, that healthcare professionals be equipped with the necessary tools to assist them manage stress and anxiety. To mitigate potential negative effects, it is essential to introduce emotional training strategies early on and embed them during their healthcare education. This will equip students with the emotional preparedness needed to navigate the more demanding realities of clinical practice. Not only should healthcare curricula be embedded with programmes or courses that facilitate stress management, interdisciplinary training in emotional regulation and resilience should also be promoted in health professions education. Such moves advocate for mental wellness necessary for healthcare students' future clinical practice.

To further safeguard mental wellness, the emotional training strategies introduced during the healthcare students' education should be continued during their working life. Hospitals and other healthcare institutions should have policies in place that mandate leadership support for mental wellness schemes. Standardised guidelines for stress management programmes should also be established.

As emotional training includes various approaches and strategies that might need to be tailored to a variety of healthcare professionals in diverse clinical settings, it is essential that the long-term effectiveness of the emotional training interventions be assessed. Additionally, future research should evaluate their impact on patient outcomes.

4.6 Conclusion

Stress and anxiety in healthcare settings are a given. They inevitably come with the highly emotionally charged clinical events that elicit stress and anxiety in healthcare professionals. To mitigate the ill effects of these emotions on patient management, and subsequently on patient outcomes, it is imperative to include emotional training strategies into health professions' curricula, and in hospital and healthcare institutions' programmes. Such a step will guarantee that the mental wellness of healthcare students and staff are prioritised as this will translate into more sound clinical decisions, satisfactory patient care and, ultimately, better patient outcomes.

References

1. Morse G, Salyers MP, Rollins AL, Monroe-DeVita M, Pfahler C. Burnout in mental health services: a review of the problem and its remediation. Adm Policy Ment Health. 2012;39(5):341–352.
2. Simpson DD, Joe GW, Rowan-Szal GA, Greener JM. The impact of organizational stress and burnout on client engagement. J Subst Abuse Treat. 2009;36(2):185–193.
3. Skinner N, Roche AM. Stress and burnout: a prevention handbook for the alcohol and other drugs workforce. Adelaide: National Centre for Education and Training on Addiction (NCETA), Flinders University; 2005.
4. Duraisingam V, Roche A, Pidd K, Zoontjens A, Pollard Y. Wellbeing, stress and burnout: a national survey of managers in alcohol and other drug treatment services. Adelaide: National Centre for Education and Training on Addiction (NCETA), Flinders University; 2007.
5. Ignacio J. Stress management in crisis event simulations for enhancing performance [dissertation]. Singapore: Maastricht University; 2017.
6. Taylor M, Hoch J, Porter K. Educational interventions to improve emotional intelligence in nursing and medical students: a systematic review. J Nurs Educ Pract. 2023;13(1):19–30.
7. Gross JJ. The emerging field of emotion regulation: an integrative review. Rev Gen Psychol. 1998;2(3):271–299.
8. Kadović M, Mikšić Š, Lovrić R. Ability of emotional regulation and control as a stress predictor in healthcare professionals. Int J Environ Res Public Health. 2022;20(1):541.
9. Pálfi K, Major J, Horváth-Sarródi A, *et al.* Adaptive emotion regulation might prevent burnout in emergency healthcare professionals: an exploratory study. BMC Public Health. 2024;24:3136.
10. Martín-Brufau R, Martin-Gorgojo A, Suso-Ribera C, Estrada E, Capriles-Ovalles ME, Romero-Brufau S. Emotion regulation strategies, workload conditions, and burnout in healthcare residents. Int J Environ Res Public Health. 2020;17(21):7816.
11. Heyhoe J, Birks Y, Harrison R, O'Hara JK, Cracknell A, Lawton R. The role of emotion in patient safety: are we brave enough to scratch beneath the surface? J R Soc Med. 2016;109(2):52–58.
12. Sattar R, Lawton R, Janes G, *et al.* A systematic review of workplace triggers of emotions in the healthcare environment, the emotions experienced, and the impact on patient safety. BMC Health Serv Res. 2024;24:603.

13. World Health Organization. Stress [Internet]. Geneva: World Health Organization; [cited 2025 Feb 20]. Available from: https://www.who.int/newsroom/questions-and-answers/item/stress
14. American Psychological Association. Anxiety [Internet]. Washington, DC: American Psychological Association; [cited 2025 Feb 20]. Available from: https://www.apa.org/topics/anxiety
15. Vetbuje BG. Burnout of nurses due to workload and long working hours during shifts: review article. Int Arch Nurs Health Care. 2023;9:191.
16. Dall'Ora C, Griffiths P, Ball J, Simon M, Aiken LH. Association of 12 h shifts and nurses' job satisfaction, burnout and intention to leave: findings from a cross-sectional study of 12 European countries. BMJ Open. 2015;5(9):e008331.
17. Maslach C, Jackson SE. The measurement of experienced burnout. J Occup Behav. 1981;2(2):99–113.
18. Shanafelt TD, Boone S, Tan L, Dyrbye LN, Sotile W, Satele D, *et al.* Burnout and satisfaction with work-life balance among US physicians relative to the general US population. Arch Intern Med. 2012;172(18):1377–1385.
19. Figley CR. Compassion fatigue: coping with secondary traumatic stress disorder in those who treat the traumatized. 1st ed. New York: Routledge; 1995.
20. Coetzee SK, Klopper HC. Compassion fatigue within nursing practice: a concept analysis. Nurs Health Sci. 2010;12(2):235–243.
21. LeBlanc VR. The effects of acute stress on performance: implications for health professions education. Acad Med. 2009;84(10 Suppl):S25–S33.
22. Pessoa L. How do emotion and motivation direct executive control? Trends Cogn Sci. 2009;13(4):160–166.
23. Porcelli AJ, Delgado MR. Stress and decision making: effects on valuation, learning, and risk-taking. Curr Opin Behav Sci. 2017;14:33–39.
24. Lewis C. The impact of interprofessional incivility on medical performance, service and patient care: a systematic review. Future Healthc J. 2023;10(1):69–77.
25. Ramsay MA. Conflict in the healthcare workplace. Proc (Bayl Univ Med Cent). 2001;14(2):138–139.
26. López-Cabarcos MA, López-Carballeira A, Ferro-Soto C. How to moderate emotional exhaustion among public healthcare professionals? Eur Res Manag Bus Econ. 2021;27(2):100140.
27. Larkin AC, Cahan MA, Whalen G, Hatem D, Starr S, Haley HL, *et al.* Human emotion and response in surgery (HEARS): a simulation-based curriculum for communication skills, systems-based practice, and professionalism in surgical residency training. J Am Coll Surg. 2010;211(2):285–292.

28. Albeshr NA, Simsekler MCE, Ugwuoke NV, Dalkilinc M, Al Qubaisi M, Campos LA, *et al.* Burnout and cardiovascular risk in healthcare professionals during the COVID-19 pandemic. Front Psychiatry. 2022;13:867233.
29. Kivimäki M, Kawachi I. Work stress as a risk factor for cardiovascular disease. Curr Cardiol Rep. 2015;17(9):630.
30. Zabin LM, Zaitoun RSA, Sweity EM, de Tantillo L. The relationship between job stress and patient safety culture among nurses: a systematic review. BMC Nurs. 2023;22(1):39.
31. Kabat-Zinn J. Bringing mindfulness to medicine: an interview with Jon Kabat-Zinn, PhD. Adv Mind Body Med. 2005;21(2):22–27.
32. Khoury B, Sharma M, Rush SE, Fournier C. Mindfulness-based stress reduction for healthy individuals: a meta-analysis. J Psychosom Res. 2015;78(6):519–528.
33. Hölzel BK, Carmody J, Vangel M, Congleton C, Yerramsetti SM, Gard T, *et al.* Mindfulness practice leads to increases in regional brain gray matter density. Psychiatry Res Neuroimaging. 2011;191(1):36–43.
34. Irving JA, Dobkin PL, Park J. Cultivating mindfulness in health care professionals: a review of empirical studies of mindfulness-based stress reduction (MBSR). Complement Ther Clin Pract. 2009;15(2):61–66.
35. Tang YY, Hölzel BK, Posner MI. The neuroscience of mindfulness meditation. Nat Rev Neurosci. 2015;16(4):213–225.
36. Hölzel BK, Lazar SW, Gard T, Schuman-Olivier Z, Vago DR, Ott U. How does mindfulness meditation work? Proposing mechanisms of action from a conceptual and neural perspective. Perspect Psychol Sci. 2011;6(6):537–559.
37. Morin A. Self-awareness part 1: definition, measures, effects, functions, and antecedents. Soc Personal Psychol Compass. 2011;5:807–823.
38. Garland EL, Gaylord SA, Fredrickson BL. Positive reappraisal mediates the stress-reductive effects of mindfulness: an upward spiral process. Mindfulness. 2011;2(1):59–67.
39. Mikkelsen K, Stojanovska L, Polenakovic M, Bosevski M, Apostolopoulos V. Exercise and mental health. Maturitas. 2017;106:48–56.
40. Anderson E, Shivakumar G. Effects of exercise and physical activity on anxiety. Front Psychiatry. 2013;4:27.
41. Dennis CL. Peer support within a health care context: a concept analysis. Int J Nurs Stud. 2003;40(3):321–332.
42. Nowell L, Norris JM, Mrklas K, White DE. Mixed methods systematic review exploring mentorship outcomes in nursing academia. J Adv Nurs. 2017;73(3):527–544.
43. Sambunjak D, Straus SE, Marušić A. Mentoring in academic medicine: a systematic review. JAMA. 2006;296(9):1103–1115.

44. Robertson IT, Cooper CL, Sarkar M, Curran T. Resilience training in the workplace from 2003 to 2014: a systematic review. J Occup Organ Psychol. 2015;88(3):533–562.
45. Codier E, Kamikawa C, Kooker BM, Shoultz J. Emotional intelligence, performance, and retention in clinical staff nurses. Nurs Adm Q. 2010;34(3):236–243.
46. Ignacio J, Dolmans D, Scherpbier A, Rethans JJ, Chan S, Liaw SY. Comparison of standardized patients with high-fidelity simulators for managing stress and improving performance in clinical deterioration: a mixed methods study. Nurse Educ Today. 2015;35(12):1161–1168.
47. Henderson C, Evans-Lacko S, Thornicroft G. Mental illness stigma, help seeking, and public health programs. Am J Public Health. 2013;103(5):777–780.
48. West CP, Dyrbye LN, Shanafelt TD. Physician burnout: contributors, consequences, and solutions. J Intern Med. 2018;283(6):516–529.

https://doi.org/10.1142/9789819817320_0005

Chapter 5

Reimagining Adolescent Mental Health in Thailand: A Nurse-Led Pathway toward Sustainable Prevention through Digital Technology "MU MyMind"

Nopporn Vongsirimas

Faculty of Nursing, Mahidol University, 999, Phuttamonthon 4 Road, Salaya, Nakhon Pathom 73170, Thailand

Nopporn.von@mahidol.ac.th

5.1 Introduction

Over the past decade, I have had the privilege of witnessing the growing urgency of adolescent mental health needs in Thailand — not only through research data, but through the lived experiences of students, families, nurses, and educators across the country. Their voices, often quiet yet unwavering, have illuminated a truth that transcends statistics: emotional suffering among youth is not a private burden, but a collective responsibility.

As a mental health nurse educator, I have walked alongside countless nursing students during their clinical placements in schools and community clinics. I vividly recall one story during my time working in one community. A teenager approached me, eyes filled with hesitation, and confided that she had recently completed an online mental health screening provided by the Department of Mental Health. The result indicated symptoms of depression. Looking uncertain and overwhelmed, she asked, "I don't know what to do next." That moment stayed with me. It reaffirmed a truth I have long believed — that behind every screening result is a young person navigating fear, confusion, and fragile hope.

It reminded me that meaningful intervention often begins not with complex protocols, but with the simple, human act of being present — listening without judgment and creating spaces of trust and dignity. These encounters quietly seeded the vision for MU MyMind — a digital mental health intervention we co-developed with the support of the National Research Council of Thailand. MU MyMind was designed to be more than a set of modules; it was envisioned as a bridge connecting adolescents to early, evidence-based support delivered with compassion and respect for their autonomy.

During the initial pilot phase of MU MyMind, I observed adolescents engaging with the "Breathe to Relieve Stress" module. One adolescent later told me, "It's the first time I felt like I had a space that belonged to me." That simple yet profound comment reaffirmed our mission. It became clear that prevention is not merely a strategy — it is a form of dignity, a recognition of each young person's inherent worth and potential.

Looking ahead, we envision MU MyMind being integrated into primary care services across Thailand, led by nurses at the frontlines of community health. Nurses are uniquely positioned to recognise early signs of emotional distress, offer timely support, and guide adolescents towards further care when needed. By embedding digital mental health interventions within nurse-led primary care settings, we aim to make mental health support more accessible, compassionate, and sustainable for future generations.

What if mental health care could begin not at the edge of crisis, but at the heart of community life? What if prevention was no longer an afterthought, but a central strategy within the healthcare system? By exploring a nurse-led model for depression prevention among adolescents — particularly through the use of digital tools and primary care infrastructure — this chapter invites a reimagination of how we design mental health services.

It is my belief that nurses, who are often the most enduring presence in both households and health systems, are uniquely equipped to lead this transformation. In writing this chapter, I am not merely advocating for a program or a platform, but for a **paradigm shift**: one that sees adolescence not as a problem to be solved, but as a possibility to be nurtured.

"True prevention in mental health begins not with systems alone, but with seeing adolescents as whole human beings — worthy of trust, belonging, and the quiet confidence that someone will walk alongside them, before crisis calls."

Note: Elements of research findings related to the "MU MyMind" have been published in Chapter 7. This chapter, therefore, does not seek to replicate the findings, but rather to **translate them into a broader discussion on system design, policy integration, and the reimagination of preventive mental health frameworks**. It is not merely a presentation of data, but the culmination of questions carried through clinical observations, policy dialogues, and countless conversations in rural community clinics.

5.2 The Mental Health and Psychiatric Landscape

Mental health has increasingly emerged as a global health priority, with a marked surge in prevalence following the COVID-19 pandemic. Within just one year of the pandemic, rates of depression and anxiety rose by more than 25% worldwide [1]. Specifically, the number of individuals experiencing depression increased from 193 million (2,471 per 100,000 population) to 246 million (3,153 per 100,000), while anxiety disorders rose from 298 million (3,825 per 100,000) to 374 million (4,802 per 100,000) [2]. The World Health Organization further reported that approximately 970 million people — or one in every eight individuals globally — are living with a mental health condition, with 82% residing in low- and middle-income countries, predominantly within Asia [3].

In the Southeast Asia region, depression and anxiety are the most commonly reported psychiatric disorders, accounting for 34.9% and 18.1% respectively — together representing 53% of all mental health conditions [4]. These disorders contribute significantly to the burden of disease, representing 23% of years lived with disability and 10% of disability-adjusted life years. Depression and self-harm are among the top 20 causes of disability-adjusted life years. Globally, suicide claims the lives of one in every 100 people, and individuals with severe mental illness tend to die 10–20 years earlier than the general population [1]. Moreover, 15% of the global working-age population experience mental health conditions, leading to the loss of 12 billion work days annually, with an estimated economic cost exceeding one trillion U.S. dollars [5].

Thailand reflects these global trends, with escalating mental health challenges evident across multiple indicators. First, there has been a sharp rise in high stress levels, risk of depression, and suicide risk. Between 2023 and 2024, high stress prevalence increased from 4.5% to 15.5%, risk of depression from 5.8% to 17.2%, and suicide risk from 3.2% to 10.6% [6]. Second, the number of psychiatric service users has grown substantially. Between 2015 and 2024, the number of individuals receiving psychiatric care rose by 123%, from 1.3 million to 2.9 million cases [7]. These findings align with the "Mental Health Check-in" project, which reports significant rates of depression symptoms (7.1%), low resilience (3.6%), suicide risk (3.3%), high stress (2.4%), and burnout (1.6%) — with adolescents and working-age adults living in Bangkok and urban municipalities identified as particularly vulnerable groups [8].

The 2023 National Epidemiological Survey on Mental Health further revealed that approximately 1.68 million Thais have experienced at least one psychotic episode during their lifetime, highlighting the potential for progression to severe psychiatric disorders [9]. Third, suicide rates have continued to rise. In fiscal year 2023, 5,172 individuals died by suicide, equating to an average of 14 deaths per day — or one life lost every two hours. Suicide attempts totalled 31,110 cases, or 85 per day. Suicide rates have risen from 6.0 per 100,000 in 2017 to 7.9 per 100,000 in 2023, with males facing nearly five times the risk of females. The highest suicide rates were observed among working-age adults (20–59 years), reflecting pressures related to economic hardship, employment, and family dynamics [10]. Fourth, data from public media and social media platforms indicate a growing societal awareness of mental health concerns in Thailand. According to Google Trends data (October 2023–October 2024), searches for terms such as "depression", "panic disorder" and "mental health" increased steadily. Content analyses of Facebook, X (formerly Twitter), and YouTube (September 2023–August 2024) identified 2,562 posts relating to mental health, with keywords such as "suicide" and "depression" appearing 451 and 385 times respectively. Posts mentioning "work stress" and "financial stress" garnered over 1.6 million engagements, suggesting that digital platforms are becoming vital spaces for individuals to express concerns and seek social validation and support [11].

Key factors contributing to the rising prevalence of mental health problems include economic and social changes, increased demand for mental health services following the pandemic, overuse of technology and social media, and environmental crises such as climate change and natural disasters [12]. Specific factors affecting mental health in Southeast Asia include poverty, economic inequality, cultural stigma surrounding mental illness, shortages of mental health professionals and services, and vulnerabilities associated with natural disasters and climate change [13]. These trends collectively underscore the urgent need for proactive mental health policy initiatives — especially those focused on prevention and health promotion — to build a responsive and resilient mental health system capable of meeting the evolving needs of populations in a digital era.

"In the face of rising global and national mental health challenges, true transformation will not come from statistics alone, but from our collective commitment to listen deeply, act compassionately, and rebuild systems that honour the dignity and resilience of every young person."

5.3 Mental Health Policy and Development Plans

The World Health Organization developed the Comprehensive Mental Health Action Plan 2013–2030 with the vision that mental health is a fundamental aspect of individual well-being. Every person should have their mental health promoted, protected, and safeguarded against mental disorders, and should be able to access quality, culturally appropriate mental health services within their communities [14]. The primary goal of the Action Plan is to encourage countries to comprehensively address mental health and uphold human rights. Its four strategic objectives are:

1. To strengthen effective leadership and governance for mental health through national health policies;
2. To provide comprehensive, integrated mental health and social care services at the community level, including through primary health-care systems;
3. To promote and protect the human rights of persons with mental health conditions and to empower individuals, families, and communities; and
4. To enhance the collection, analysis, and dissemination of mental health data of high quality.

Despite global advocacy efforts, the World Mental Health Report 2022 highlights persistent challenges in management, resources, service provision, information systems, and technology [15]. Although many countries have adopted policies promoting community-based mental health services, the development and delivery of primary care mental health services remain slow and uneven. A significant proportion of the population, particularly in low- and middle-income countries, continues to face barriers to accessing services. Several structural factors contribute to this gap, including inadequate budget allocation and a shortage of trained personnel. Mental health funding typically accounts for less than 2% of national health budgets, with the majority directed towards large psychiatric hospitals. Less than 20% of mental health funding is allocated to general hospitals and community mental health services [15].

The shortage of human resources is equally critical, with an average of only one mental health worker per 100,000 population, most of whom are concentrated in secondary and tertiary care settings [15]. The limited availability of mental health professionals at the primary care level restricts the provision of psychosocial interventions that are essential for early intervention and prevention. Access to essential psychiatric medications also remains a significant barrier, particularly in low- and middle-income countries, where availability is limited and costs are often prohibitive [15].

Moreover, the development of robust mental health information systems remains incomplete. Current data largely originate from psychiatric hospitals and fail to capture service utilisation at the primary and secondary care levels [15].

Finally, limited internet access among large segments of the population further constrains the ability to disseminate information, deliver online counselling services, and expand digital mental health interventions. These realities highlight the urgent need for systemic reforms that not only address service gaps but also build sustainable, community-centred mental health systems responsive to diverse needs [15].

"A truly responsive mental health system cannot be built through infrastructure alone; it must be cultivated through relationships, equity, and the unwavering belief that every community holds the seeds of its own healing."

5.4 Thailand's Mental Health Landscape and the Role of Primary Care Clinics

Thailand's adolescent mental health crisis mirrors global patterns but is further complicated by unique structural challenges. National data indicate that approximately 1.5 million Thais suffer from depressive symptoms, with over 30% of adolescents at risk of depression and nearly one in five having contemplated suicide [16, 17]. These are not abstract numbers — they are a call for urgent, system-level innovation.

Despite long-standing efforts from the Ministry of Public Health, such as nationwide school-based screening initiated in 2007, service delivery has struggled to keep pace with rising needs. The asymmetrical distribution of mental health professionals — only 295 child and adolescent psychiatrists across the country, a third of whom are based in Bangkok — presents a profound barrier to equitable care [18]. For youth in rural provinces, professional psychiatric support often remains out of reach, if not entirely invisible. This is where primary care clinics emerge not only as alternative service points — but as potential transformation nodes within the healthcare system. With over 5,000 community clinics and thousands of professional nurses distributed throughout the country, there exists an untapped workforce that is already embedded in the daily lives of Thai families. These nurses are not just service providers — they are cultural interpreters, trusted community members, and frontline agents of early detection. Recognising this, our research team collaborated with the National Research Council to integrate a digital tool, MU MyMind, into primary care workflows. The tool was not designed to replace human care, but to amplify it — to extend reach, enhance early identification, and offer adolescents a sense of privacy and ownership over their mental health journey. But even with promising results from pilot studies showing significant reductions in stress, anxiety, and depressive symptoms, the question remains: can we evolve from pilot to policy? Can nurse-led clinics be officially recognised and resourced as mental health gateways for young people? The answer, we argue, lies not merely in technology or protocol, but in redefining what mental health infrastructure looks like in the Thai context. It is not built from buildings and budgets alone — it is built from relationships, trust, and the capacity to care early, locally, and continuously.

"The future of adolescent mental health in Thailand will not be shaped solely by technology or institutions, but by the quiet, enduring presence of nurses who meet young people early, listen without judgment, and build care systems from the ground up — one relationship at a time."

5.5 Innovation in Action

As an illustrative case, one youth-centred digital intervention — MU MyMind — offers insight into how culturally attuned, nurse-integrated tools can support mental health promotion. Co-designed by nurses, adolescents, and mental health experts, MU MyMind was developed not merely as a set of online modules but as a bridge between early emotional distress and accessible support within community health systems. Its design reflected principles of privacy, autonomy, and emotional resonance, all of which are essential for adolescent engagement.

Rather than examining the technical components or evaluating outcomes already addressed in Chapter 7, this section considers MU MyMind as a prototype for how nurse-led digital tools can integrate into prevention frameworks. It serves as a proof of concept that relational care, technological access, and community-based delivery can intersect effectively when guided by trusted professionals — particularly nurses embedded in the primary care landscape.

This example supports the argument that meaningful prevention is not merely about tools, but about how those tools are situated within relationships, policies, and systems that reflect the lived realities of youth and frontline providers.

5.5.1 *Stakeholder Engagement: Voices Informing System Design*

To ensure that the proposed model aligns with the lived realities of those involved in adolescent mental health, extensive stakeholder engagement was conducted. Rather than repeating direct quotations or detailed narratives presented in Chapter 7, this section distils cross-cutting themes that emerged from conversations with adolescents, parents, teachers, nurses, and mental health professionals. Stakeholders consistently emphasised five thematic priorities:

1. **Confidential and Trustworthy Spaces** — Adolescents value environments where they can seek help without fear of judgment or breach of privacy.
2. **Cultural and Visual Relevance** — Youth expressed a preference for materials and interventions that reflect their context, use simple language, and incorporate relatable visuals.
3. **Autonomy and Self-Directed Access** — Both adolescents and providers supported systems that allow young people to initiate help-seeking, especially through digital platforms.
4. **Timely and Tiered Support** — Teachers and nurses highlighted the need for a stratified support system — one that responds differently to varying levels of distress.
5. **Relational Continuity** — Families and frontline staff pointed to the importance of sustained, trusting relationships over one-time interventions.

These themes form the ethical and practical foundation for the Nurse-Led Depression Prevention Clinic (NDPC) model. They also reinforce the proposition that meaningful prevention requires relational sensitivity, cultural humility, and systemic coordination across the diverse actors involved in adolescent care.

5.5.2 *Pilot Results*

Preliminary findings from the initial pilot and subsequent controlled trials of the MU MyMind application — detailed extensively in Chapter 7 — indicated promising trends in adolescent emotional resilience, reduced depressive symptoms, and improved stress management. These outcomes were supported not only by quantitative metrics, but also by qualitative feedback that underscored the application's potential to foster trust and early engagement.

Rather than repeating specific data points here, this chapter emphasises the implications of those findings for broader system design. Specifically, the pilot results validate the feasibility of integrating nurse-led digital interventions into community-based mental health care. They also reinforce the value of culturally relevant, adolescent-centred tools in promoting timely and personalised mental health support within primary care settings.

Informed by this pilot phase, the next section explores how these insights were translated into the structural elements of the NDPC model.

5.6 Designing the Model: Nursing-Led Systems for Adolescent Mental Health Prevention

To address the mental health needs of adolescents in a sustainable and meaningful way, it is necessary to move beyond isolated interventions and toward the development of an integrated, preventive, and community-engaged system of care. Nurses, situated at the vital intersection of health-care delivery, community life, and long-term relationship-building, are uniquely positioned to lead such initiatives. Their accessibility, continuity of care, and trusted presence within communities make them central to the development of a responsive mental health infrastructure.

Drawing from both empirical evidence and field-based insights, this section proposes a conceptual framework for the NDPC model, specifically adapted to the Thai healthcare and cultural context. The model aims to strengthen preventive services, promote early identification and intervention, and foster a holistic approach to adolescent mental health within community settings.

5.6.1 *Nurse-Led Depression Prevention Clinic Framework Diagram*

To visually represent the conceptual structure of the NDPC model, this section introduces a framework diagram that illustrates the flow from systemic context to adolescent outcomes. Unlike the tables and graphs of pilot findings detailed in Chapter 7, this figure focuses on the integration of design principles, stakeholder-informed priorities, and implementation mechanisms.

5.6.2 *Conceptual Framework of the Nurse-Led Depression Prevention Clinic Model*

- **Input Layer:** Stakeholder insights, pilot findings (Chapter 7), adolescent needs, nurse capacity
- **Process Layer:** Digital tool co-creation, screening protocols, referral pathways, youth engagement strategies
- **Structural Supports:** Integration with community health systems, policy alignment, data governance
- **Expected Outcomes:** Improved emotional resilience, early identification of distress, enhanced access to care

This framework encapsulates the relational and contextual factors that drive the NDPC model, ensuring it aligns with both community realities and scalable system design. It reflects the shift from program-specific outputs to a replicable and sustainable mental health prevention architecture (Figure 5.1).

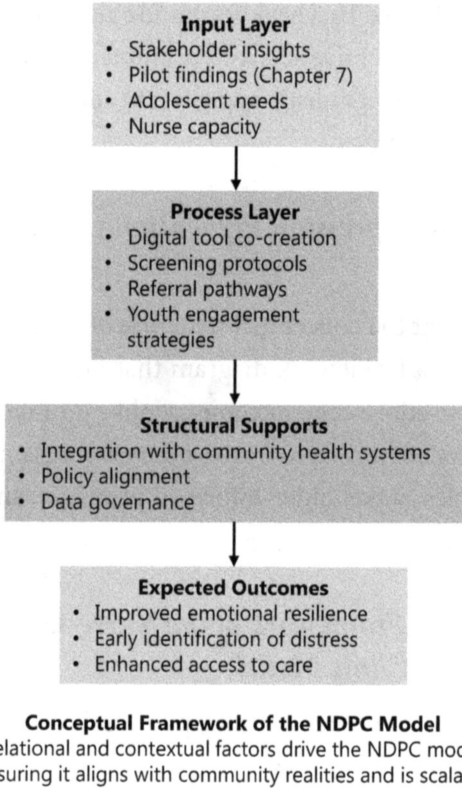

Figure 5.1 Conceptual framework of the NDPC model.

5.6.3 *Proposed Model for Implementation: Advancing a Nurse-Led, Community-Based System for Adolescent Mental Health Prevention*

Adolescent mental health care must move beyond fragmented, reactive systems toward community-embedded, relational models led by trusted local actors. Drawing from field experience, stakeholder engagement, and early program prototyping, this proposal outlines the NDPC model designed to integrate early identification, empowerment, and system-level supports within the fabric of Thai communities.

Table 5.1 The NDPC model.

Component	Description	System Implications
Early Identification	Screening using digital tools (DASS) in schools and clinics, stratified by risk.	Enables timely, differentiated care; reduces over-reliance on tertiary services.
Safe Access Pathways	Adolescents ≥18 can self-refer for counselling without parental gatekeeping.	Promotes youth autonomy; requires legal and policy adaptations.
Tiered Nursing Intervention	Tier 1: Psychoeducation; Tier 2: Brief Counselling; Tier 3: Referral Coordination.	Utilises and expands existing nursing workforce; requires certification and supervision.
Community Integration	Engages families, teachers, volunteers, and spiritual leaders in the care process.	Builds a culturally grounded, relational system of support.
Digital Support System	Use of MU MyMind for screening, tracking, exercises, and follow-up.	Extends accessibility; requires IT infrastructure and data privacy safeguards.
Policy and Financing Enablers	UHC inclusion, payment for services, short-course certifications.	Ensures sustainability; reduces financial barriers to access.

The model is structured around five interconnected components that collectively address the realities and aspirations of adolescents, families, and frontline providers (Table 5.1):

1. Early Identification and Risk Stratification

Adolescents are screened confidentially within schools and community clinics using validated tools such as the DASS modules embedded in the MU MyMind platform. Rather than a binary "at-risk/not-at-risk" framework, screening outcomes are stratified by risk level and readiness for engagement, enabling tailored follow-up pathways.

2. Safe Access Pathways

Acknowledging legal and cultural considerations, the model promotes age-appropriate self-referral mechanisms. Adolescents aged 18 years and above are empowered to seek mental health consultations with nurses independently, in alignment with global best practices on youth autonomy.

3. Nursing Interventions

Nurses are trained and certified in a three-tiered support system:

- Part 1: Psychoeducation and emotional support for low-risk youth.
- Part 2: Structured counselling using brief interventions such as Problem-Solving Therapy (PST) and Satir-based techniques for mild- to moderate-risk adolescents.
- Part 3: Coordination and referral for high-risk or complex cases requiring specialist input. All tiers are enhanced by digital platforms, which extend but do not replace the human connection central to care.

4. Community and Family Integration

Recognising the relational dimensions of adolescent well-being, the model embeds families, teachers, community health volunteers, and local spiritual leaders into the prevention and care processes. Care moves beyond institutional boundaries to cultivate a supportive ecosystem rooted in cultural and relational strengths.

5. Policy and System Enablers

For sustainability, the model requires formal recognition and financing within Thailand's Universal Health Coverage (UHC) system. Payment structures for nurse-led counselling, digital service use, and mobile outreach must be defined. Furthermore, scalable training pipelines — including short courses and e-certification programs — are critical to expand the model beyond pilot sites.

5.6.4 *Strategic Enablers for Implementation*

To realise the full potential of this model, the following systemic supports are essential:

1. **Targeted Training and Capacity-Building**
Comprehensive, context-sensitive training in screening, early intervention, youth engagement, and trauma-informed care must be provided to nurses. Mentorship networks and reflective practice opportunities will sustain professional growth.

2. **Policy Frameworks and Institutional Recognition**
Formal policy frameworks must articulate the scope, roles, and standards for nurse-led mental health services, accompanied by sustainable funding channels within national health insurance systems.

3. **Decentralised and Flexible Funding Models**
Resource allocation should be localised and responsive to community needs, supporting adaptive service models and fostering innovation at the frontline level.

4. **Robust Data Systems**
Ethical, real-time data systems are critical for monitoring service quality, evaluating outcomes, and supporting continuous learning and improvement.

5.7 Draft: Nurse-Led Depression Prevention Clinic Model

5.7.1 *Expanded Conceptual Flow*

1. **Initial Screening**
   - Digital screening via MU MyMind (DASS modules)
   - Risk stratification (low, moderate, high)

2. **Tiered Nursing Support**
   - **Tier 1:** Psychoeducation, emotional first aid for low-risk adolescents
   - **Tier 2:** Brief, structured counselling (e.g., PST, Satir techniques) for moderate-risk adolescents
   - **Tier 3:** Collaborative referral to psychiatrist/social worker for high-risk adolescents

3. **Community and Family Engagement**
   - Involvement of teachers, village health volunteers, and parents
   - Psychoeducation workshops and digital resources

4. **Sustained Support System**
   - Regular digital check-ins (via MU MyMind)
   - Scheduled nurse follow-ups every 1–3 months based on risk profile
   - Data-driven monitoring and evaluation

Visual Summary Description: The NDPC model visualises a seamless continuum where adolescents are first screened digitally, stratified by risk, engaged through tiered nursing interventions, and integrated into a supportive community framework — all leading toward sustained mental health and resilience. Each phase builds relational trust and enables early, personalised care.

5.7.2 *Proposed Operational Plan: Translating the Nurse-Led Depression Prevention Clinic Model into Practice*

1. **Workforce Preparation**
   - Develop a short-course certification program in adolescent mental health nursing (30 hours, hybrid model)
   - Core modules: adolescent development, early detection tools (DASS, risk indicators), psychoeducation techniques, brief intervention methods (PST, Satir model), digital health communication, ethics and confidentiality
   - Certification renewal every three years with refresher courses

2. **Screening and Engagement**
   - Standardise digital screening implementation in participating primary care clinics and selected secondary schools
   - Training on risk stratification algorithms integrated into MU MyMind
   - Establish consent protocols, especially for adolescents aged under 18, respecting autonomy within legal frameworks

3. **Service Delivery Model**
   - Embed nurse-led mental health consultations as part of routine health checks for adolescents (opt-in system)
   - Provide private, youth-friendly counselling spaces within clinics
   - Implement structured care pathways based on risk tier

4. **Referral System**
   - Formalise referral mechanisms to psychiatric services for Tier 3 cases
   - Create partnership Memorandums of Understanding with nearby psychiatric hospitals and mental health specialists

5. **Community and Family Integration**
   - Conduct biannual community workshops on adolescent mental health literacy
   - Develop parent toolkits and online modules to support resilience building at home
   - Engage youth peer leaders to act as mental health ambassadors in schools

6. **Monitoring and Evaluation**
   - Establish a real-time digital dashboard (aggregated, de-identified data) for monitoring engagement, follow-up compliance, and symptom trajectory
   - Quarterly quality assurance reviews and annual external evaluations
   - Key Performance Indicators: Percentage of adolescents screened, proportion receiving follow-up support, reduction in moderate-to-severe depressive symptoms at 6 months

7. **Policy Advocacy and Sustainability**
   - Work with the Ministry of Public Health and local governments to integrate nurse-led adolescent mental health services into the Universal Coverage Scheme
   - Advocate for reimbursement codes for digital counselling, psychoeducation, and mobile follow-up
   - Pilot funding secured through Health Systems Research Institute with scaling proposals for broader national rollout by year three

5.8 Policy Reflections and System Implications

The broader value of the NDPC model lies not only in its pilot-level outcomes but in its potential for scale, sustainability, and alignment with national health priorities. Translating nurse-led digital innovations into national programs requires policy support in several key domains:

- **Scaling Pathways:** Integration into Thailand's primary care system via community health clinics, leveraging existing nurse networks.
- **Financing Models:** Options include capitation-based models under Universal Coverage Scheme, or earmarked mental health prevention funds.
- **Governance:** Multi-sectoral coordination among Ministry of Public Health, Ministry of Education, and community-based organisations.
- **Data Governance and Ethics:** Policies must ensure youth privacy, consent, and ethical digital health standards.

These reflections highlight that prevention cannot be the sole responsibility of frontline providers. Strategic policymaking and infrastructure investment are essential to institutionalise models like NDPC and to ensure equitable access for all Thai adolescents.

5.8.1 *Reflection*

This model does not propose abstract reforms. It is grounded in real experiences, real needs, and the quiet leadership of nurses who have long acted at the frontlines of care. By investing in structures that honour relationships, foster resilience, and bridge gaps in access, Thailand has the opportunity to reimagine adolescent mental health care — not as a crisis response, but as a community commitment to nurture the next generation.

"We do not need to build new buildings. We need to build trust — within systems, and between people."

5.8.2 *Policy Momentum for Adolescent Mental Health*

The proposed NDPC model represents more than a clinical intervention — it is a call to reimagine mental health prevention as an integrated, scalable, and nurse-led public health strategy. The findings and design insights presented in this chapter reinforce three strategic imperatives:

1. **Institutionalise Prevention as a Core Mandate**: Mental health promotion for adolescents must shift from fragmented projects to a system-wide commitment embedded in primary care policy and budgeting.
2. **Empower Nurses as Community Innovators**: Nurses are not only frontline providers but also system architects. Policy frameworks must enable their leadership in designing, adapting, and scaling interventions.
3. **Align Digital Innovation with Equity and Ethics**: Digital tools like MU MyMind must be deployed not as isolated apps, but as integrated solutions backed by governance, data protection, and cultural relevance.

To catalyse real-world change, these imperatives must be anchored in national strategies — through financing mechanisms, cross-sectoral governance, and long-term investment in youth well-being. The NDPC model offers a pragmatic pathway forward, but its promise can only be fulfilled through sustained policy action and collaborative system transformation.

5.9 Comparative Analysis: International Perspectives on Nurse-Led Mental Health Services

To design an effective and contextually appropriate adolescent mental health service model, it is crucial to examine existing international frameworks. Comparative analysis enables identification of best practices, lessons learned, and contextual nuances that inform the adaptation of a nurse-led model in Thailand. Drawing insights from established systems in the United Kingdom and Australia provides valuable direction for enhancing the feasibility, sustainability, and cultural sensitivity of the proposed NDPC model (Table 5.2).

United Kingdom (UK): Primary Mental Health Worker Model

- Focus: Nurses and allied health professionals deliver early mental health interventions within schools and general practitioner (GP) clinics.
- Strengths: Integrated into National Health Service (NHS) pathways; emphasis on early identification and multi-agency collaboration [19].
- Challenges: Workforce shortages and variable service quality between regions.

Australia: Headspace Youth Mental Health Services

- Focus: Multidisciplinary centres offering mental health, physical health, vocational, and drug/alcohol services for youths aged 12–25.
- Strengths: Community-driven model; youth participation in service design; accessible "no wrong door" policy [20].
- Challenges: Service demand outpacing capacity; urban-rural service inequity.

Thailand: Proposed NDPC Model

- Focus: Nurse-led digital-enabled screening, tiered support, and community/family integration embedded within primary care.
- Strengths: Utilises existing nursing workforce; culturally adapted digital tools; emphasises relational and preventive approaches.
- Anticipated Challenges: Policy recognition, sustainable funding, and scaling nurse certification programs.

Table 5.2 Comparative models.

Country	Model Name	Focus	Strengths	Challenges	Key Success Factors	Critical Barriers
United Kingdom	Primary Mental Health Worker Model	Early intervention by nurses in schools and GP clinics	NHS integration; multi-agency collaboration	Workforce shortages; regional disparities	Early detection embedded in education system	Inconsistent funding and regional variability
Australia	Headspace Youth Mental Health Services	Multidisciplinary youth services centres	Community-driven; youth-led design; accessible services	Service demand vs. capacity; rural gaps	Youth engagement in service design	Workforce burnout and service saturation
Thailand	NDPC Model (Proposed)	Nurse-led digital-enabled adolescent mental health support	Embedded in primary care; culturally tailored; emphasis on relational prevention	Need for policy support; sustainable funding	Integration into community healthcare; relational trust	Lack of formal policy recognition; resource limitations

While models like those in the UK and Australia provide valuable blueprints for early intervention and integrated care, the NDPC model distinguishes itself through its strategic emphasis on digital innovation, nurse leadership, and deep community engagement tailored to Thai socio-cultural contexts. Embedding prevention within primary care and prioritising relational trust-building positions the NDPC model as a contextually grounded and scalable innovation for adolescent mental health promotion.

5.10 Lessons Learned and Future Directions

The development and piloting of the NDPC model for adolescents has illuminated not only service gaps, but also systemic potential. Within a healthcare landscape often shaped by top-down mandates, limited budgets, and fragmented responsibility, this initiative offered a contrasting vision — one grounded in trust, collaboration, and the lived expertise of those closest to the work. What emerged from this process, particularly through direct engagement with nurses, teachers, adolescents, and families, were not abstract ideas, but relational truths — insights born from experience rather than instruction. These formed the basis for a model that is not only feasible, but deeply relevant to the Thai context.

5.10.1 *Lessons Learned*

1. Local Wisdom Precedes System Design

Sustainable solutions are seldom imported; they are cultivated. Nurses, school personnel, and even adolescents themselves demonstrated a clear understanding of what support looks like within their context. The role of system designers is not to impose external frameworks, but to listen attentively, curate emergent practices, and amplify what already works.

2. Technology Must Be Grounded in Trust and Context

Digital tools such as MU MyMind can extend the reach of care, but their effectiveness depends on how they are introduced and experienced.

Adolescents responded positively not because the platform was new, but because it was designed to be safe, respectful, and reflective of their lived realities.

3. Fragmentation Dilutes Impact

Mental health care cannot rely on any single actor. The absence of coordinated referral systems, shared language, and cross-sectoral communication places undue burden on individual providers — who often operate in silos without adequate institutional support. Integrated pathways and collective accountability are essential for meaningful change.

4. Nurses Are Ready, But Under-Recognised

This initiative revealed a workforce ready to lead — with adaptability, empathy, and skill. However, it also surfaced the persistent absence of institutional support structures. Without formal recognition, protected time, and financial mechanisms, nurse-led mental health care remains under-leveraged despite its promise.

5.10.2 *Future Directions*

To translate these lessons into sustained progress, several strategic pathways are proposed:

1. Policy Integration and UHC Alignment

For nurse-led adolescent mental health services to be scalable, they must be formally recognised within the Universal Coverage Scheme. This includes establishing billing codes, reporting mechanisms, and standard protocols that position prevention as a reimbursable, essential service.

2. Certification and Workforce Development

A national short-course certification in adolescent mental health for generalist nurses should be developed, with flexible formats — including hybrid and online options — to ensure accessibility. Competency-based training will ensure quality while accommodating diverse learning needs across regions.

3. Strengthening Multi-Sector Partnerships
Future implementation should prioritise co-creation with educational institutions, youth-led organisations, and community-based groups. Mental health promotion must be relational and intergenerational, with adolescents positioned not only as recipients, but as collaborators in system design.

4. Research and Evaluation at Scale
To build legitimacy and guide continuous improvement, implementation research is needed across multiple sites. Key metrics should include not only health outcomes and cost-effectiveness, but also user satisfaction and cultural fit — particularly from adolescents themselves.

5. Ethical and Cultural Adaptation
As the model expands, attention must be paid to consent, confidentiality, and the ethical use of digital tools. Content and delivery approaches must be sensitive to cultural and religious diversity across Thailand. Prevention efforts will only be meaningful if they are experienced as respectful, safe, and contextually relevant.

"We cannot afford to wait for perfection before we act. But we also cannot afford to act without listening."

5.11 Closing Reflection

The journey of this chapter has not been one of invention, but of recognition — recognising what is already alive in the quiet corners of clinics, in the steady hands of nurses, in the unspoken questions of adolescents, and in the deep resolve of families who refuse to give up hope. What we have learned is simple, yet profound: systems do not heal people — people do. And when systems are designed to reflect the dignity, complexity, and context of those they serve, healing becomes not just possible, but probable. We do not need to create new heroes. We need to honour the ones already among us — nurses who stay after hours, teachers who notice the quiet child, parents who listen before reacting, and young people who, despite everything, still hope. Let this work be not a conclusion, but a compass — a way to navigate uncertainty with structure, and to meet suffering not only with skill, but with soul.

"Let us always remember: prevention is not just a policy — it is a heartfelt promise. A promise to recognise the earliest signs, to respond with understanding and care, and to hold an unwavering belief that every adolescent deserves not only to survive but to grow, to flourish, and to thrive with dignity."

5.12 Executive Summary

The increasing prevalence of adolescent mental health issues in Thailand demands innovative, community-centred responses. Building on evidence from the MU MyMind initiative, this work proposes the NDPC model that strategically embeds early identification, risk stratification, and tiered interventions within primary care settings. Central to the model is the empowerment of nurses — trusted figures within communities — to lead prevention and early intervention efforts, supported by digital tools and relational frameworks.

Drawing from comparative analyses with international models such as the UK's Primary Mental Health Worker Model and Australia's Headspace network, the NDPC model emphasises cultural adaptation, digital accessibility, and relational trust as core pillars. Pilot studies indicate promising reductions in stress, anxiety, and depressive symptoms, alongside enhanced engagement and satisfaction among adolescents.

The operationalisation plan outlines critical components, including workforce preparation, community integration, structured referral systems, and sustainable policy support under Thailand's Universal Coverage Scheme. Lessons learned affirm that prevention must be proactive, relational, and contextually anchored — not reactive or institutionally distant. This model offers a blueprint for scalable, nurse-led mental health services that honour the lived experiences of young people, ensuring that mental health care becomes not an exception but an expected, enduring part of community life.

References

1. Su Z, McDonnell D, Li X, et al. Post-COVID mental health crises: globally minded for solutions and solidarity. Disaster Med Public Health Prep. 2024 Dec 2;18:e295.
2. World Health Organization. The impact of COVID-19 on mental, neurological and substance use services: results of a rapid assessment. Geneva: WHO; 2022. Available from: https://iris.who.int/handle/10665/335838
3. World Health Organization. Mental health atlas 2020. Geneva: WHO; 2022. Available from: https://iris.who.int/handle/10665/345946
4. World Health Organization, Regional Office for South-East Asia (SEARO). Mental health status of adolescents in South-East Asia: evidence for action. New Delhi: WHO-SEARO; 2022. Available from: https://iris.who.int/handle/10665/254982
5. World Health Organization. Mental health and work: impact, issues and good practices. Geneva: WHO; 2022. Available from: https://iris.who.int/handle/10665/42346
6. Office of the National Economic and Social Development Council (NESDC). Social situation and outlook report Q1 2024. Bangkok: NESDC; 2024. Available from: https://www.nesdc.go.th/main.php?filename=social_outlook
7. Department of Mental Health, Ministry of Public Health. Annual mental health service report 2024. In: NESDC, editor. Bangkok: NESDC; 2024. Available from: https://fliphtml5.com/aumvq/shcc
8. Dechkhong T, Tienchai T, Chomchoey N. Mental health check-in: insights from big data analysis. Bangkok: Health Systems Research Institute; 2023.
9. Jutha W, Terdudom T, Boonchutima S. 2023 national epidemiological survey on mental health. Nonthaburi: Department of Mental Health; 2023.

10. Health Promotion Office, Department of Mental Health. National suicide statistics FY2023. Nonthaburi: Ministry of Public Health; 2024.
11. Google. Google Trends: Thailand mental health search analysis Oct 2023–Oct 2024. 2024 [cited 2025 May 16]. Available from: https://trends.google.com
12. Juraszek P, Sobczyk K, Działach E, Krupa-Kotara K, Grajek M. The impact of the COVID-19 pandemic on the demand for publicly funded mental health services in Poland (data report 2018–2023). Front Public Health. 2025 Apr 23;13:1499628.
13. World Health Organization. Climate change and mental health: risks, impacts and opportunities. Geneva: WHO; 2023. Available from: https://iris.who.int/handle/10665/359755
14. World Health Organization. Comprehensive mental health action plan 2013–2030. Geneva: WHO; 2021. Available from: https://www.who.int/publications/i/item/9789240031029
15. World Health Organization. World mental health report: transforming mental health for all. Geneva: WHO; 2022. Available from: https://www.who.int/publications/i/item/9789240049338
16. Department of Mental Health. Annual report on adolescent mental health status in Thailand. Nonthaburi: Ministry of Public Health; 2021.
17. Department of Health. National adolescent health behavior survey report 2022. Nonthaburi: Ministry of Public Health; 2022.
18. Child and Adolescent Mental Health Rajanagarindra Institute. Workforce and service distribution report: child and adolescent psychiatrists in Thailand. Nonthaburi: Ministry of Public Health; 2022.
19. Department of Health and Social Care. Transforming children and young people's mental health provision: a green paper. London: UK Government; 2017. Available from: https://www.gov.uk/government/publications/transforming-children-and-young-peoples-mental-health-provision
20. Rickwood DJ, Telford NR, Mazzer KR, Parker AG, Tanti CJ, McGorry PD. The services provided to young people by headspace centres in Australia. Med J Aust. 2015;202(10):533–536.

https://doi.org/10.1142/9789819817320_0006

Chapter 6*

Impact of Technology-Based Perinatal Interventions on Paternal Outcomes: A Mixed Methods Systematic Review

Jacquelaine Tan[1], Annabelle Lim[1], and Piyanee Klainin-Yobas[2,*]

[1]*National University Hospital, 5 Lower Kent Ridge Road, Main Building 1, Singapore 119074*

[2]*Alice Lee Centre for Nursing Studies, Yong Loo Lin School of Medicine, National University of Singapore, Level 5, Centre of Translational Medicine, Block MD6, 14 Medical Drive, Singapore 117599*

**Corresponding author: nurpk@nus.edu.sg*

6.1 Introduction

Most parents face many challenges during the perinatal period and they are at risk for psychological problems [1]. Evidence shows that many parents developed perinatal anxiety and depression [2–7]. The transition theory postulated [8] that fatherhood can be a dynamic process, which involves social, physical and emotional phases during the perinatal period. Some of the challenges faced by fathers were unpreparedness without a sense of reality, leading to informational and emotional needs [9]. These might lead to unfavourable implications on child development, mother-infant interaction, and conjugal and family interactions [10]. Most fathers were tech-savvy, with the internet being their key informational support [11]. Since some fathers may not feel comfortable seeking help in person due to social stigma, virtual support groups were proposed to alleviate depressive symptoms [12, 13]. Technology presents the opportunity for a good source of tailored and accessible information.

---

* Appendices to this chapter are available for download at https://www.worldscientific.com/worldscibooks/10.1142/14420#t=suppl.

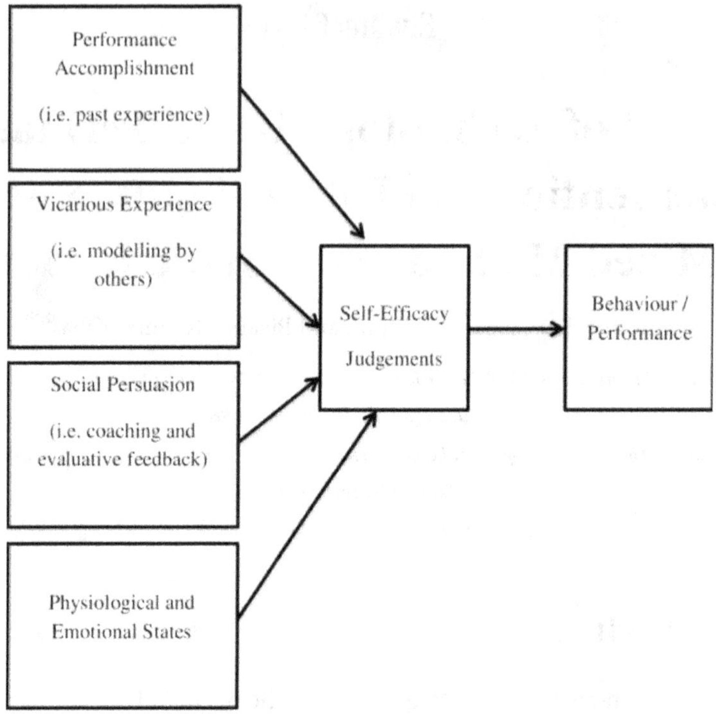

Figure 6.1 Bandura's theory of self-efficacy [15].

Technology-enhanced healthcare is linked with outcomes, including parenting self-efficacy (PSE), postnatal anxiety (PNA), postnatal depression (PND), stress, social support and parent-child bonding [14]. According to Bandura's theory of self-efficacy (Figure 6.1), parents with higher PSE had higher motivation to seek help and possess greater perseverance [15]. Approximately 10% of new fathers experienced significant perinatal depression and anxiety. They had loss of interest, lowered mood, changes in appetite, difficulty sleeping, feelings of worthlessness and self-harm [16]. High PSE has demonstrated to be a shield against perinatal anxiety and depression [17]. Besides, good emotional well-being (low anxiety and depression) and high PSE brought about children with better health outcomes via increased parent-child bonding [17–20]. Social support refers to the interpersonal skill that aids in relieving stress and emotional assistance [21].

6.1.1 *Gaps in Existing Literature*

Studies examining the postnatal needs of fathers are scarce. Technology-based interventions are a promising and modern approach for mental health and ten systematic reviews were identified. Five reviews did not involve paternal-specific outcomes [14, 22, 24–26]. Six reviews did not focus on the use of technology. Therefore, they could not provide distinct insights regarding the effectiveness and/or experiences of technology-based perinatal interventions [14, 27–29]. Three reviews examined limited outcomes compared to this review's objectives [27–29]. One review focused on technologies used in perinatal depression screening [24].

In view of literature gaps, this systematic review aimed to consolidate and appraise evidence based on these questions:

1. In comparison with control, will technology-based interventions be effective in improving PSE, anxiety, depression, stress, social support and parent-child bonding among fathers during the perinatal period?
2. What strategies underpin the implementation of technology-based interventions targeting PSE, anxiety, depression, stress, social support and parent-child bonding among fathers during the perinatal period?

6.2 Methods

The review was conducted in accordance with the Joanna Briggs Institute (JBI)'s methodology for mixed methods systematic reviews [30]. The integration of quantitative, qualitative and mixed methods studies complements the strengths and limitations of each other for in-depth understanding [31–33]. Review findings were reported according to the Preferred Reporting Items for Systematic Reviews and Meta Analyses (PRISMA) guidelines [34]. Selection process, quality assessment and data extraction were carried out by two independent reviewers. Any disagreement that arose between the reviewers at each stage was resolved through discussion, or with a third reviewer when consensus was not reached.

6.2.1 *Eligibility Criteria*

Concerning participants (P), we considered studies conducted on fathers aged 18 years and above, whose partner was a pregnant woman or had a baby up to one year of age, regardless of sociological background. Studies that involved both parents would be included if separate data for fathers were available. Fathers, whose spouse had miscarriage, stillbirth or abortion, would not be included, as they may require interventions specific to their psychological needs [14]. For phenomena of interest (I), we considered studies exploring fathers' experiences on utilising technology-based interventions during the perinatal period. Quantitative outcomes (O) included PSE, depression, anxiety, stress, social support and parent-child bonding. Types of studies included qualitative, quantitative and mixed methods research, both published and unpublished, reported in English language only. No restriction was set on the year of publication.

6.2.2 *Search Strategy and Information Sources*

A three-step search strategy was utilised [30]. An initial search of Cochrane and PubMed identified relevant articles. Keywords and index terms of these articles were used to develop a full search strategy under the advice of an experienced librarian (Appendix A). A second comprehensive search was conducted across seven electronic databases for published articles: PubMed, Embase, Cochrane, CINAHL, Scopus, MEDLINE and IEEE Xplore. Unpublished and grey literature involved four electronic databases: ProQuest Dissertations and Theses, Google Scholar, ClinicalTrials.gov and ISRCTN Registry. Mainstay journals such as *International Journal of Mental Health* were screened through for relevant articles. Reference lists of selected studies were screened for additional studies via backward searching. Authors were contacted to obtain full texts of potentially relevant but inaccessible studies.

6.2.3 *Selection Process*

All identified citations were loaded into the EndNote X9 software and duplicates were removed. Titles and abstracts were first screened against the eligibility criteria. Full texts of eligible studies were then retrieved for thorough reviewing.

6.2.4 *Methodological Quality Assessment*

All included studies were critically appraised using the Mixed Methods Appraisal Tool (MMAT) version 2018 [33]. The tool covers study methodologies, study selection bias, study design, data collection methods, sample size, intervention integrity and analysis. Studies were given a methodological rating of low (0%/20%), fair (40%/60%) and good (80%/100%). Risk of bias (ROB) assessment using Cochrane's Collaboration Tool 2 for was conducted for randomised controlled trials (RCTs) [34]. ROB was scored as high, medium or low and includes selection, performance, detection, attrition and reporting biases. Studies would be included regardless of their MMAT or ROB scores.

To grade the strength of the quantitative evidence, GRADEpro software version 3.6 was used for Grading of Recommendations, Assessment, Development, and Evaluation (GRADE) [35]. The factors include limitations, inconsistencies, indirectness, inaccuracy and publication bias. Level of evidence quality was expressed as high, medium, low, or very low [36]. GRADE-CERQual Interactive Summary of Qualitative Findings (iSoQ) Version 1.0 [37] was used to ascertain the strength of qualitative evidence. It includes methodological limitations, relevance, coherence and adequacy of data [38]. The level of evidence quality expressed was similar to GRADE.

6.2.5 *Data Extraction*

Quantitative data were extracted from quantitative components of mixed methods studies. Similarly, qualitative data were extracted from qualitative components of mixed methods studies. These were performed using the standardised quantitative and qualitative data extraction tool modified based on JBI-MAStARI and JBI-QARI [39]. Data extracted include methodology, interventions, populations and outcomes of significance to the review questions. The tool was piloted to ensure consistency [40].

6.2.6 *Data Synthesis and Integration*

A convergent segregated approach to data synthesis and integration [30] was conducted. Quantitative and qualitative syntheses were conducted separately first, followed by integration of both findings (Figure 6.2) [32].

Quantitative synthesis. Meta-analysis was performed for four outcomes using Review Manager Version 5.4 [41]. Heterogeneity was calculated using I^2 statistics and chi-square test. For outcome(s) with low heterogeneity (less than 60%), pooled effect size was used. Where meta-analysis was not possible, narrative reporting was conducted. Cohen's d was used to interpret the effect size (Table 6.1) [42].

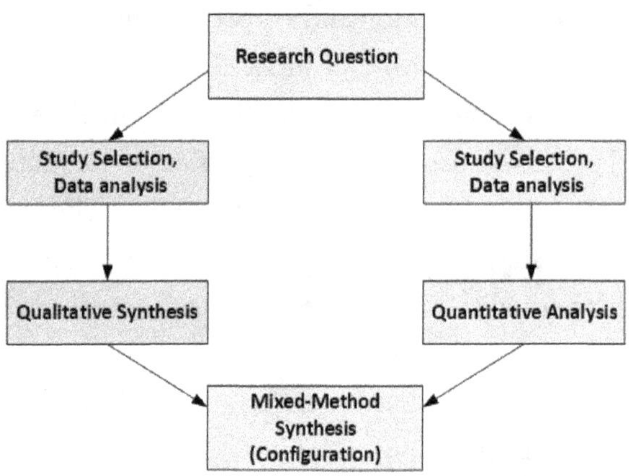

Figure 6.2 Convergent segregated approach [39].

Table 6.1 Interpretation of Cohen's d.

d	**Effect Size**
$d < 0.2$	Very small
$0.2 \leq d < 0.5$	Small
$0.5 \leq d < 0.8$	Moderate
$d \geq 0.8$	Large

Qualitative synthesis. A three-step thematic synthesis [43] was conducted. First, we performed line-by-line coding on transcriptions, and we then generated initial inductive codes. Next, we created descriptive themes, after comparing and categorising the initial codes. Finally, we developed analytical themes, after comparing the descriptive themes with textual data of the included studies.

6.3 Results

6.3.1 *Search Outcomes*

A total of 12,750 records were retrieved. Upon removing duplicates, 6,543 were screened based on titles and abstracts, and 138 full-text articles were identified for further review. Finally, 25 studies were included in this review. The selection process is illustrated in Figure 6.3.

6.3.2 *Study Characteristics*

Among the 25 studies, there were 17 quantitative studies, three qualitative studies, and five mixed methods studies (Appendix B). Most studies were conducted in Asia, encompassing Iran (n = 2), Turkey (n = 2), Singapore (n = 4), Taiwan (n = 1), and Japan (n = 1). Some were in Europe, including Finland (n = 1), Sweden (n = 2), Denmark (n = 1), and the United Kingdom (n = 1). The rest were in Canada (n = 2), the United States of America (n = 3) and Australia (n = 5). One study was conducted during an antenatal period, 14 in postnatal period and 10 across the perinatal

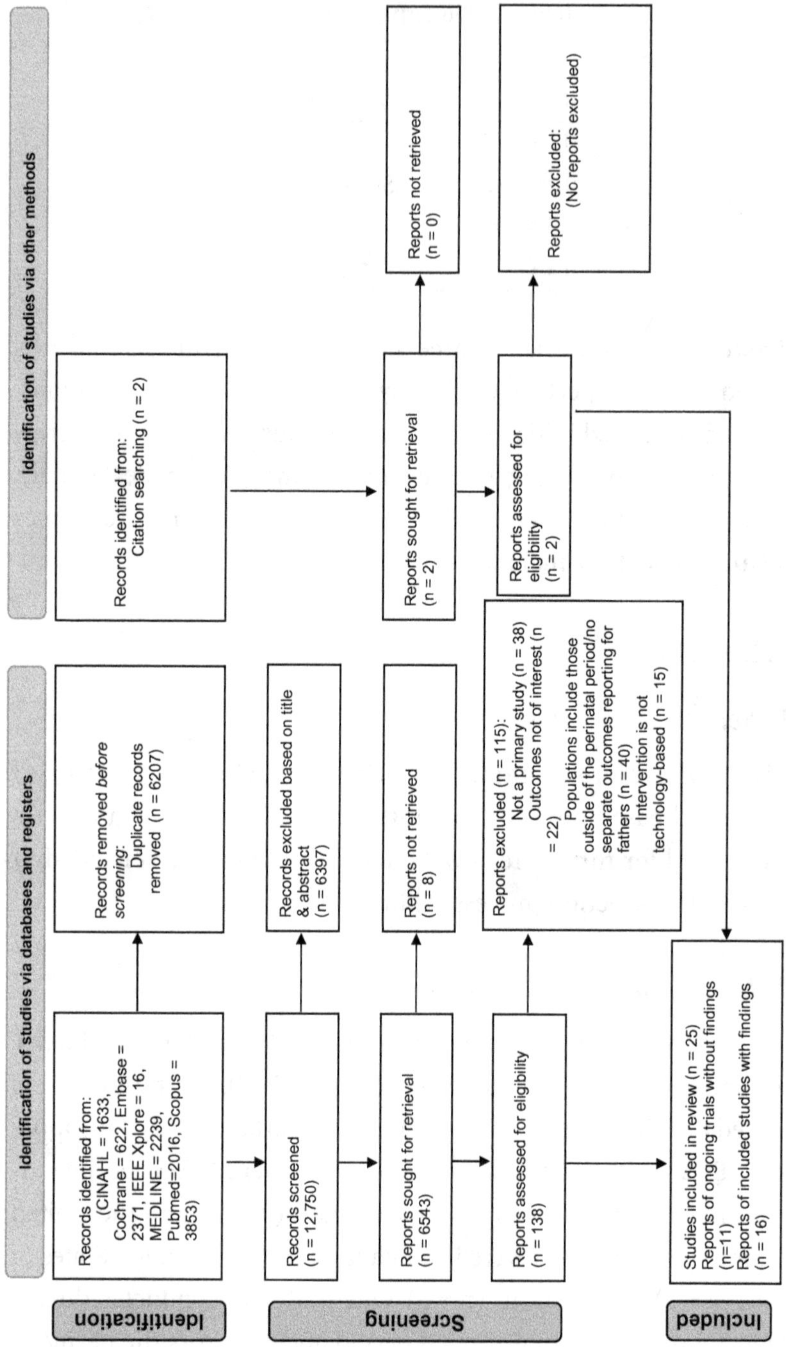

Figure 6.3 PRISMA flow diagram.

periods. Quantitative studies used varied measurement tools and most qualitative studies conducted focus groups. Table 6.2 provides a summary. Out of the 25 studies, 11 studies are ongoing clinical trials and excluded in results as they do not have findings.

Table 6.2 Summary of studies.

Characteristics	Classification	No. of studies	Percentage
Type of study design	Descriptive qualitative	2	8%
	Randomised controlled trial	15	60%
	Mixed methods studies	4	16%
	Quasi-experimental design	3	12%
	Single-group longitudinal pre-post design	1	4%
Type of intervention	Mobile health application	6	24%
	Videoconferencing support	1	4%
	Internet resource (information database, peer discussion forum, contact nurse/midwife if needed)	12	48%
	Telephone-based educational support	1	4%
	Short message service (SMS)	3	12%
	Telegram/WhatsApp social media application	2	8%
Outcome measured	Experiences, views, perceptions	6	10.5%
	Parenting self-efficacy	12	21.1%
	Social support	10	17.5%
	Postnatal depression	13	22.8%
	Postnatal anxiety	8	14.1%
	Perceived stress	2	3.5%
	Parental bonding/attachment	6	10.5%
Device used	Mobile phone/tablet	11	44%
	Video camera	1	4%
	Devices capable of connecting to the Internet	13	52%

6.3.3 *Quality Ratings*

The overall MMAT methodological quality of the studies was relatively good. Most studies had good scores except for one that was low and another average. Most qualitative studies had clear themes/subthemes (findings) with acceptable interpretation, except some studies did not mention data saturation.

6.3.4 *Qualitative Synthesis*

Qualitative findings were organised into three main themes and eight subthemes (Table 6.3). Preliminary synthesis with illustrative quotes are in Appendix C. These themes are related to strategies underpinning the implementation of technology-based interventions for fathers to achieve positive paternal outcomes.

6.3.4.1 *Theme 1: Gaining Personalised Informational Support Easily and Timely*

Subtheme 1.1 Comprehensive, professional and reliable informational support. Five studies mentioned that fathers found technology

Table 6.3 Summary of themes for qualitative findings.

Main themes	1. Gaining personalised informational support easily and timely	2. Finding social support within a virtual community and beyond	3. Understanding one's mental health
Subthemes	1.1 Comprehensive, professional and reliable informational support 1.2 Sharing personal experiences 1.3 Receiving timely reminders 1.4 Ease of access, convenience and comfort	2.1 Befriending within a virtual community 2.2 Forming connections for offline interactions	3.1 Being aware of the challenges of fatherhood 3.2 Alleviating stress and gaining confidence

useful when they provided comprehensive, professional and reliable informational support to answer their specific queries and improve PSE (in Table 6.1, studies 4, 6, 9, 14, 20). For instance, fathers from two studies [44, 45] highlighted how prompt replies from the nurse/midwife provided them instant reassurance. Other sources of professional informational support included notifications and knowledge banks curated by the healthcare teams.

Subtheme 1.2 Sharing personal experiences. Informational support was also enhanced with fellow users sharing personal experiences so that fathers who are facing the same difficulties can relate, find solutions and be reassured [9, 20, 27]. Fathers felt that online forums created a culture of giving and receiving feedback on parenting habits. In fact, fathers mentioned how this feature made informational support feel more personalised and relatable.

Subtheme 1.3 Receiving timely reminders. Four studies mentioned that receiving timely reminders could increase the chance of fathers reflecting on their parenting behaviours and receive reassurance [4, 6, 9, 27]. This is because the notifications came at times when fathers were struggling and provided tips to inspire them to improve their parenting skills, support their spouses and look after their mental well-being.

Subtheme 1.4 Ease of access, convenience and comfort. Participants in four studies pointed out that technology is coupled with ease of access, convenience and comfort to fathers who are preoccupied with work or live in rural areas that make face-to-face visits time-consuming and inaccessible [4, 9, 14, 20]. A father from a study [46] mentioned that the videoconferencing intervention with the nurse during postpartum follow-up felt natural. With most online interventions accessible via mobile phones, this was a key feature that encouraged fathers to be more involved in perinatal care.

6.3.4.2 *Theme 2: Finding Social Support within a Virtual Community and Beyond*

Subtheme 2.1 Befriending within a virtual community. Fathers from two studies highlighted how they were able to befriend other fathers and they found this an essential source of social support during fatherhood [6, 27]. With most fathers juggling with work, they felt that the user-based online forums provided the chance for fathers to bond with other like-minded individuals. One father from one study [47] highlighted the use of humour to form social connection with other fathers.

Subtheme 2.2 Forming connections for offline interactions. In fact, fathers from one study [48] explained how they hoped to meet some of the new online friends in real life once in a while. According to them, this improves the engagement between fathers on the technology-based interventions by building a stronger social support network via the proposed occasional get-togethers.

6.3.4.3 *Theme 3: Understanding One's Mental Health*

Subtheme 3.1 Being aware of the challenges of fatherhood. Four studies have shared that the technology has allowed fathers to utilise the platforms to become more open and aware of the emotional and physical challenges of fatherhood [6, 9, 20, 27]. The online forums have provided fathers the opportunity to be honest about their own well-being. Some used them as platforms to vent their frustrations to process their emotions.

Subtheme 3.2 Alleviating stress and gaining confidence. Fathers from the same four studies [6, 9, 20, 27] then mentioned that upon awareness, they were able to take steps to alleviate stress and anxiety, gain confidence and improve their PSE. Fathers mentioned that identifying their emotions via the online forums or notifications reminders helped them to realise their knowledge gaps. This encouraged them to seek informational or emotional support via the same technology-based interventions respectively to "stay on track" and alleviate stress during fatherhood.

6.3.4.4 *Certainty of Qualitative Evidence*

The strength of the qualitative findings was assessed using GRADE-CERQual [35] and a summary can be found in Appendix G. Gaining personalised informational support easily and timely, finding social support and understanding one's mental health were met with moderate confidence due to moderate concerns regarding adequacy of the studies.

6.3.5 *Quantitative Synthesis: Effects of Technological-Based Interventions on Outcomes*

6.3.5.1 *Parenting Self-Efficacy*

Six studies used PSE as an outcome, involving 1,012 participants. Two RCTs and two controlled clinical trials were submitted into meta-analysis, while two RCTs were reported in narrative synthesis. Results of meta-analysis (Figure 6.4) indicated substantial heterogeneity ($I^2 = 99\%$, chi-square = 372.93, $p < 0.00001$) and therefore the pooled effect size was not used. An examination of individual effect size across six studies showed the range of −4.69 to 1.12. One study with the strongest effect size (SMD = 1.12) examined the web-based intervention that lasted for six months postpartum [49] while other studies had interventions that lasted from four to eight weeks. Subgroup analysis was not conducted due to limited studies.

Narrative Reporting. One RCT [50] examined the effectiveness of a telephone-based education with mHealth application. Spouses of fathers ranged from 28 weeks pregnancy to four weeks postpartum. Differences in PSE between the intervention (n = 59) and control group (n = 59) increased from baseline (OR = −0.40, CI = −0.91, 0.11) to three months postpartum (OR = 0.51, CI = 0.03, 0.99). Another RCT [51] examined the effectiveness of a supportive parenting application

Study or Subgroup	Experimental Mean	Experimental SD	Experimental Total	Control Mean	Control SD	Control Total	Weight	Std. Mean Difference IV, Random, 95% CI
Hudson et al., 2003	0.87	0.2	14	0.24	0.968	20	24.7%	0.81 [0.10, 1.53]
Kavanagh et al., 2021	11.4	1	124	16.1	1	124	25.0%	-4.69 [-5.17, -4.20]
Salonen et al., 2010	0.21	0.361	53	0.28	0.268	234	25.2%	-0.24 [-0.54, 0.06]
Shorey et al., 2017	11.6	24.8	63	-15.4	23.1	62	25.1%	1.12 [0.74, 1.50]
Total (95% CI)			**254**			**440**	**100.0%**	**-0.75 [-3.14, 1.64]**

Heterogeneity: Tau² = 5.88; Chi² = 372.93, df = 3 (P < 0.00001); I² = 99%
Test for overall effect: Z = 0.62 (P = 0.54)

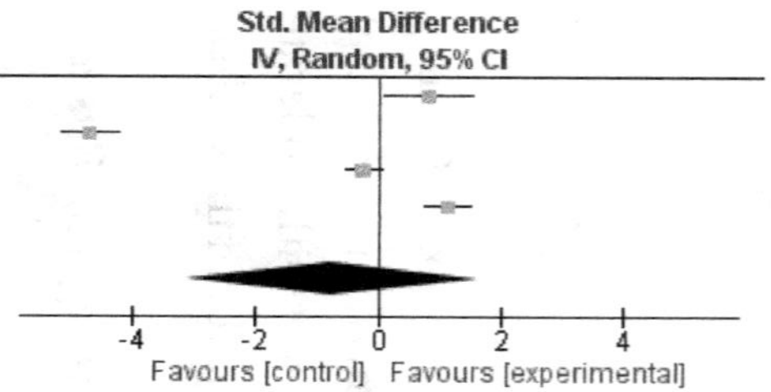

Figure 6.4 Effectiveness of technological-based interventions of PSE.

Study or Subgroup	Experimental Mean	Experimental SD	Experimental Total	Control Mean	Control SD	Control Total	Weight	Std. Mean Difference IV, Random, 95% CI
Canbay & Seker, 2021	5.2	4.071	75	-4.59	4.352	75	24.3%	2.31 [1.90, 2.73]
Kavanagh et al., 2021	0	0.367	124	-0.4	0.273	124	26.6%	1.23 [0.96, 1.50]
Shorey et al., 2017 (A)	0.59	12.3	63	-31.6	20.8	62	24.2%	1.88 [1.45, 2.30]
Shorey et al., 2017 (B)	3.9	26.3	63	-23.8	21.5	62	24.9%	1.15 [0.77, 1.52]
Total (95% CI)			**325**			**323**	**100.0%**	**1.63 [1.10, 2.15]**

Heterogeneity: Tau² = 0.25; Chi² = 24.69, df = 3 (P < 0.0001); I² = 88%
Test for overall effect: Z = 6.08 (P < 0.00001)

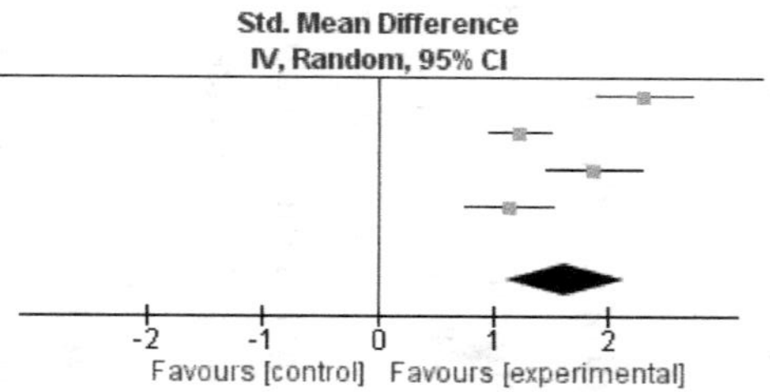

Figure 6.5 Effectiveness of technological-based interventions on social support.

Note: Shorey *et al.* 2017 (A) and (B) belong to one study.

a. Shorey *et al.*, 2017 (A): 4-item Perceived Social Support for Parenting Scale — Spouses [53].

b. Shorey *et al.*, 2017 (B): 4-item Perceived Social Support for Parenting Scale — Other sources [53].

(psychoeducational content and forums), which lasted from pregnancy to six months postpartum. Father's PSE in the intervention group (n = 100) increased at the 12-month assessment point (mean = 32.59, SD = 4.68) in comparison with that at baseline (mean = 29.97, SD = 5.23). Overall, technology-based interventions showed positive effects on PSE among fathers in four studies.

6.3.5.2 *Social Support*

Six studies examined social support as an outcome (involving 871 participants). Three RCTs were submitted into meta-analysis (Figure 6.5), while the rest used narrative synthesis. Results indicated substantial heterogeneity ($I^2 = 88\%$, chi-square = 24.69, $p < 0.0001$), and therefore the pooled effect size was not used. An examination of individual effect size across six studies showed the range of 1.15–2.31. One RCT [52] with the strongest effect size (SMD = 2.31) delivered the intervention across the perinatal period while other RCTs took place during postpartum. Subgroup analysis was not conducted due to limited studies.

Narrative Reporting. In one RCT [50], differences in social support between the intervention (n = 59) and control group (n = 59) increased from baseline (OR = −0.22, CI = −0.62, 0.18) to three months postpartum (OR = 0.81, CI = 0.16, 1.45). Nevertheless, one RCT [51] reported that fathers' support in the intervention group (n = 100) decreased from baseline (mean = 12.04, SD = 4.65) to 12 months (mean = 10.84, SD = 4.78). A single group, quasi-experimental research was conducted to examine the effectiveness of a 12-week text-massaging intervention based on cognitive-behavioural therapy. Surprisingly, fathers' (n = 30) social support decreased slightly from baseline (mean = 60.9, SD = 14.3) to six months (mean = 59.3, SD = 13.7). Overall, four out of six studies reported a positive effect of technology-based interventions on social support among fathers.

6.3.5.3 *Postnatal Depression*

Five studies examined PND as an outcome (involving 721 participants). Two RCTs were submitted into meta-analysis (Figure 6.6), while the rest were reported in narrative summary. Results indicated substantial heterogeneity ($I^2 = 99\%$, chi-square = 114.79, $p < 0.00001$) and therefore the pooled effect size will not be used. An examination of individual effect size across six studies ranged from −0.14 to −2.87. The study [54] with the strongest effect size (SMD = −2.87) used a web-based program that lasted for six months postpartum, while another study lasted for four weeks postpartum.

Narrative Reporting. In one study [50], estimated PND differences between the intervention (n = 59) and control group (n = 59) decreased from baseline (OR = 0.13, CI = −0.23, 0.49) to three months postpartum (OR = −1.09, CI = −1.68, −0.49). In another study [51], fathers' PND in the intervention group (n = 100) decreased from baseline (mean = 8, SD = 6) to 12 months (mean = 5, SD = 4). Moreover, fathers' (n = 30) PND decreased from baseline (mean = 6.5, SD = 6.6) to six months (mean = 3.6, SD = 5.1) [55]. Overall, technology-based interventions may have positive effects on PND among fathers.

6.3.5.4 *Parent-Child Bonding*

Four studies examined parent-child bonding as an outcome (involving 426 participants). Two RCTs were submitted into meta-analysis (Figure 6.7), while the rest went into narrative synthesis. Results indicated low heterogeneity ($I^2 = 10\%$, chi-square = 1.11, $p < 0.04$) and a small pooled effect size (SMD = 0.43, 95% CI = 0.02,0.84). The study with the strongest effect (SMD = 0.58) was an intervention on prenatal care education.

Narrative Reporting. In one study [50], estimated parent-child bonding differences intervention (n = 59) and control group (n = 59) decreased

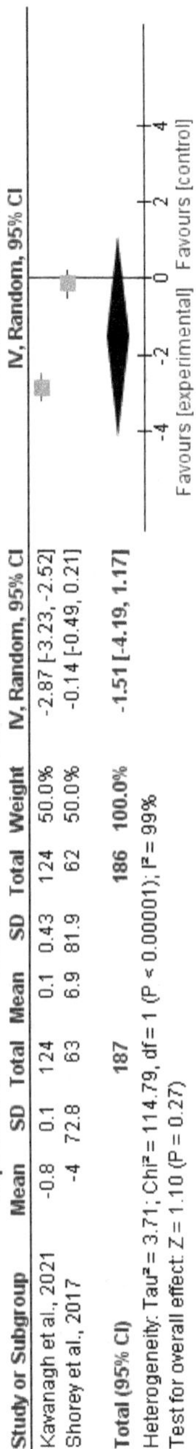

Figure 6.6 PND forest plot.

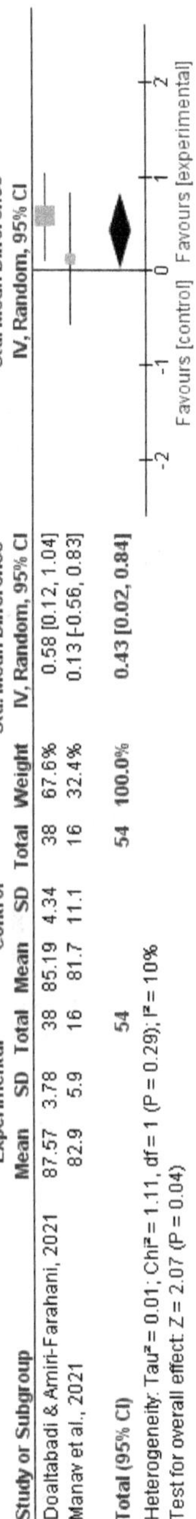

Figure 6.7 Parent-child bonding forest plot.

from baseline OR = −0.04, CI = −0.49, 0.41 to three months postpartum OR = −1.48, CI = −2.22, −0.75. Fathers' parent-child bonding for Shorey *et al.* (2023)'s study in the intervention group (n = 100) decreased from baseline mean (SD) = 3.46(3.40) to 12 months mean (SD) = 2.64(2.74). Overall, effects of technology-based interventions on parent-child bonding among fathers are inconclusive.

6.3.5.5 *Postnatal Anxiety*

Three studies examined PNA as an outcome (involving 348 participants). One RCT [50] suggested an insignificant difference in PNA between the intervention (n = 59) and control group (n = 59) at three months postpartum (OR = −1.09, CI = −1.57, −0.61). Another RCT [51] found a decrease in fathers' PNA at six months (mean = 35.83, SD = 9.62), when compared with baseline (mean = 36.71, SD = 8.64). Similarly, another study [55] reported decreased PNS at six months (mean = 2.8, SD = 3.2) in comparison with baseline (mean = 4.1, SD = 4.5). Overall, technology-based interventions might have positive effects on PNA among fathers.

6.3.5.6 *Perceived Stress*

Only one RCT [55] measured perceived stress as an outcome and showed positive effects. Specifically, fathers' (n = 30) perceived stress decreased at six months (mean = 10.9, SD = 9.1) in comparison to baseline (mean = 14.9, SD = 7.6).

6.3.5.7 *Certainty of Quantitative Evidence*

The strength of the quantitative findings was assessed using GRADE (Appendix H) and ROB. PSE, PND and PNA were assessed to be of high certainty, social support of moderate certainty, parent-child bonding of low certainty and stress to be of very low certainty. Low certainty was mostly due to serious ROB and inconsistency in findings.

6.3.5.8 *Integration of Findings*

Three themes emerged through integrating findings from both syntheses: curating perinatal knowledge, building a virtual community, and gaining self-awareness on one's mental health. Figure 6.8 illustrates the process of integration. These themes describe the main features that underpin the implementation of technology-based interventions and validate the positive quantitative effects on paternal outcomes.

Fathers in qualitative findings have pointed out that they feel more confident in their parenting skills upon timely and accessible information provided by both professionals and fellow fathers. Quantitative findings validated this theme with an increase in PSE. Thus, curating a good perinatal knowledge bank was a key feature for technology-based interventions to be effective as fathers could easily gain access to personalised information.

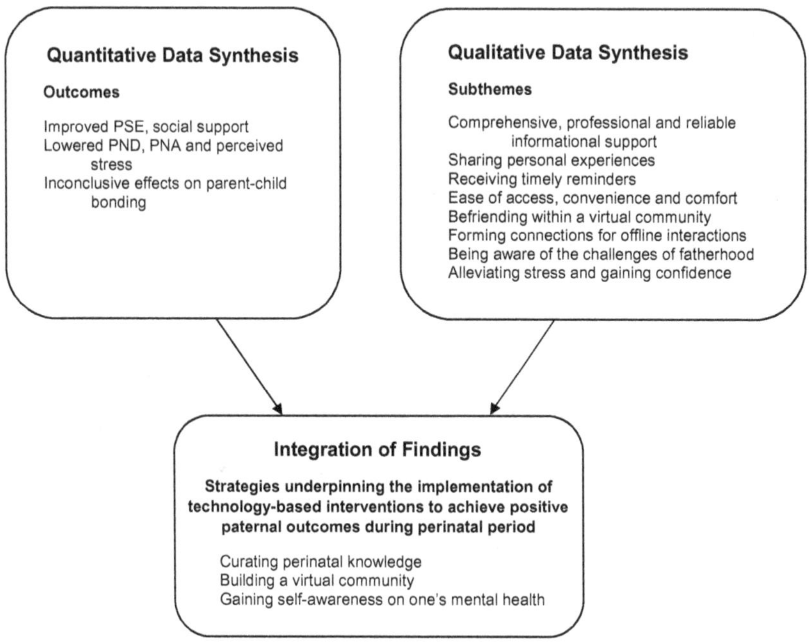

Figure 6.8 Integration of qualitative and quantitative findings.

Besides information sharing, qualitative findings have also highlighted that online forums have allowed fathers to connect and find social support. This qualitative finding was substantiated with the improvement in social support from quantitative studies. Technology-based interventions should include features such as online forums to allow user-based sharing and the building of virtual communities to boost social support for fathers.

Qualitative synthesis suggested that fathers have gained the self-awareness to understand the emotional challenges behind fatherhood and take steps to alleviate stress and anxiety. This justifies the quantitative findings of lowered PND, PNA and stress. Content curation of technology-based interventions should be geared towards psychosocial education to ensure that fathers are mindful of their mental well-being.

6.4 Discussion

This review incorporated findings from 14 studies, across nine countries, on 2,156 fathers' experiences and effectiveness of utilising technology-based interventions during the perinatal period. Upon integration of quantitative and qualitative findings, the final themes developed in this review are curating perinatal knowledge, building a virtual community, and gaining self-awareness on one's mental health.

6.4.1 *Curating Perinatal Knowledge*

One of the key strategies that underpin implementation of technology-based interventions to increase PSE was the curation of a reliable and comprehensive knowledge bank. This finding is consistent with previous reviews, which suggested that online delivery of educational programs have demonstrated efficacy to improve access to relevant content [56, 57].

The mechanism behind this can be explained using Bandura's self-efficacy theory (Figure 6.1), whereby the search and retrieval of information via technology assist fathers during decision making and encourage them to act autonomously [15, 58]. According to the theory, professional support provides verbal persuasion via coaching and evaluative feedback. Participating in online forums allows the sharing of vicarious experiences provided by social models, i.e., fellow users. This allows fathers to believe that they too possess the capabilities to succeed. With the high certainty and moderate confidence for quantitative and qualitative findings via the respective GRADE assessments, integrating a comprehensive perinatal knowledge bank in technology-based interventions will greatly improve paternal outcomes.

6.4.2 *Building a Virtual Community*

Another important technology feature that brought about positive effects on paternal outcomes was building a virtual community to enhance social support. Fatherhood can be a lonely journey with most fathers juggling between work and family life [59]. There is a compelling body of evidence on the utilisation of peer support network to manage mental health issues during the perinatal period [12, 60].

The Bowlby's theory of attachment postulated that social support, PSE and parental mental well-being (less stress, anxiety, and depression) give rise to strong parent-child bonds [61]. Therefore, cultivating a virtual community give rise to participants finding commonalities in challenging experiences. This enhances shared understanding and a sense of belonging [27]. Fatherhood becomes less lonely and daunting when fathers befriend and form connections with like-minded people. This encourages fathers to improve their PSE, find time and strengthen parent-child bonds. In this review, although the GRADE certainty of quantitative and qualitative findings for social support and parent-child bonding ranges from low to moderate, this was due to the lack of adequate studies. It is suggested that the contradictory results in parent-child bonding could be due to response-shift bias [51]. The intervention changed the parents' understanding of what good parent-child bonding entails and thus fathers could become more critical of this outcome. More research is needed to focus on and define these areas when examining the effectiveness of online forums for fathers.

6.4.3 *Gaining Self-Awareness of One's Mental Health*

Findings in this review highlighted the importance on how technology-based interventions had the potential for fathers to open up and gain self-awareness on their mental health. This is consistent with previous studies that highlighted the issue on how social stigma and poor mental health-seeking behaviours remain prevalent among fathers [13, 57]. However, technology-based interventions have greatly encouraged fathers to feel more comfortable seeking help [12].

Most of the content related to fathers included psychosocial components to remind fathers to take care of their mental well-being. Qualitative findings in this review have revealed how fathers gradually became aware, acknowledge and articulate their emotional needs during fatherhood [47, 48]. Bandura's theory of self-efficacy also postulates that PSE is affected by physiological and emotional states (Figure 6.1). Upon recognition of their mental state, they were then able to find targeted solutions to alleviate stress and anxiety. This corresponds to the positive quantitative effects on PSE, PND, PNA and perceived stress in this review. Another possible explanation is that the essence of anonymity on such platforms may come in handy as fathers are welcomed to ask questions openly.

Surprisingly, there was only one study that used a validated stress measurement tool to measure stress outcome [55]. This was unexpected and caused the GRADE assessment for stress outcome to be very low. As stress plays a huge part that could affect other outcomes examined in this review [62, 63], it is essential for future research to measure stress as a primary outcome.

6.4.4 *Strengths and Limitations*

This review was conducted using a rigorous approach to ensure high quality of evidence. It provides a holistic view on current technology-based evidence across the perinatal period, which helps to set the direction for future research on paternal well-being. The findings have contributed meaningful evidence and strengthened existing concepts proposed by other scholars. Although not used in the eligibility criteria, the methodological quality of evidence was discussed in relation to the potential impact of the findings' interpretations.

A limitation for this review includes the language restriction of only English, which might have resulted in some relevant studies to be left out. Most studies took place in developed countries and thus it might not be representative of the general population. Results could not be pooled in a meaningful manner due to the high heterogeneity of interventions and participants. Lastly, most of the recruitment strategies involved approaching mothers first to take part in the studies together with their spouses. This means that single fathers or fathers themselves who are keen to participate in the interventions may have been missed out.

6.4.5 *Implications on Clinical Practice*

This review establishes the start to build more definitive conclusions about similar future interventions. Fathers need more support to improve family mental health outcomes. Like new mothers, healthcare providers should not rely on new fathers as caregivers without foreseeing a need for support. Therefore, healthcare institutions should encourage more fathers to be involved. Nurses should provide clinical advice to both parents whenever possible. Healthcare policy makers and corporations alike need to relook into granting sufficient paternity leaves.

6.4.6 *Implications on Future Research*

Larger quantitative effect sizes of studies with longer intervention durations [52, 54] mean that more longitudinal research is needed to investigate similar outcomes to enhance the trustworthiness of evidence from this review. In fact, given the 11 ongoing clinical trials, this calls for the need for future synthesis of evidence to better inform healthcare policymakers.

6.5 Conclusion

This review explored the effectiveness and experiences of fathers who used technology-based interventions during the perinatal period. Technology has the potential to address issues like accessibility, affordability and patient acceptance by facilitating modes of communication, data collection and patient experience [56]. Given the scarcity of literature, the benefits and strategies highlighted in this review is an incentive for more in-depth research to improve research rigor and clinical outcomes for new and expectant fathers.

References

1. Vismara L, Rollè L, Agostini F, Sechi C, Fenaroli V, Molgora S, Neri E, Prino LE, Odorisio F, Trovato A, Polizzi C, Brustia P, Lucarelli L, Monti F, Saita E, Tambelli R. Perinatal parenting stress, anxiety, and depression outcomes in first-time mothers and fathers: a 3- to 6-months postpartum follow-up study. Front Psychol. 2016;7:938. https://doi.org/10.3389/fpsyg.2016.00938
2. Cameron EE, Sedov ID, Tomfohr-Madsen LM. Prevalence of paternal depression in pregnancy and the postpartum: an updated meta-analysis. J Affect Disord. 2016;206:189–203. https://doi.org/10.1016/j.jad.2016.07.044
3. Dennis C-L, Falah-Hassani K, Shiri R. Prevalence of antenatal and postnatal anxiety: systematic review and meta-analysis. Br J Psychiatry. 2017;210(5): 315–23. https://doi.org/10.1192/bjp.bp.116.187179
4. Grigoriadis S, VonderPorten EH, Mamisashvili L, Tomlinson G, Dennis C-L, Koren G, Steiner M, Mousmanis P, Cheung A, Radford K, Martinovic J, Ross LE. The impact of maternal depression during pregnancy on perinatal outcomes:

a systematic review and meta-analysis. J Clin Psychiatry. 2013;74(4):e321–41. https://doi.org/10.4088/JCP.12r07968

5. Leiferman JA, Farewell CV, Jewell J, Lacy R, Walls J, Harnke B, Paulson JF. Anxiety among fathers during the prenatal and postpartum period: a meta-analysis. J Psychosom Obstet Gynaecol. 2021;42(2):152–61. https://doi.org/10.1080/0167482X.2021.1885025
6. Wong O, Nguyen T, Thomas N, Thomson-Salo F, Handrinos D, Judd F. Perinatal mental health: fathers — the (mostly) forgotten parent. Asia-Pac Psychiatry. 2016;8(4):247–55. https://doi.org/10.1111/appy.12204
7. Woody CA, Ferrari AJ, Siskind DJ, Whiteford HA, Harris MG. A systematic review and meta-regression of the prevalence and incidence of perinatal depression. J Affect Disord. 2017;219:86–92. https://doi.org/10.1016/j.jad.2017.05.003
8. Draper J. Men's passage to fatherhood: an analysis of the contemporary relevance of transition theory. Nurs Inquiry. 2003;10(1):66–78.
9. Shorey S, Dennis C L, Bridge S, Chong YS, Holroyd E, He H-G. First-time fathers' postnatal experiences and support needs: a descriptive qualitative study. J Adv Nurs. 2017;73(12):2987–96. https://doi.org/10.1111/jan.13349
10. Field T. Postpartum depression effects on early interactions, parenting, and safety practices: a review. Infant Behav Dev. 2010;33(1):1–6. https://doi.org/10.1016/j.infbeh.2009.10.005
11. Koh YLM, Tan LCA, Shorey S. Perceptions of distressed fathers in the early postpartum period: a descriptive qualitative study. J Fam Issues. 2021;42(10):2397–2417. https://doi.org/10.1177/0192513X20980042
12. Breuer L, Barker C. Online support groups for depression: benefits and barriers. SAGE Open. 2015;5(2):2158244015574936. https://doi.org/10.1177/2158244015574936
13. Cole BP. An exploration of men's attitudes regarding depression and help-seeking [PhD thesis]. University of Nebraska; 2013.
14. Chua JYX, Shorey S. Effectiveness of mobile application-based perinatal interventions in improving parenting outcomes: a systematic review. Midwifery. 2022;114:103457. https://doi.org/10.1016/j.midw.2022.103457
15. Bandura A. Self-efficacy: the exercise of control. New York: W.H. Freeman; 1997.
16. Goodman JH. Paternal postpartum depression, its relationship to maternal postpartum depression, and implications for family health. J Adv Nurs. 2004;45(1):26–35. https://doi.org/10.1046/j.1365-2648.2003.02857.x
17. Albanese AM, Russo GR, Geller PA. The role of parental self-efficacy parent and child well-being: a systematic review of associated outcomes. Child Care Health Dev. 2019;45(3):333–63. https://doi.org/10.1111/cch.12661

18. Biehle SN, Mickelson KD. Personal and co-parent predictors of parenting efficacy across the transition to parenthood. J Soc Clin Psychol. 2011;30(9):985–1010. https://doi.org/10.1521/jscp.2011.30.9.985
19. Jones TL, Prinz RJ. Potential roles of parental self-efficacy in parent and child adjustment: a review. Clin Psychol Rev. 2005;25(3):341–63. https://doi.org/10.1016/j.cpr.2004.12.004
20. Sanders MR, Woolley ML. The relationship between maternal self-efficacy and parenting practices: implications for parent training. Child Care Health Dev. 2005;31(1):65–73. https://doi.org/10.1111/j.1365-2214.2005.00487.x
21. Haslam DM, Pakenham KI, Smith A. Social support and postpartum depressive symptomatology: the mediating role of maternal self-efficacy. Infant Ment Health J. 2006;27(3):276–91. https://doi.org/10.1002/imhj.20092
22. Attard R, Iles J, Satherley R-M. How acceptable do parents experiencing mental health challenges find e-Health interventions for mental health in the postnatal period: a systematic review. BMC Pregnancy Childbirth. 2022;22(1):763. https://doi.org/10.1186/s12884-022-05070-7
23. Hong QN, Fàbregues S, Bartlett G, Boardman F, Cargo M, Dagenais P, Gagnon M-P, Griffiths F, Nicolau B, O'Cathain A, Rousseau M-C, Vedel I, Pluye P. The mixed methods appraisal tool (MMAT) version 2018 for information professionals and researchers. Educ Inform. 2018;34(4):285–91. https://doi.org/10.3233/EFI-180221
24. Martínez-Borba V, Suso-Ribera C, Osma J. The use of information and communication technologies in perinatal depression screening: a systematic review. Cyberpsychol Behav Soc Netw. 2018;21(12):741–52. https://doi.org/10.1089/cyber.2018.0416
25. Siani SA, Dol J, Campbell-Yeo M. Impact of parent-targeted ehealth on parent and infant health outcomes: a scoping review. J Perinat Neonatal Nurs. 2017;31(4):332–40. https://doi.org/10.1097/JPN.0000000000000265
26. Silang KA, Sohal PR, Bright KS, Leason J, Roos L, Lebel C, Giesbrecht GF, Tomfohr-Madsen LM. eHealth interventions for treatment and prevention of depression, anxiety, and insomnia during pregnancy: systematic review and meta-analysis. JMIR Ment Health. 2022;9(2):e31116. https://doi.org/10.2196/31116
27. Fisher ML, Sutcliffe P, Southern C, Grove AL, Tan BK. The effectiveness of interventions for the prevention or treatment of paternal perinatal anxiety: a systematic review. J Clin Med. 2022;11(22):6617. https://doi.org/10.3390/jcm11226617
28. Goldstein Z, Rosen B, Howlett A, Anderson M, Herman D. Interventions for paternal perinatal depression: a systematic review. J Affect Disord. 2020;265:505–10. https://doi.org/10.1016/j.jad.2019.12.029

29. Rodrigues AL, Ericksen J, Watson B, Gemmill AW, Milgrom J. Interventions for perinatal depression and anxiety in fathers: a mini-review. Front Psychol. 2022;12:744921. https://doi.org/10.3389/fpsyg.2021.744921
30. Aromataris E, Munn Z, editors. Joanna Briggs Institute Manual for Evidence Synthesis. Adelaide (AU): Joanna Briggs Institute; 2020. https://doi.org/10.46658/JBIMES-20-01
31. Almalki S. Integrating quantitative and qualitative data in mixed methods research–challenges and benefits. J Educ Learn. 2016;5(3):288. https://doi.org/10.5539/jel.v5n3p288
32. Hong QN, Pluye P, Bujold M, Wassef M. Convergent and sequential synthesis designs: implications for conducting and reporting systematic reviews of qualitative and quantitative evidence. Syst Rev. 2017;6(1):61. https://doi.org/10.1186/s13643-017-0454-2
33. Tariq S, Woodman J. Using mixed methods in health research. J R Soc Med Short Rep. 2013;4(6). https://doi.org/10.1177/2042533313479197
34. Moher D, Liberati A, Tetzlaff J, Altman DG, The PRISMA Group. Preferred reporting items for systematic reviews and meta-analyses: the PRISMA statement (Reprinted from Ann Intern Med). Phys Ther. 2009;89(9):873–80. https://doi.org/10.1093/ptj/89.9.873
35. GRADE-CERQual Interactive Summary of Qualitative Findings (iSoQ). Version 1.0 [computer software]. Oslo: Norwegian Institute of Public Health; 2022. Available at https://isoq.epistemonikos.org
36. Atkins D, Best D, Briss P. Grading quality of evidence and strength of recommendations. BMJ. 2004;328(7454):1490. https://doi.org/10.1136/bmj.328.7454.1490
37. GRADEpro Guideline Development Tool. Version 3.6 [computer software]. Hamilton (ON): McMaster University and Evidence Prime; 2022. Available at https://gradepro.org
38. Lewin S, Bohren M, Rashidian A, Munthe-Kaas H, Glenton C, Colvin CJ, Garside R, Noyes J, Booth A, Tunçalp Ö, Wainwright M, Flottorp S, Tucker JD, Carlsen B. Applying GRADE-CERQual to qualitative evidence synthesis findings-paper 2: how to make an overall CERQual assessment of confidence and create a summary of qualitative findings table. Implement Sci. 2018;13 (Suppl 1):10. https://doi.org/10.1186/s13012-017-0689-2
39. Joanna Briggs Institute. Joanna Briggs Institute Reviewers' Manual: 2014 edition/Supplement. The Joanna Briggs Institute; 2014.
40. Li T, Higgins JPT, Deeks JJ, editors. Collecting data. In: Higgins JPT, Thomas J, Chandler J, Cumpston M, Li T, Page MJ, Welch VA, editors. Cochrane Handbook for Systematic Reviews of Interventions version 6.3. The Cochrane Collaboration; 2022. Available from www.training.cochrane.org/handbook

41. Review Manager. RevMan Version 5.4 [computer software]. Copenhagen: The Cochrane Collaboration; 2020. Available at https://revman.cochrane.org
42. Cohen J. Statistical power analysis for the behavioral sciences. 2nd ed. Hillsdale (NJ): Lawrence Erlbaum Associates; 1988.
43. Thomas J, Harden A. Methods for the thematic synthesis of qualitative research in systematic reviews. BMC Med Res Methodol. 2008;8:45. https://doi.org/10.1186/1471-2288-8-45
44. Danbjørg DB, Wagner L, Kristensen BR, Clemensen J. Intervention among new parents followed up by an interview study exploring their experiences of telemedicine after early postnatal discharge. Midwifery. 2015;31(6):574–81. https://doi.org/10.1016/j.midw.2015.02.007
45. Shorey S, Ang L, Goh ECL, Lopez V. Paternal involvement of Singaporean fathers within six months postpartum: a follow-up qualitative study. Midwifery. 2018;70:7–14. https://doi.org/10.1016/j.midw.2018.12.003
46. Lindberg I, Christensson K, Ohrling K. Parents' experiences of using videoconferencing as a support in early discharge after childbirth. Midwifery. 2009;25(4):357–65. https://doi.org/10.1016/j.midw.2007.06.002
47. White BK, Giglia RC, Scott JA, Burns SK. How new and expecting fathers engage with an app-based online forum: qualitative analysis. JMIR mHealth uHealth. 2018;6(6):e144. https://doi.org/10.2196/mhealth.9999
48. Hamil J, Gier E, Garfield CF, Tandon D. The development and pilot of a technology-based intervention in the United States for father's mental health in the perinatal period. Am J Mens Health. 2021;15(5). https://doi.org/10.1177/15579883211044306
49. Shorey S, Lau YY, Dennis CL, Chan YS, Tam WWS, Chan YH. A randomized-controlled trial to examine the effectiveness of the 'Home-but not Alone' mobile-health application educational programme on parental outcomes. J Adv Nurs. 2017;73(9):2103–11. https://doi.org/10.1111/jan.13293
50. Shorey S, Ng YPM, Ng ED, Siew AL, Mörelius E, Yoong J, Gandhi M. Effectiveness of a technology-based supportive educational parenting program on parental outcomes (part 1): randomized controlled trial. J Med Internet Res. 2019;21(2):e10816. https://doi.org/10.2196/10816
51. Shorey S, Law E, Thilagamangai Mathews J, Lim SH, Shi L, Chua JS, Du R, Chan YH, Tan TC, Chee C, Chong YS. Evaluating the effectiveness of the supportive parenting app on parental outcomes: randomized controlled trial. J Med Internet Res. 2023;25:e41859. https://doi.org/10.2196/41859
52. Çitil Canbay F, Şeker S. The effect of web based training given to fathers on their functional status after birth: a randomized controlled trial. Am J Fam Ther. 2021;1–18. https://doi.org/10.1080/01926187.2021.1967225

53. Higgins JPT, Altman DG, Gøtzsche PC, Jüni P, Moher D, Oxman AD, Savović J, Schulz KF, Weeks L, Sterne JAC. The Cochrane Collaboration's tool for assessing risk of bias in randomised trials. BMJ. 2011;343(7829):889–93. https://doi.org/10.1136/bmj.d5928
54. Kavanagh DJ, Connolly J, Fisher J, Halford WK, Hamilton K, Hides L, Milgrom J, Rowe H, Scuffham PA, White KM, Wittkowski A, Appleton S, Sanders D. The baby steps web program for the well-being of new parents: randomized controlled trial. J Med Internet Res. 2021;23(11):e23659. https://doi.org/10.2196/23659
55. Tandon SD, Hamil J, Gier EE, Garfield CF. Examining the effectiveness of the fathers and babies intervention: a pilot study. Front Psychol. 2021;12:668284. https://doi.org/10.3389/fpsyg.2021.668284
56. Novick AM, Kwitowski M, Dempsey J, Cooke DL, Dempsey AG. Technology-based approaches for supporting perinatal mental health. Curr Psychiatry Rep. 2022;24(9):419–29. https://doi.org/10.1007/s11920-022-01349-w
57. Shorey S, Ang L, Tam WWS. Informational interventions on paternal outcomes during the perinatal period: a systematic review. Women Birth. 2018;32(2):e145–58. https://doi.org/10.1016/j.wombi.2018.06.008
58. Shorey S, Yang YY, Dennis C-L. A mobile health app-based postnatal educational program (Home-but not Alone): descriptive qualitative study. J Med Internet Res. 2018;20(4):e119. https://doi.org/10.2196/jmir.9188
59. Cooklin AR, Giallo R, Strazdins L, Martin A, Leach LS, Nicholson JM. What matters for working fathers? job characteristics, work-family conflict and enrichment, and fathers' postpartum mental health in an Australian cohort. Soc Sci Med. 2015;146:214–22. https://doi.org/10.1016/j.socscimed.2015.09.028
60. Li Y, Long Z, Cao D, Cao F. Social support and depression across the perinatal period: a longitudinal study. J Clin Nurs. 2017;26(17–18):2776–86. https://doi.org/10.1111/jocn.13817
61. Bowlby J. Attachment and loss. Vol no. 79, 95, 109; 1969.
62. Chen CV, George SA, Liberzon I. Stress and anxiety disorders. In: Pfaff DW, Joels M, editors. Hormones, Brain and Behavior. Elsevier Inc; 2017. p. 251–74.
63. Kinser PA, Goehler LE, Taylor AG. How might yoga help depression? A neurobiological perspective. Explore (NY). 2012;8(2):118–26. https://doi.org/10.1016/j.explore.2011.12.005
64. Carlos HP. Brief internet-based acceptance and commitment therapy intervention for parents in the postpartum. Identifier NCT05173285. ClinicalTrials.gov; 2020 Jun 3-2022 Mar 28. https://clinicaltrials.gov/show/NCT05173285

65. Doaltabadi Z, Amiri-Farahani L. The effect of in-person and virtual prenatal care education of the spouses of primiparous women on the father and mother's attachment to infant: a quasi-experimental and controlled study. Trials. 2021;22(1):588. https://doi.org/10.1186/s13063-021-05559-0
66. Fletcher R, Knight T, Macdonald JA, St George J. Process evaluation of text-based support for fathers during the transition to fatherhood (SMS4dads): mechanisms of impact. BMC Psychol. 2019;7(1):63. https://doi.org/10.1186/s40359-019-0338-4
67. Garfield C, Santiago J. Baby2Home (B2H) mobile health application. Identifier NCT05595486. ClinicalTrials.gov; 2022 Nov 9-2024 Aug 1. https://clinicaltrials.gov/ct2/show/NCT05595486
68. Gemmill A, Holt C. DadBooster: a randomised controlled trial of an online depression treatment for new fathers. Identifier ACTRN12622001029785. ANZCTR; 2022 Aug 15. https://anzctr.org.au/ACTRN12622001029785.aspx
69. Hudson DB, Campbell-Grossman C, Fleck MO, Elek SM, Shipman A. Effects of the new fathers network on first-time fathers' parenting self-efficacy and parenting satisfaction during the transition to parenthood. Issues Compr Pediatr Nurs. 2003;26(4):217–29. https://doi.org/10.1080/01460860390246687
70. Ivers N. Proactive, personalized postpartum mental healthcare (P3MH). Identifier NCT03803189. ClinicalTrials.gov; 2019 Mar 14-2021 Apr 24. https://clinicaltrials.gov/ct2/show/NCT03803189
71. Lawrence C, Brotto LA. The SUPPORT study: effectiveness and usability of a web-enabled resource for postpartum mental health (SUPPORT). Identifier NCT05382884. ClinicalTrials.gov; 2022 Apr 20-2023 Feb. https://clinicaltrials.gov/ct2/show/NCT05382884
72. Manav AI, Gozuyesil E, Tar E. The effects of the parenting education performed through WhatsApp on the level of maternal-paternal and infant attachment in Turkey. J Pediatr Nurs. 2021;61:e57. https://doi.org/10.1016/j.pedn.2021.04.018
73. Nakajima A. Internet-based, randomized, 28 weeks (from 28th weeks of pregnancy to 100 days after childbirth) intervention, parallel-group, superiority study to compare the efficacy of text messaging (NCNP kizuna mail) group to non-intervention group for father's mental health assessed by the general health questionnaire-12 (GHQ12). Identifier UMIN000040172. UMIN CTR; 2020 Apr 17-. https://center6.umin.ac.jp/cgi-open-bin/ctr_e/ctr_view.cgi?recptno = R000045750
74. Salonen AH, Kaunonen M, Astedt-Kurki P, Järvenpää AL, Isoaho H, Tarkka MT. Effectiveness of an internet-based intervention enhancing Finnish parents'

parenting satisfaction and parenting self-efficacy during the postpartum period. Midwifery. 2011;27(6):832–41. https://doi.org/10.1016/j.midw.2010.08.010

75. Shakibi N. Investigating the effect of fathers tele counseling on spouse social support and postpartum quality of life in primiparous women. Identifier IRCT20211206053295N1. IRCT; 2022 Jan 15-. http://en.irct.ir/trial/61292
76. Shorey S, Chua JYX. Effect of 'Parentbot — a Digital Healthcare Assistant (PDA)' in improving parenting outcomes during the perinatal period (PDA). Identifier NCT05463926. ClinicalTrials.gov; 2022 Nov-2023 Dec. https://clinicaltrials.gov/ct2/show/NCT05463926
77. Shu YK. The development and evaluation of a web-based childbirth and parenting intervention program. Identifier NCT04981730. ClinicalTrials.gov; 2022 Dec-2023 Jun. https://clinicaltrials.gov/ct2/show/NCT04981730
78. Teague S. Harnessing social media and mHealth to manage adjustment to parenthood in fathers. Identifier ACTRN12621000275864. ANZCTR; 2021 Mar 24-Nov 13. https://anzctr.org.au/ACTRN12621000275864.aspx

https://doi.org/10.1142/9789819817320_0007

Chapter 7

Reimagining Adolescent Mental Health through Digital Compassion: The MU MyMind Experience

Nopporn Vongsirimas[1,*] and Piyanee Klainin-Yobas[2]

[1]*Faculty of Nursing, Mahidol University, 999, Phuttamonthon 4 Road, Salaya, Nakhon Pathom 73170, Thailand*

[2]*Alice Lee Centre for Nursing Studies, Yong Loo Lin School of Medicine, National University of Singapore, Level 5, Centre of Translational Medicine, Block MD6, 14 Medical Drive, Singapore 117599*

**Corresponding author: nopporn.von@mahidol.ac.th*

7.1 Introduction

As a psychiatric nursing educator and adolescent mental health researcher, we have spent over a decade working closely with schools, communities, and young people across Thailand. Our professional journey has been grounded in the conviction that adolescent mental health must be nurtured through culturally resonant, developmentally sensitive, and ethically guided interventions.

Building on these lived experiences and long-standing commitments, this chapter extends upon previously published work by offering theoretical reflections, ethical framing, and practice-based insights from the implementation of the MU MyMind mobile application — a digital intervention co-designed to promote psychological well-being among secondary school students. Rooted in participatory design and informed by the lived experiences of youth, the app was not merely developed for adolescents, but with them.

We believe that meaningful digital mental health innovation must be more than technically sound — it must be human-centred. When grounded in compassion, cultural attunement, and relational ethics, technology becomes a bridge that connects theory with practice, and science with lived experience. In writing this chapter, our aspiration is not only to report findings, but to invite readers into a deeper contemplation of what it means to care for youth in a rapidly changing world.

This work would not have been possible without the generous collaboration of fellow researchers, school leaders, teachers, students, and parents who co-owned this journey. We hope that the reflections offered here will serve as a source of inspiration for those committed to advancing adolescent mental health through innovations that are accessible, meaningful, and grounded in the dignity and potential of every young person.

This chapter builds upon the system-level framework introduced in Chapter 5, which outlined the Nurse-Led Depression Prevention Clinic (NDPC) model for adolescent mental health in Thailand. While Chapter 5 focused on policy design, service integration, and strategic implementation, this chapter offers an in-depth exploration of the MU MyMind application — its development, theoretical foundations, and practical outcomes. Together, the two chapters offer complementary perspectives on how digital innovation and nurse-led care can be integrated to support youth mental well-being at both system and practice levels.

7.2 Setting the Stage: The Context of Adolescent Mental Health

The global rise in adolescent mental health challenges is acutely mirrored in Southeast Asia, with Thailand experiencing disproportionately high rates of depressive symptoms among its youth. Recent studies reveal that approximately 37.8% of Thai adolescents are at risk for depression, while 22% report suicidal ideation [1]. These concerning trends are often attributed to multifaceted psychosocial factors, including excessive smartphone use, diminished self-esteem, and insufficient resilience — with female students appearing particularly vulnerable [2].

Despite increasing awareness, adolescents in Thailand continue to face systemic barriers in accessing mental health services. These barriers include entrenched stigma surrounding mental illness, limited knowledge about available support, geographic inaccessibility, and a critical shortage of youth-focused mental health professionals. Traditional care models, reliant on in-person consultations, can be intimidating or uninviting to adolescents who may feel hesitant to disclose emotional difficulties in formal environments. This limited access to supportive services not only leaves emotional needs unmet but also directly undermines adolescents' psychological well-being, making it harder for them to develop essential capacities such as emotional regulation, autonomy, and connectedness [3].

Psychological well-being, a multidimensional construct encompassing autonomy, emotional regulation, purpose, and connectedness, remains under-addressed within both educational and healthcare frameworks. Although digital platforms have gained momentum as scalable solutions, few interventions are adequately tailored to the nuanced socio-cultural realities of Thai adolescents. A recent study by Metheekul [4] demonstrated that a well-structured digital intervention can significantly enhance both digital literacy and psychological well-being among Thai early adolescents.

Within this landscape, digital interventions are emerging not merely as technical tools, but as culturally adaptable and developmentally sensitive pathways toward equitable mental health support. When grounded in mindfulness practices, cognitive-behavioural strategies, and emotional learning, digital tools can bridge the accessibility gap and resonate deeply with adolescents' lived experiences. Importantly, centring adolescents as co-creators — rather than passive recipients — ensures that such tools remain relevant, empowering, and ethically aligned.

Guided by this vision, the present chapter frames adolescent mental health through the lens of compassionate technology. It proposes that healing lies not in the technology itself, but in its intentional, ethically attuned design. By cultivating trust, engagement, and agency, digital interventions such as MU MyMind may help foster emotional resilience and promote holistic well-being for Thai youths across diverse contexts.

7.3 Conceptualising the Intervention: MU MyMind App

The MU MyMind mobile application emerged from a collaborative and interdisciplinary design process driven by a shared purpose: to strengthen the psychological well-being of Thai adolescents through evidence-informed, culturally grounded, and ethically sensitive approaches. Developed by psychiatric nursing educators in partnership with technology specialists, the app was built not merely as a digital product, but as a reflection of lived experience and relational care.

To ensure contextual relevance, the design process was informed by qualitative insights gathered from four key stakeholder groups: adolescents aged 12–18 years, classroom teachers, guidance counsellors, and parents. These diverse voices shaped the development of features, aesthetics, and content, ensuring alignment with the psychosocial realities of youth in Thailand. This work was supported by a research grant from the National Research Council of Thailand in the fiscal years 2019–2020 (B.E. 2562–2563), awarded to the lead author for the development and evaluation of the MU MyMind intervention.

7.3.1 *Stakeholder Perspectives*

Students' perspectives: Adolescents described mental well-being as deeply rooted in their inner world — comprising emotions, thoughts, and interpersonal stressors. They identified familial pressures, peer conflicts, and environmental stress as key challenges to their emotional balance. In coping with distress, students often turned to self-guided strategies such as listening to music, journaling on their phones, or talking to trusted peers or parents. A recurring theme was their desire for a digital mental health space that was confidential, visually engaging, non-intrusive, and offered tools for optional self-assessment — features they felt would enhance trust and autonomy.

Teachers' perspectives: Teachers emphasised emotional regulation as a critical determinant of students' mental health. They observed that academic overload and heightened parental expectations created undue stress for learners. In response, they advocated for upstream school-based initiatives that provide emotional scaffolding, including teacher-led support, peer group activities, and early home visits. Teachers also noted the importance of equipping educators with tools and training to identify emotional distress before it escalates.

Guidance Teachers' perspectives: Guidance teachers pointed to a recurrent pattern of emotional strain linked to peer dynamics, family expectations, and systemic academic pressures. While their current interventions — such as individual counselling and financial support — were helpful, they acknowledged the need for a shift toward preventive approaches. Strategies to promote self-esteem, goal setting, and emotional self-awareness were highlighted. For digital solutions, counsellors encouraged the integration of animated and interactive elements to create a sense of relatability and reduce psychological barriers to engagement.

Parents' perspectives: Parents, reflecting on their children's emotional landscape, noted the significance of family dynamics, peer relationships, and academic stress. Many expressed concerns about their own limited capacity to identify early signs of emotional distress. They recommended that digital platforms include colourful, playful, and developmentally appropriate content, framed in a way that invites dialogue within the family. They also emphasised the importance of emotional education that is both accessible and enjoyable to sustain adolescent engagement.

The synthesis of stakeholder insights provided the foundational blueprint for translating adolescent needs into tangible app functionalities. In direct response to their voices, the MU MyMind application integrated a number of key components that reflect user-centred, culturally grounded, and developmentally appropriate mental health design.

First, the app incorporated confidential and user-driven mental health screening tools to allow adolescents to assess their emotional state privately and at their own pace. These tools were carefully calibrated to be non-invasive and optional, aligning with the participants' desire for autonomy and safety.

Second, to sustain engagement and emotional investment, interactive features such as animated avatars, gamified challenges, and visually rich interfaces were embedded. These features not only captured attention but also fostered emotional exploration in a playful and non-threatening manner.

Third, the platform delivered psychoeducational content that was accessible, evidence-based, and youth-oriented. This content focused on cultivating self-esteem, resilience, and emotional regulation — skills repeatedly emphasised across stakeholder interviews.

Fourth, the interface was designed to be visually appealing and intuitively navigable. Its use of vibrant colours, local cultural motifs, and modern aesthetics ensured relatability and ease of use, regardless of the adolescent's digital literacy level.

Lastly, the app provided built-in pathways to help-seeking, including links to mental health professionals and hotlines, reinforcing the normalisation of accessing support.

Through this integrative and evidence-based approach, MU MyMind is positioned as a culturally competent and ethically attuned digital mental health intervention for Thai adolescents. The following section introduces the structured framework that underpins the MU

MyMind mobile application, detailing its components, theoretical foundations, and educational media. This comprehensive design serves as both a curriculum for emotional development and a medium for accessible, youth-oriented care. Drawing upon evidence-informed principles and direct input from Thai adolescents and their communities, the MU MyMind program exemplifies how participatory digital innovation can operationalise compassionate, relational support in practice.

7.3.2 *Structure, Theoretical Foundations, and Learning Media*

The MU MyMind mobile application is a comprehensive digital intervention designed to promote psychological well-being among Thai adolescents (Figure 7.1). Developed collaboratively by psychiatric nursing educators and technology developers, the program integrates evidence-based psychological theories with practical, culturally relevant activities. The design of MU MyMind draws upon extensive qualitative

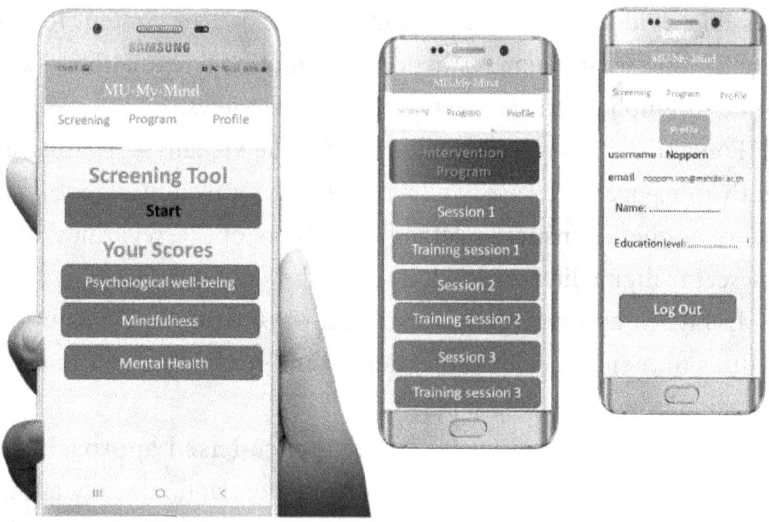

Figure 7.1 Sample screenshots of the MU MyMind Mobile Application.

data gathered through focus groups with adolescents and key stakeholders (classroom teachers, guidance counsellors, and parents). Based on these insights, the program employs engaging video animations depicting real-life situations that adolescents face, fostering high relevance and emotional connection. The intervention is organised into four sequential programs, each underpinned by a robust theoretical foundation. These programs are integrated within three core functional systems of the MU MyMind platform, which work synergistically to guide users through assessment, skill-building, and emotional growth. The following sections describe each system in detail and how they operationalise the theoretical and practical elements of the intervention.

7.3.2.1 *System 1: Initial Registration and Emotional Self-Check*

Upon first accessing the application, students register their basic information and perform an initial emotional check-in. Emotional awareness is assessed through a visual-based self-rating system, combining emotional literacy promotion with data-driven tracking of psychological states. In addition to the initial check-in, standardised and validated psychological assessment tools are embedded into the system to comprehensively evaluate users' psychological status across three domains: well-being, emotional distress, and mindfulness. These assessments include:

- **Scales of Psychological Well-Being:** Developed by Ryff, this instrument evaluates key dimensions of psychological well-being, including autonomy, personal growth, purpose in life, environmental mastery, positive relations with others, and self-acceptance [5].
- **Depression Anxiety Stress Scales-21 (DASS-21):** A shortened form of the original DASS developed by Lovibond and Lovibond, this tool measures the severity of symptoms related to depression, anxiety, and stress [6].

- **Mindful Attention Awareness Scale:** Developed by Brown and Ryan, this scale assesses trait mindfulness, focusing on the frequency of open, receptive attention to and awareness of present-moment experiences [7].

The use of these tools enables early identification of emotional distress and psychological vulnerabilities, allowing the intervention to be tailored to better meet the individual needs of users.

7.3.2.2 *System 2: Core Psychological Skills Training Modules*

Program 1: Breathe to Relieve Stress

This program introduces adolescents to fundamental mindful breathing techniques grounded in the principles of Mindfulness-Based Stress Reduction, with the aim of reducing physiological arousal and promoting emotional self-regulation [8]. Through a series of structured activities — including educational videos explaining the neurophysiological basis of breath, *Episode 1: The Remarkable Benefits of Breathing Correctly* [9], *Episode 2: Breathing to Release Stress* [10], and *Episode 3: Mastering Correct Breathing to Reduce Stress* [11] — students learn to recognise their body's stress responses and regulate them through intentional diaphragmatic breathing. Participants are also encouraged to observe changes in physiological indicators such as blood pressure and heart rate, as well as subjective emotional states, before and after the practice. By fostering present-moment awareness and calming the autonomic nervous system, mindful breathing serves as a practical and evidence-based tool for stress management in adolescent populations.

Program 2: Observing the Body

This program is grounded in the practice of body scan meditation, a core component of mindfulness-based interventions, and aims to cultivate adolescents' non-judgemental awareness of bodily sensations as a foundation for emotional regulation [12]. Through the use of animated educational videos and guided practices, students are introduced to systematic techniques for directing attention across various regions of the body, thereby anchoring their focus in the present moment. The session includes exposure to materials such as *Episode 4: Body Scan Meditation — Mindfulness for Beginners* [13], along with structured body scan exercises that promote interoceptive awareness. Participants are encouraged to observe and record physiological responses (e.g., heart rate, blood pressure) and subjective emotional states before and after each session, reinforcing the link between bodily awareness and emotional experiences. By enhancing sensitivity to internal cues, this program supports the early detection of stress responses and contributes to more adaptive self-regulation, in alignment with mindfulness-based theoretical frameworks.

Program 3: Emotional Awareness

This program focuses on enhancing adolescents' emotional literacy through daily mood tracking and reflective exercises, aimed at fostering deeper self-awareness and emotional regulation. Grounded in the integration of mindfulness principles and theories of self-awareness development, the session guides students to identify, label, and rate their emotional responses in relation to everyday experiences. Utilising animated scenarios and educational videos — such as *Episode 5: Understanding the Nature of Emotions* [14] and *Episode 6: Emotional Awareness — Continuation and Practice* [15] — students are encouraged to reflect on both positive and negative emotional events, assign intensity scores, and build the habit of observing emotions with non-judgemental awareness. These practices promote an understanding of emotional patterns and triggers, which serves as a foundation for cultivating resilience and adaptive coping strategies. By developing the capacity to recognise and articulate emotions in real time, adolescents are better equipped to manage emotional challenges and engage in mindful decision-making.

Program 4: Adjust Your Thoughts...Conquer the Sadness

This program is grounded in the principles of cognitive behavioural therapy and aims to help adolescents identify, challenge, and reframe negative automatic thoughts, thereby fostering more adaptive and balanced cognitive patterns. Through a series of structured activities and animated instructional videos — such as *Episode 7: Becoming Aware of Your Thoughts and Managing Them* [16] — students are introduced to the interconnected nature of thoughts, emotions, and behaviours. The session guides participants in recognising unhelpful thinking patterns and engaging in cognitive restructuring techniques, including thought-challenging exercises and guided cognitive reappraisal practices. By developing metacognitive awareness and the ability to reinterpret distressing thoughts, adolescents enhance their emotional resilience and reduce susceptibility to prolonged sadness, anxiety, and depressive symptoms. The integration of cognitive behavioural therapy-based strategies in this program supports the development of healthier mental frameworks essential for psychological well-being.

Learning Media: Video Animation Integration

Across all four intervention programs, video animations are employed as the primary instructional medium to enhance engagement, comprehension, and skill application among adolescents. These animations are grounded in qualitative data derived from focus group discussions, depicting relatable adolescent experiences and modelling effective emotional and behavioural responses. By integrating storytelling elements and visual cues, the animations promote active engagement and facilitate experiential learning, while supporting knowledge retention and the generalisation of learned skills to real-life contexts. This multimedia approach, as implemented through the MU MyMind platform, ensures that the interventions are accessible, contextually relevant, and developmentally appropriate, thereby increasing their effectiveness in promoting emotional awareness, self-regulation, and psychological resilience.

7.3.2.3 *System 3: Help-Seeking and Support Notification*

This system incorporates a built-in help-seeking mechanism designed to promote early intervention and normalise mental health support behaviours among adolescents. When users' responses to screening tools indicate elevated distress, the app generates supportive and non-alarming messages that gently encourage users to connect with mental health professionals. These messages are paired with direct access to external counselling services and national crisis hotlines, reinforcing the app's commitment to user safety and timely support.

Moreover, the app was designed for Android platforms with user-friendly navigation, gamified reflective activities, and embodied mindfulness practices — all features intended to meet adolescents where they are. The seamless integration of help-seeking resources into the app emphasises that mental health support should be as mobile, responsive, and accessible as the digital environments that youths routinely engage with.

7.3.3 *Methodology and Implementation*

To assess the feasibility and initial effectiveness of the MU MyMind application, a pilot study was conducted using a single-group, pre-posttest quasi-experimental design. The study involved 30 secondary school students in Bangkok, Thailand and received ethical approval from the institutional review board (IRB-NS2019/526.0912). Informed consent was obtained from all participants prior to data collection.

The evaluation encompassed both quantitative and qualitative outcome indicators. Quantitative measures included psychological well-being, mindfulness, and symptoms of depression, anxiety, and stress — assessed using standardised instruments integrated within the app. Qualitative data were derived from open-ended responses embedded into the platform, allowing participants to express personal reflections on their experiences.

Data collection was conducted entirely through the MU MyMind mobile platform, reinforcing its capacity for seamless digital integration in real-world educational settings. Statistical analysis was performed using paired t-tests to compare pre- and post-intervention outcomes. Thematic analysis was applied to qualitative responses to identify patterns of experience, insight, and change. This mixed-methods approach enabled a nuanced understanding of both the measurable impact and the subjective experience of adolescents engaging with the intervention.

7.3.4 *Participant Characteristics*

A total of 30 participants completed the pre-posttest and none of them dropped out from the study. The students average age was 15.33 years old (standard deviation (SD) = 1.97). Most students were female (66.7%, n = 20) and Buddhist (93.3%, n = 28), and all of them (100%, n = 30) had grade point average higher than 3.0 (out of 4.0) (Table 7.1).

Table 7.1 Baseline participant characteristics (n = 30).

Age (year)	**n (%)**
Mean (SD)	15.33 (1.97)
Gender	
Male	10 (33.3)
Female	20 (66.7)
Level of education	
Junior high school	14 (46.7)
High school	16 (53.3)
Grade point average	
Lower than 3.00	—
Above 3.00	30 (100.0)
Religion	
Buddhism	28 (93.3)
Christianity	1 (3.3)
Islam	1 (3.3)

7.3.5 *Results*

Quantitative findings revealed statistically significant improvements across multiple psychological domains following participation in the intervention programs. Participants demonstrated a notable increase in psychological well-being, with mean scores rising from M = 78.37 to M = 81.50 (p = .01), indicating enhanced overall mental health functioning. Similarly, levels of mindfulness improved significantly, with mean scores increasing from M = 61.67 to M = 65.07 (p = .01), suggesting greater present-moment awareness and emotional regulation capacity. In addition, measures of depression, anxiety, and stress showed significant reductions ($p < .05$), highlighting the efficacy of the intervention in mitigating internalising symptoms and promoting psychological resilience among adolescents (Table 7.2).

7.3.6 *Students' Reflections*

Upon completion of the pilot implementation of the MU MyMind mobile application, participants were invited to provide qualitative feedback regarding their experiences with the intervention. The responses

Table 7.2 Comparisons of mean between pre-test and post-test across outcome variables (n = 30). * denotes statistically significant differences, indicating that the observed changes between pre- and post-test were unlikely to have occurred by chance.

	Pre-test			Post-test				
	Mean	**SD**	**SE**	**Mean**	**SD**	**SE**	***t***	***p***
Psychological well-being	78.37	9.34	1.71	81.50	12.26	2.24	−2.72	0.01*
Mindfulness	61.67	10.34	1.89	65.07	12.40	2.26	−2.98	0.01*
Mental health problems	22.27	12.20	2.23	17.77	13.90	2.54	3.19	<0.001*
— depression	6.17	5.02	0.92	4.37	4.75	0.87	3.14	<0.001*
— anxiety	7.73	4.53	0.83	6.30	5.13	0.94	2.70	0.01
— stress	8.37	4.11	0.75	7.10	5.10	0.93	2.30	0.03*

indicated a generally favourable perception across several domains. Students particularly appreciated the clarity and brevity of the video-based content, describing it as engaging and accessible. The breathing exercises introduced in the initial program were frequently cited as highly beneficial, with students reporting that these techniques effectively facilitated emotional regulation both personally and among peers.

The initial program within the MU MyMind application introduced students to foundational mindful breathing techniques aimed at enhancing emotional regulation. Participants consistently reported that this component was particularly effective in managing acute emotional responses such as anger and anxiety. Through short, engaging video segments, students were guided to practice mindful breathing, resulting in observable improvements in emotional self-control. To reinforce this practice, the program integrated additional multimedia resources, including YouTube videos such as *Episodes 1–3,* which offer concise, evidence-based instruction on deep breathing. The clarity and brevity of such materials were cited by participants as key factors facilitating understanding and real-world application. Beyond breathing exercises, Programs 3 and 4 — focused on emotional awareness and cognitive reframing — were praised for promoting perspective-taking and cognitive flexibility. Several participants reflected on a transformative shift in their interpretation of social experiences, including increased empathy toward marginalised individuals. Others described substantial gains in emotional self-awareness and impulse control, particularly in interpersonal and academic contexts. One student highlighted the ability to mitigate anger through consistent breathing practice, while others noted greater resilience in response to academic setbacks. The cumulative effect of daily engagement with the application fostered improvements in students' capacity to identify, articulate, and manage emotional states. Many expressed appreciation for the self-guided nature of the intervention, which offered accessible emotional support without requiring formal psychological services. Notably, participants suggested that the program could be further enhanced by incorporating a broader range of emotion regulation strategies to address diverse emotional needs.

7.3.7 *Acceptability*[1]

After completion of the application, the students were asked to provide comments based on the open-ended questions, which can be summarised into six topics: (a) Overall feedback of the program, (b) Learning to manage stress and challenges, (c) Elevating relaxation responses and calmness, (d) Heightened mindfulness and concentration, (e) Increased awareness and management of emotions, and (f) Altering perspectives and managing thoughts. Most comments were positive, suggesting that the application is well-received by the students.

7.3.7.1 *Topic 1: Overall Feedback to the Program*

Most participants complimented the MU MyMind app as useful, smooth, user friendly, easy to understand and well-functioned. Videos were useful for daily living, interesting, cute, and easy to understand. Students learned about managing thoughts, emotion and stress.

"This program allows us to know about our own emotions. Sometimes we feel that emotions go before our thoughts. I listened to several video clips in the program in mobile application and I repeated it for 3 days, it allowed us to know what we were thinking. This thinking can come out to be a sentence. For example, if we have feelings but we don't think, right? But when we know our feelings, we will say we're frustrated right now. We can stop our emotion. It makes us more conscious. I think this program is pretty good for people who don't want to consult a doctor." (P1, female).

"Videos are easy to understand, interesting and very cute. I learned and improved myself in managing emotions. I had less mood swing and

[1] Publisher's Note: The quotes in this section were not copyedited for language errors to retain originality.

quarrelled less with friends. Playing games helped me aware of my emotions." (P10, female).

"Thank you teachers for making this program for us. Given that we will be able to know our emotions, we will know ourselves. I think it really helps and I can see the results. I can confirm that it's ok. It really relieves my stress." (P6, female).

7.3.7.2 *Topic 2: Learning to Managing Stress and Challenges*

Some participants mentioned that the application helped them manage stress in general and stress related to examinations. Furthermore, the program helped calm the body and increased awareness of self.

"I think the program is very good; however, there is a bug that need to be managed. Contents can be used to improved myself. In terms of stress management, I gave 100% satisfaction towards the programme." (P9, male).

"Session two is very good as it makes us rest our mind and the body. Thinking about the body and our mind, which does not wander, make me calm down, not stress. Practicing mindful breathing helped clear my head, relaxed my body, and relieved stress when doing my homework." (P5, male).

7.3.7.3 *Topic 3: Elevating Relaxation Responses and Calmness*

The first session of the program was perceived to be useful to many participants. The video guided them to practice mindful breathing, which helped them to be aware of the current moment, relax and calm down.

"I really liked the first session about "Breathe to relieve stress." I showed it to my friends, everyone instantly calmed down. The short video clip is good, not boring and it makes me wish to watch it." (P6, female).

"The first session made me relaxed. Before the practice, the heart was beating fast. After the practice, the heart was more relaxed and I could sleep better." (P14, male).

7.3.7.4 *Topic 4: Heightened Mindfulness and Concentration*

Some participants testified that the mindful breathing helped increase concentration, focus on their tasks and control emotion. This technique can be applied to daily activities.

"The first session makes me more mindful and control emotions better. I just broke up with my boyfriend. Practicing the first session helped me a lot. I wish that my friends can use it and practice it before taking examinations. That will help increase concentration." (P13, male).

"The program helped to perform meditation, making the mind less distracted. It is a systematic meditation that is practical, not just closing the eyes. It helped manage thoughts better and it can be integrated into daily activities, just like the video mentioned." (P9, male).

7.3.7.5 *Topic 5: Increased Awareness and Management of Emotions*

Most students felt that the MU MyMind app helped them recognise and manage emotions better. They also learned about symptoms of depression and how to prevent it.

"[The program]...helped me understand and manage my emotions better. I perceived my emotions more. When I was not in a good mood, I followed instruction guided by the videos. Then, I felt more relaxed and my mood became better quickly. The videos had contents that I have never seen before. I recognised my emotions and learned how to make myself into a better mood." (P16, male).

"The program made us know emotions. It is useful and makes know if we are at a risk of developing depression." (P3, female).

"Even the research project is completed, I wish that everyone can try the program because it contains a test to determine if we are depressed. If so, we can do practice to fix our problems. For me, the test showed that I am mildly and moderately depressed. Then, I am aware of my depression and I practice to manage my thoughts...positive thinking...do not think so much because that

leads to poor mental health. Wish that everyone takes care of his/her mental health because there are news talking about stress every day." (P29, male).

7.3.7.6 *Topic 6: Altering Perspectives and Managing Thoughts*

The fourth session of the application addressed how to recognise and manage negative thoughts. Some participants appreciated the session and stated that it helped them be aware of their own perspectives and changed some thoughts that are not useful.

"The contents of the videos in session 3 and 4 allowed us to know that our thought will depend on the point of view. What we think, it depends on our point of view. For example, I met a beggar, in the past, I might have thought that they are ugly and I might have walked away. But when I changed my perspective…They're human being." (P2, 07).

"I failed a chemistry exam. At first, I couldn't take it, it was so sad. However, after I practiced in the program in mobile application, I could accept the failure. So, I regret it for only a short time." (P3, 13).

"I'm quite satisfied, especially session 1, because I feel better after using it… I'm a person who talks without thinking, causing problems with my friends. After practicing in the program in mobile application, when I am mad, then I told to myself that I can't think of anything like this. I will stop and then I will breathe, then I can talk to my friends." (P4, 02).

7.3.8 ***Feasibility***

All 30 students who enrolled in the pilot successfully completed the four core sessions and corresponding pre- and post-test assessments within the designated four-week timeline. The modules — Breathe to Relieve Stress, Observing the Body, Emotional Awareness, and Adjust Your Thoughts — were completed without attrition, suggesting strong adherence. The smooth delivery and usability of the mobile platform further underscore its feasibility for broader implementation within school-based mental health initiatives. This preliminary evidence affirms that MU MyMind is both acceptable and feasible for promoting mental health engagement in adolescent populations.

7.3.9 *Discussion: Technology with a Human Face*

This pilot study underscores both the potential and responsibility inherent in developing digital mental health innovations. The MU MyMind application, though limited in scope, demonstrates that a well-designed mobile intervention can serve as both a mirror — reflecting adolescents' emotional states — and a guide — supporting their psychological growth. The observed improvements in well-being and reductions in psychological symptoms align with global evidence on the benefits of mindfulness-based digital interventions.

A key factor contributing to these outcomes is the incorporation of mindfulness into the intervention. Mindfulness encourages individuals to focus on the present moment with openness and non-judgment. For adolescents, this can enhance emotional regulation, reduce stress, and promote self-awareness. By supporting young users to better understand and manage their emotions, mindfulness becomes an essential part of the therapeutic process.

In addition, the participatory design and culturally relevant approach play an important role in the app's acceptability. Rather than treating adolescents as passive recipients of care, the intervention engaged them as active participants in shaping their own mental health journey. This co-creative process, combined with mindfulness-based strategies, helps create a more meaningful and effective user experience.

Moreover, the app's emphasis on social support aligns with findings that underscore its role in mitigating perceived stress and improving mental health outcomes [17]. By providing resources and guidance on seeking support, MU MyMind facilitates the development of a supportive network, which is crucial for adolescents navigating complex emotional landscapes.

Overall, the success of the MU MyMind app suggests that digital tools for mental health should not only be evidence-based but also grounded in mindfulness practices and tailored to the cultural and developmental needs of the target population. By integrating theoretical frameworks like Lazarus and Folkman's stress and coping model [18], and emphasising participatory design, such interventions can offer comprehensive support that resonates with adolescents' experiences and promotes lasting well-being.

7.3.10 *Practice and Policy Implications*

The findings from this intervention suggest strong practical and policy-level implications for enhancing adolescent mental health support, particularly through nurse-led, technology-mediated initiatives within educational settings.

First, the integration of **mental health mobile applications into school curricula** is essential. This means that mental health education, including the use of digital tools like MU MyMind, should not be treated as an optional or extracurricular activity, but as a structured part of students' learning experiences. Embedding such content into health education or homeroom sessions ensures that all students are routinely exposed to evidence-based strategies for managing stress, recognising emotions, and seeking help when needed.

Second, **professional development for school personnel** — particularly teachers and school nurses — plays a crucial role in sustaining such initiatives. Educators and nurses need training not only to understand how to use digital mental health tools, but also to identify warning signs of psychological distress and to facilitate meaningful conversations about mental health. Training programs should cover key areas such as adolescent psychological development, digital literacy, and ethical considerations in digital health interventions.

Third, at the **policy level**, national endorsement and support from health and education ministries can significantly strengthen the implementation and reach of such programs. When digital mental health platforms receive recognition within national mental health strategies or school health policies, they are more likely to receive funding, technical support, and institutional buy-in. This formal recognition helps to move such interventions from isolated pilot projects to sustainable, scalable components of youth mental health care.

Lastly, **the long-term sustainability of digital mental health interventions** depends not only on their technological design but also on the broader policy and social ecosystem. Even the most innovative apps require supportive environments — such as clear referral pathways, data privacy protections, and cross-sector collaboration — to function effectively. Therefore, building strong partnerships between schools, healthcare institutions, and policymakers is vital for ensuring that digital tools are not just available, but meaningfully embedded into the daily lives of young people.

7.3.11 *Limitations*

The pilot implementation of the MU MyMind application offers promising preliminary evidence for the role of mobile-based psychosocial interventions in enhancing adolescent psychological well-being. However, as with all early-stage research, this study carries certain limitations that must be transparently acknowledged to inform both academic interpretation and future application.

First, the **limited sample size** reduces the statistical power and scope of the conclusions that can be drawn. While meaningful trends were observed, the small cohort may not fully represent the diversity of adolescent experiences in Thailand. Important differences — such as those based on gender identity, socioeconomic background, or family structure — may have been underrepresented or obscured within the available data.

Second, the **lack of a control group** makes it difficult to attribute the observed outcomes solely to the intervention. Without a comparative baseline, it remains possible that improvements in psychological well-being could be partially explained by unrelated developmental changes, seasonal shifts, or external support systems not accounted for within the study design. Future iterations should prioritise randomised controlled trials to strengthen internal validity.

Third, the **geographic concentration of participants**, primarily from a limited number of regions, may reduce the applicability of the findings across the broader national or regional context. Thailand's adolescents live in culturally and economically diverse environments — from urban Bangkok to rural northern provinces — and each context brings its own unique psychosocial dynamics. A scalable intervention must be tested across these varied landscapes to ensure cultural sensitivity and systemic feasibility.

Despite these limitations, one of the key strengths of this study lies in its **novelty and innovation**. To date, there have been few, if any, structured mobile interventions in Thailand that integrate validated assessment tools, mindfulness-based psychoeducation, and built-in help-seeking mechanisms — all within a culturally contextualised framework designed specifically for adolescents. MU MyMind represents an important step forward in the country's mental health landscape, introducing a **locally developed, youth-centred, and technology-mediated model** that aligns with both global trends and local needs.

7.3.12 *Future Pathways*

To strengthen the evidence base and enhance practical implementation, several future research directions are recommended:

- **Scalability and Adaptability:** Future studies should examine whether the MU MyMind app can be scaled to reach a broader population of adolescents across different regions and educational settings, and whether the content can be adapted to suit specific cultural or developmental needs.

- **Long-term Effectiveness:** It is important to assess whether the benefits of the intervention are sustained over time. Longitudinal studies following users for several months — or even years — after participation can help determine the durability of outcomes such as improved emotional regulation and reduced psychological distress.
- **Integration with Multi-Tiered Systems of Care:** Rather than functioning as a standalone tool, future versions of the app should be explored as part of a broader mental health support system, involving school-based counselling, referral pathways to mental health professionals, and community-based support networks.
- **Co-Design with Stakeholders:** Involving key stakeholders such as **parents, teachers, school nurses, and mental health professionals** in the design and evaluation of future interventions can improve their relevance, cultural sensitivity, and acceptance. Co-design ensures that the intervention meets real-world needs and fosters shared ownership among those supporting adolescent mental health.
- **Controlled Efficacy Trials:** To increase the scientific credibility of the MU MyMind intervention, future research should include controlled trials with appropriate comparison groups. Randomised controlled trials or quasi-experimental designs can help isolate the intervention's true effects by controlling for potential confounding variables, thereby strengthening causal inferences.

In summary, while this pilot demonstrates the potential of mobile mental health interventions for youth, further research is essential to enhance its rigour, reach, and real-world integration.

7.3.13 *Lessons Learned*

The development and implementation of the MU MyMind mobile application offered several key lessons for future digital mental health interventions targeting adolescents:

1. **Compassionate Design is Foundational**: Adolescents respond positively to interventions that not only educate but also respect their emotional complexity. The emphasis on a non-judgemental tone, visual storytelling, and self-guided reflection demonstrated the power of designing with empathy.
2. **Participatory Development Enhances Relevance**: Involving adolescents, parents, and educators during development allowed the app to directly reflect the cultural, linguistic, and social realities of its users. This ensured the content was not only age-appropriate but also culturally meaningful.
3. **Mindfulness is More Than a Technique**: Framing mindfulness as a life skill rather than a therapeutic tool deepened its resonance with students. When embedded in relatable, daily scenarios, mindfulness became an accessible, sustainable form of self-care.
4. **Multi-modal Learning Builds Engagement**: The integration of animations, gamified elements, and reflection tools supported multiple learning styles and helped sustain user engagement. These interactive features made emotional learning both enjoyable and impactful.
5. **Early Help-Seeking Pathways Matter**: By embedding non-intrusive, accessible help-seeking features, the app normalised reaching out for support and promoted mental health literacy. This proactive structure empowered users before distress escalated.
6. **Digital Tools Must Reflect Real-World Use**: Adolescents navigate digital spaces intuitively. The app's mobile-first design, short-form content, and flexible access mirrored their daily habits, reinforcing integration rather than disruption.

Together, these lessons affirm that ethical, participatory, and context-sensitive approaches are not optional — they are essential in building digital mental health tools that genuinely serve and empower young people.

7.4 Conclusion

MU MyMind is more than just a mobile application — it represents a new way of thinking about mental health promotion for adolescents. At its core, this intervention embodies a pedagogical and ethical stance: that young people deserve not only access to support, but access that is grounded in respect, cultural relevance, and scientific credibility.

By integrating validated assessment tools, mindfulness-based practices, cognitive-behavioural techniques, and stress-coping strategies within a digital format, MU MyMind bridges the often-disconnected worlds of evidence-based care and real-world accessibility. It responds directly to the pressing need for adolescent mental health support in Thailand and Southeast Asia, where traditional services remain difficult to access, particularly for those in remote or underserved communities.

More than delivering content, MU MyMind offers a relational experience — one that recognises adolescents as active agents in their own emotional development. The app does not prescribe solutions from above; instead, it walks alongside users, inviting them into a process of reflection, self-awareness, and emotional growth. This orientation reflects a deep commitment to ethical engagement: one that views mental health not merely as symptom reduction, but as the cultivation of well-being, resilience, and agency.

The implementation findings and reflections shared in this chapter offer a micro-level complement to the macro-level system design presented in Chapter 5. Readers seeking further insights into how nurse-led digital mental health services can be embedded within national policy frameworks and community-based primary care are encouraged to refer to Chapter 5 for a comprehensive discussion.

As mental health systems across the region look for scalable and sustainable models, MU MyMind serves as a prototype for what is possible when digital innovation is guided by both science and story — by rigorous methodology, and by an attuned listening to the voices of those it seeks to serve.

> "Innovation in mental health care is not only about doing something new — it's about doing something meaningful, especially when it reaches those who have long remained unseen."

References

1. Patanavanich R, et al. The experience of Thai adolescents with depression: a qualitative study. Nurs Open. 2022;9(1):2161.
2. Ratanasiripong P, Hanklang S, Nungdanjark W, Thongthammarat Y. Predictors of mental health among secondary school students in Thailand: the roles of grit, self-esteem, and smartphone addiction. Thai J Public Health. 2024;54(2): 903–13.
3. Ryff CD. Happiness is everything, or is it? Explorations on the meaning of psychological well-being. J Pers Soc Psychol. 1989;57(6):1069–81.
4. Metheekul P. The development and effectiveness of digital well-being intervention on enhancing digital literacy and psychological well-being of Thai adolescents. J Behav Sci. 2024;19(2):89–102.
5. Ryff CD. Happiness is everything, or is it? Explorations on the meaning of psychological well-being. J Pers Soc Psychol. 1989;57(6):1069–81.
6. Lovibond SH, Lovibond PF. Manual for the Depression Anxiety Stress Scales. 2nd ed. Sydney: Psychology Foundation; 1995.
7. Brown KW, Ryan RM. The benefits of being present: mindfulness and its role in psychological well-being. J Pers Soc Psychol. 2003;84(4):822–8.
8. Kabat-Zinn J. Full catastrophe living: using the wisdom of your body and mind to face stress, pain, and illness. New York: Delta; 1990.
9. MU MyMind Episode 1: The Remarkable Benefits of Breathing Correctly. Available from: https://youtu.be/xUB-oFom0u4

10. MU MyMind Episode 2: Breathing to Release Stress. Available from: https://youtu.be/rp-i4c8q1ls
11. MU MyMind Episode 3: Mastering Correct Breathing to Reduce Stress. Available from: https://youtu.be/JkUxhnJqhVQ
12. Kabat-Zinn J. Full catastrophe living: using the wisdom of your body and mind to face stress, pain, and illness. New York: Delta; 1990.
13. MU MyMind Episode 4: Body Scan Meditation — Mindfulness for Beginners. Available from: https://youtu.be/pjTOTg4ns7E
14. MU MyMind Episode 5: Understanding the Nature of Emotions. Available from: https://youtu.be/wwFgC2p5Y4U
15. MU MyMind Episode 6: Emotional Awareness — Continuation and Practice. Available from: https://youtu.be/8UXbSnJBlTY
16. MU MyMind Episode 7: Becoming Aware of Your Thoughts and Managing Them. Available from: https://youtu.be/7GIgNp65-aE
17. Liu RT, Alloy LB. Stress generation in depression: a systematic review of the empirical literature and recommendations for future study. Clin Psychol Rev. 2010;30(5):582–93.
18. Lazarus RS, Folkman S. Stress, appraisal, and coping. New York: Springer Publishing Company; 1984.

https://doi.org/10.1142/9789819817320_0008

Chapter 8*

Effectiveness of Pu'er Tea in Reducing Cardiometabolic Risk Factors of Metabolic Syndrome and Promoting Weight Loss in Adults: A Systematic Review and Meta-Analysis of Clinical Trials

Xiu Fang Tai[1], Ho Xinn[2], and Jeanette Ignacio[3,*]

[1]*Khoo Teck Puat Hospital, Singapore, 90 Yishun Central, Singapore 768828*

[2]*National University Hospital, 5 Lower Kent Ridge Road, Main Building 1, CCU, Singapore 119074*

[3]*Alice Lee Centre for Nursing Studies, Yong Loo Lin School of Medicine, National University of Singapore, 10 Medical Drive, Singapore 117597*

**Corresponding author: nurimjj@nus.edu.sg*

8.1 Introduction

Tea, the second most consumed beverage after drinking water, is produced from the leaves and buds of tea plant *Camellia sinensis* [1]. Over two billion cups of tea are consumed daily, with approximately 78% being black tea [2, 3]. Tea consumption is not only part of many people's daily routine, but is also used as a therapeutic aid for illnesses [4]. Pu'er tea (PET), a fully fermented Chinese black tea from Yunnan province of China, possesses numerous health benefits. Research on cell lines,

* Appendices to this chapter are available for download at https://www.worldscientific.com/worldscibooks/10.1142/14420#t=suppl.

rodents and humans have shown that PET possesses weight loss [5], antihypercholesterolemic [6] and antihyperglycemic properties [7].

8.1.1 *Obesity and Metabolic Syndrome*

Rising prevalence of obesity is a global threat as excess weight gain leads to increased risk of chronic diseases; most notably cardiovascular disease and type 2 diabetes mellitus [8]. Obesity is most commonly classified by body mass index (BMI) [9]. The introduction of weight loss medications, paired with lifestyle adjustments, is a prospective area of research for pharmacological management of obesity [10]. Several drugs, such as phentermine and orlistat, have been approved by the U.S. Food and Drug Administration for the management of obesity. However, these drugs come with side effects [11]. Alternatively, natural products have been shown to promote weight reduction with little to no side effects [12–14].

Metabolic syndrome is a major public health problem globally that encompasses a set of metabolic disorders such as dyslipidemia and insulin resistance. Commonly associated with central fat accumulation, it comprises numerous cardiometabolic risk factors which lead to chronic diseases like diabetes mellitus and cardiovascular disease [15].

8.1.2 *Pu'er Tea*

Teas are classified into three types: (i) 'non-fermented' tea, (ii) 'semi-fermented' tea and (iii) 'fermented' tea. Depending on its processing methods, six Chinese teas can be produced [16–18]. The various types can be identified by the colour of the resulting brew: green, yellow, white, blue-green, red and dark, with dark tea being a fully fermented tea which PET is categorised under. Bioactive composition of PET includes tea polysaccharides and tea polyphenols [19].

Increasing evidence points to the theory that phytochemicals from tea may produce anti-obesity effects through fat, glucose and lipid absorption as well as thermogenesis [20, 21]. A review of tea and weight reduction suggests a budding role for tea in weight control [22]. Furthermore, tea is a popular choice in weight control planning as it is a non-caloric beverage, ranking second in value after water [23]. Kuo *et al.* [24] and Sano *et al.* [25] demonstrated lipid-lowering effects of PET in Wistar rats and Sprague-Dawley rats. A meta-analysis by Mahdavi-Roshan *et al.* [26] found that consistent tea consumption in people with elevated blood pressure (BP) causes reduced systolic and diastolic blood pressure (SBP; DBP). Yang *et al.* [27] found that PET has a significant impeding effect on alpha-amylase and alpha-glucosidase located on the luminal surface of enterocytes, consisting of maltase/glucoamylase and sucrase/isomaltose action. Additionally, alpha-glucosidase blocker favourably influenced some cardiovascular actions.

8.1.3 *Research Rationale*

As the second most consumed beverage worldwide [28], tea could have large implications for public health [29]. However, there is still inconclusive evidence from interventional and observational studies of PET consumption on clinical metabolic syndrome and obesity endpoints. Available reviews regarding tea's effect on metabolic syndrome and obesity were conducted on animal studies and mostly on green tea. Currently, no systematic review on the effect of PET on metabolic syndrome and obesity in humans is available. A systematic review is needed to clarify the association between PET consumption with metabolic syndrome and obesity to better inform relevant government bodies, agencies and the public on the health benefits of PET as a health-promoting beverage. This systematic review will add to the knowledge of complementary medicines to benefit the increasing prevalence of metabolic syndrome and obesity.

8.1.4 *Objectives*

This systematic review aims to synthesise the best available evidence to determine the effectiveness of PET consumption for the primary prevention of metabolic syndrome risk factors and weight reduction in adults, in comparison to non-consumers of PET. The review question is: What is the effectiveness of consuming PET on reducing the cardiometabolic risk factors (anthropometry, body fat percentage, glucose metabolism, blood lipids and BP) for metabolic syndrome and obesity, as compared to placebo, and their adverse effects in adults?

8.2 Methods

8.2.1 *Protocol Registration*

In conformity with the Cochrane Handbook for Systematic Reviews of Interventions [30], this systematic review was performed based on an *a priori* protocol.

8.2.2 *Eligibility Criteria*

Type of studies. All randomised trials that examined the effectiveness of PET on weight loss and cardiometabolic risk factors were included in this systematic review. No limit was set on publication status.

Type of participants. Studies examining the adult population, with or without pre-existing health conditions, were included. Studies conducted on overweight or obese individuals or those with metabolic syndrome were included.

Type of intervention. Studies wherein the participants were asked to take PET, black tea or theaflavin in any form were included. No restriction was set on the dosage, frequency, and duration of PET consumed.

Type of comparator. Trials with placebo as a control were included. Studies comparing varying dosages of PET were included. Trials with multifactorial interventions were excluded to prevent confounding.

8.2.3 *Type of Outcome Variables*

Primary outcomes. Outcomes considered included body weight, BMI, waist circumference, waist-hip ratio, body fat percentage, blood lipids (low-density lipoprotein [LDL], high-density lipoprotein [HDL], triglyceride, total cholesterol), SBP, DBP, and blood glucose.

Secondary outcomes. Adverse effects of consuming PET were included when identified.

8.2.4 *Type of Publications*

Trials published in commercial scientific databases and documents not published in commercial databases were considered. Only English publications with human subjects were included. No limits were set on the publication date.

8.2.5 *Context*

Studies that use black tea or its bioactive components without specifying the type of black tea used were included because PET is a type of black tea (fully fermented).

8.2.6 *Information Sources*

All studies on PET and their active components used in the treatment of obesity and metabolic syndrome were searched and reviewed. Databases searched include the Cochrane Library, PubMed, EMBASE, CINAHL, ProQuest, Scopus, Web of Science and Science Direct. To obtain ongoing clinical trials, metaRegister of controlled trials, Clinicaltrials.gov, and the WHO International Clinical Trials Registry platform were searched. Google Scholar was searched to identify relevant grey literature. To ensure literature saturation, hand-searching of reference lists of all eligible studies were done. All searching was done from December 2021 to January 2022.

8.2.7 *Search Strategy*

A detailed search strategy of all databases, registries and grey literatures was conducted.

8.2.8 *Selection Process*

All search records were uploaded to EndNote to serve as a reference manager. Search records were uploaded to Rayyan to facilitate collaboration among reviewers during the study selection process. Two reviewers pilot-tested screening titles and abstracts on three articles. The two reviewers then independently screened the titles and abstracts yielded by the search against the predetermined inclusion criteria. Full-text articles that met the inclusion criteria or were deemed potentially eligible upon initial screening were retrieved for further assessment. Reviewers pilot-tested screening questions and forms on three studies based on the inclusion and exclusion criteria. Two reviewers then independently screened the full-text reports and decided whether they were eligible. Any disagreements were resolved by consensus between the two reviewers and a third reviewer was consulted when disagreement persisted. Reasons for excluding trials were recorded together in the PRISMA flow diagram (Figure 8.1) that illustrates the selection process.

8.2.9 *Data Extraction*

Two reviewers extracted data independently from included trials according to a predefined data extraction sheet. To ensure consistency across reviewers, calibration exercises (pilot forms for 3–5 articles) were conducted before starting the extraction. Reviewers resolved disagreements by consensus and consulted a third reviewer if disagreement persisted. Additional information from study authors were sought where necessary to resolve questions about eligibility, but information was not obtained. WebPlotDigitizer [31] was used to approximate means and measures of dispersion from figures in the reports.

Individual studies consisting of multiple intervention groups, such as different genders, were combined into a single arm to avoid the possibility of introducing bias caused by multiple statistical comparisons with one control group.

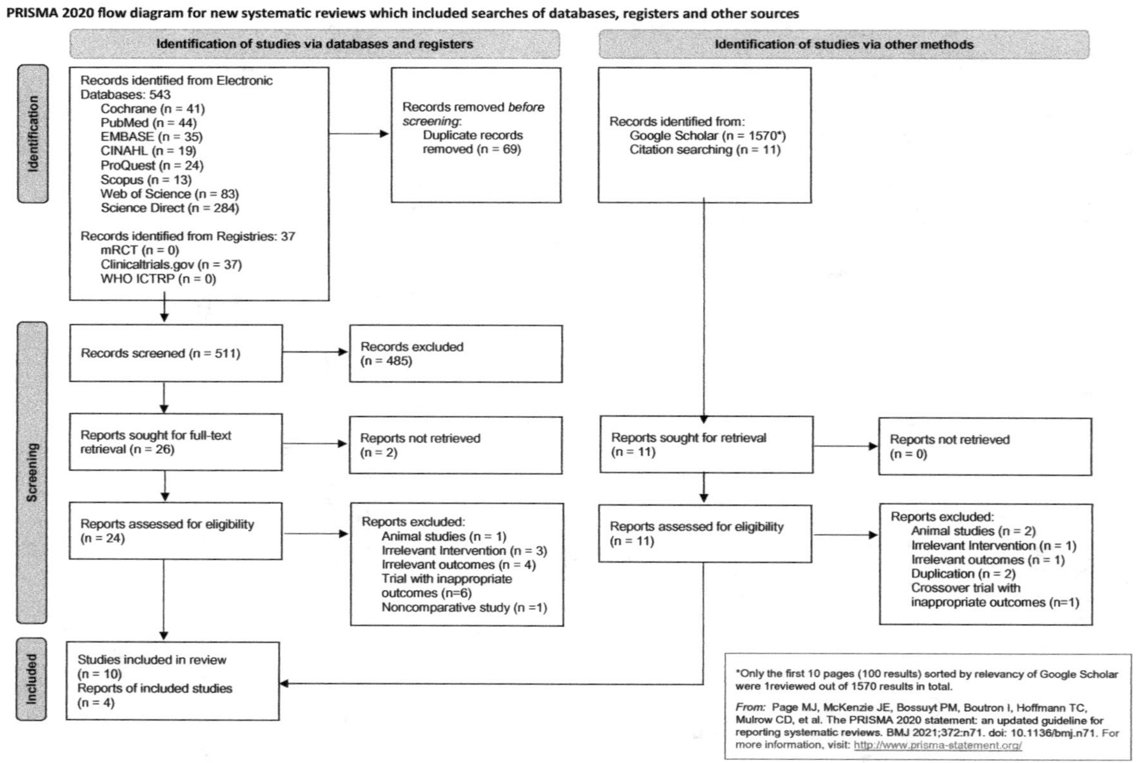

Figure 8.1 PRISMA flow diagram. Only the first 10 pages (100 results) sorted by relevancy in Google Scholar were reviewed, out of 1,570 results in total.

8.2.10 *Risk of Bias Assessment*

Risk of bias of included randomised trials were assessed independently by two reviewers with the Cochrane Risk of Bias Tool in Review Manager 5.4.1. Risk of bias of included studies were rated as low, high or unclear for each domain [30]. Possible biases were computed using RevMan graphically.

8.2.11 *Data Analysis and Synthesis*

Summary measures. To measure treatment effects of continuous outcomes, standardised mean difference (SMD) and their 95% confidence interval (CI) calculated were used for analysis. Non-quantitative data were presented descriptively.

Methods of combined results. For studies with study design and comparators that are sufficiently homogenous, meta-analysis using a random-effects model was conducted. RevMan was used to pool data for statistical meta-analysis. Outcomes for papers included in the meta-analysis were as follows: anthropometric, blood lipids and blood glucose.

Assessment of heterogeneity. Chi-squared and I^2 tests were used to determine heterogeneity.

Sensitivity analysis. Sensitivity analysis was used to determine the effects of risk of bias on important outcomes. It was conducted to verify the robustness of our primarily given assumptions of the review process. The principal decision nodes concluded the methodological quality, sample size, and the effect of missing data. The reviewer repeated the meta-analysis with the exclusion of low-quality studies. The results were compared and interpreted in the context of findings from previous studies.

Subgroup analysis. Subgroup analyses were conducted for outcomes with significant heterogeneity based on (1) type of tea used (PET vs black tea extract [BTE]), (2) ethnicity (Asian vs non-Asian), (3) length of study (≤3 months vs >3 months), and (4) health condition of participants (healthy vs those with metabolic syndrome/obesity). Outcomes with subgroup analyses reported were blood lipids and blood glucose.

Reporting bias assessment. There were inadequate numbers of studies to produce a funnel plot to distinguish symmetry [32].

Assessing certainty in findings. GRADEpro [33] was used to generate a Summary of Findings table for important meta-analysis findings. GRADE approach for quality assessment was performed. Anthropometric, blood lipids and blood glucose were considered important outcomes for representation in the Summary of Findings table.

8.3 Results

8.3.1 *Study Selection*

580 potential studies were identified from electronic databases and registers. After screening, nine randomised controlled trials (RCTs) and one randomised trial were included.

Additionally, 1,581 potentially relevant studies were identified via citation searching and grey literature. Out of the 1,570 results, only the first 10 pages sorted by relevance on Google Scholar were reviewed, as subsequent entries were deemed largely irrelevant. 11 studies were sought for retrieval. After screening, four RCTs were included.

8.3.2 *Study Characteristics*

All included studies were published in English, with publication years ranging from 2007 to 2017. Appendix A provides a summary of the main characteristics of the included studies.

8.3.3 *Study Settings*

Four studies recruited their participants from the general population, six from hospitals and two from production companies. It was unclear in which setting two studies recruited their participants from.

Seven of the included studies were conducted in Asian countries like Japan, China, Iran and Taiwan. The remaining seven studies were conducted in the United States, Australia, Switzerland and the Netherlands.

8.3.4 *Participants*

Thirteen RCTs and one randomised trial analysed a total of 810 participants. BMI range of participants were reported in three studies. Nine other studies reported mean BMI. Three studies compared results between male and female participants. Four studies recruited healthy participants, two studies recruited patients with metabolic syndrome, three studies recruited obese participants, three studies recruited participants with diabetes mellitus, and two studies recruited participants with borderline hypercholesterolemia. One study included participants with cardiovascular disease risks in their RCT.

8.3.5 *Interventions and Comparators*

Source of tea used for intervention varied across all studies. Harvested leaves of categorised fenhai broad-leaf tea cultivated in the Yunan highlands of China were used in three studies. Other sources of PET were used in two studies. Four studies sourced their black tea from Unilever. Other teas used were theaflavin extract from Yaizu Suisankagaku Industry Co Ltd, and black tea from Mauritius Corson Tea Estate Co Ltd, Templar Food Products and Nooshineh Chaay.

Placebo used by studies included dextrin, cellulose, caffeine, hot water and water. It is important to note that Neyestani *et al.* [34] used 150 mL (1 tea bag) of BTE per day as control. Mahmoud *et al.* [35] did not have a control group as the study compared the effect between high intake and low intake of black tea.

Tea and its extract, and placebo were given to participants in the form of tea bags, powder, capsules and tablets.

8.3.6 *Follow-Up and Measurement Intervals*

Follow-up periods differed: 4 weeks, 10 weeks, 11 weeks, 3 months, 5 months and 6 months.

8.3.7 *Outcomes*

Anthropometric. Seven studies reported body weight as an outcome. Aizawa *et al.* [36] and Oi and Fujita [37] reported body weight in graphical presentations while the others reported mean body weight with SD/SE. Pre- and post-intervention BMI was reported in seven studies, of which five studies reported means and its ranges, two reported graphically and one descriptively. Waist circumference was reported in four studies, of which three studies reported means and its ranges and one reported descriptively. Waist-hip ratio was reported by Bøhn *et al.* [38] and Chu *et al.* [39] in means and its ranges. Body fat percentage was reported by Aizawa *et al.* [36] and Jensen *et al.* [40] graphically.

Appetite. Bahorun *et al.* [41] and Jensen *et al.* [40] reported black tea's effect on appetite descriptively.

Blood lipids. Blood lipids including LDL, HDL and triglycerides were reported in 11 studies in means and its ranges, and graphically. Total cholesterol was similarly reported in abovementioned studies except one.

Blood pressure. SBP and DBP were reported in four studies.

Blood glucose. Blood glucose was reported by 10 studies, of which nine reported means and its ranges and one reported graphically. Chu *et al.* [39] reported fasting and two-hour postprandial blood glucose monitoring, which were combined into one arm during analysis.

Adverse effects. Presence or absence of adverse effects were disclosed in six studies.

8.3.8 *Risk of Bias in Studies*

Two studies [34, 35] had three or more high risk of bias. They were considered of poor methodological quality and were excluded in sensitivity analysis.

Mahmoud *et al.* [35] and Neyestani *et al.* [34] did not have control groups in their study and there was no blinding during the trial, resulting in a lower quality study design. Moreover, Neyestani *et al.* [34] did not have a negative control group as the control group was given one tea bag of black tea to consume daily throughout the intervention period. Despite the authors explaining that drinking 150 mL of tea had no significant short-term effect, exposing participants in the control group to the bioactive component of black tea may affect outcomes of the study when the intervention group is compared to the control group.

8.3.9 *Effect of Pu'er Tea Extract on Anthropometric Data*

8.3.9.1 *Body Weight and Body Mass Index*

PET showed statistically significant efficacy in reducing body weight compared to placebo in six studies with daily consumption of 0.1 g theaflavin for ten weeks [36], 1 g BTE for three months [6, 37, 42], 3 g of PET for five months [40] and three cups of powdered BTE [38] for three months. However, Bøhn *et al.* [38] noted that the effect was insignificant at six months.

Four studies found statistically significant efficacy in BMI reduction when PET is compared to placebo with daily consumption of 1 g of PET water extract (19% extraction rate) for three months [39], 1 g of BTE for three months [37, 42], and 3 g of PET for five months [40]. Lastly, Yang *et al.* [27] found significant reduction in body weight and BMI within the intervention group (BTE 1 g/day) when comparing baseline and three months.

Five studies investigating the effect of PET compared with placebo on body weight were included in a meta-analysis (Figure 8.2). A statistically non-significant difference (SMD = −0.14, 95% CI: −0.58, 0.30, p-value = 0.53) was found in the reduction of body weight in the tea group compared to placebo. PET did not demonstrate significant efficacy in reducing body weight and there is substantial heterogeneity ($I^2 = 68\%$). Subgroup analysis was unable to explain heterogeneity as there were no statistical differences between subgroups (p-value > 0.1). Sensitivity analysis was conducted, where a study [34] with more than three 'high risk of bias' were excluded (Figure 8.3). Results showed low heterogeneity ($I^2 = 0\%$) and insignificant difference (p-value 0.55) in body weight reduction in the tea group compared to placebo (SMD = 0.08, 95% CI: −0.13, 0.82).

Meta-analysis conducted on five studies on BMI demonstrated a significant effect (p-value = 0.02) favouring the tea group (SMD = −0.51, 95% CI: −0.95, 0.07) (Figure 8.4). There was substantial heterogeneity ($I^2 = 73\%$). Subgroup analysis was unable to explain heterogeneity. There was no heterogeneity in the sensitivity analysis ($I^2 = 0\%$), and effect was significant but reduced (SMD = −0.29, 95% CI: 0.53, −0.05, p-value = 0.02) (Figure 8.5).

8.3.9.2 *Waist and Hip Circumference*

Both Bøhn *et al.* [38] and Kubota *et al.* [42] found statistically significant reduction in waist circumference compared to placebo with daily consumption of three cups of BTE and 1 g BTE, respectively for three months. Bøhn *et al.* [38] noted that the effect was insignificant at six months. Furthermore, two studies found statistical significance in waist-hip ratio reduction when 1 g of PET [39] or three cups of BTE [38] were consumed daily for three months compared to placebo. Bøhn *et al.* [38] noted that the effect was insignificant at six months.

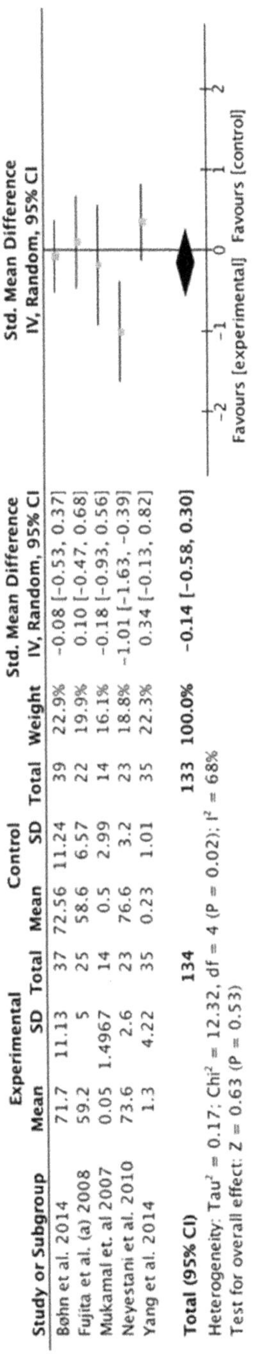

Figure 8.2 Meta-analysis of body weight.

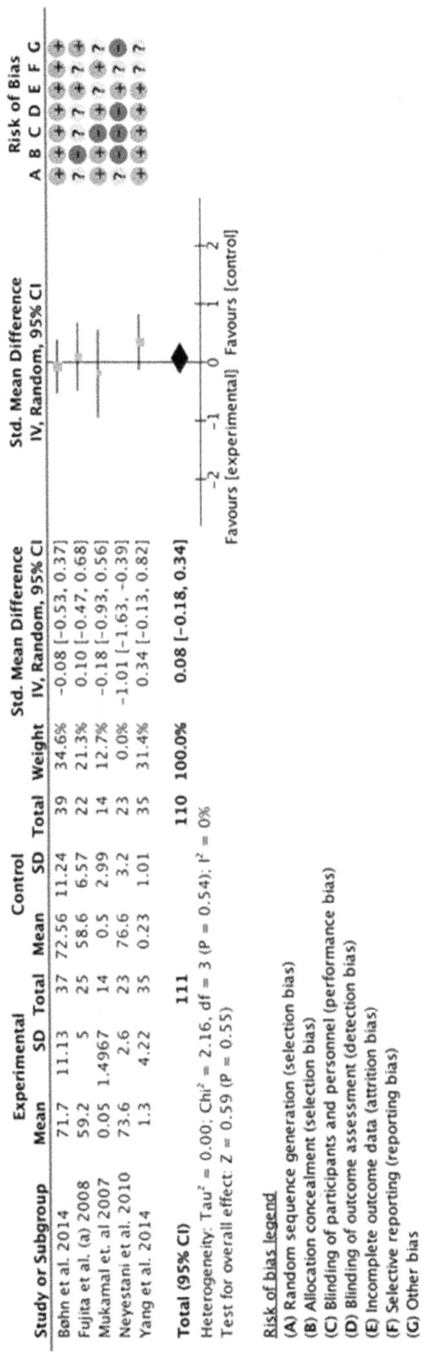

Figure 8.3 Sensitivity analysis for body weight.

Study or Subgroup	Experimental Mean	Experimental SD	Experimental Total	Control Mean	Control SD	Control Total	Weight	Std. Mean Difference IV, Random, 95% CI
Bøhn et al. 2014	24.94	3.22	37	25.02	3.25	39	21.5%	-0.02 [-0.47, 0.43]
Chu et al., 2011	26.86	3.17	59	28.49	3.74	30	21.6%	-0.48 [-0.92, -0.03]
Fujita et al. (a) 2008	22.7	1.5	25	23.4	2.81	22	18.8%	-0.31 [-0.89, 0.27]
Neyestani et al. 2010	29.2	1	23	30.9	1.1	23	16.9%	-1.59 [-2.26, -0.92]
Yang et al. 2014	-0.47	1.51	35	-0.09	0.39	35	21.1%	-0.34 [-0.81, 0.13]
Total (95% CI)			**179**			**149**	**100.0%**	**-0.51 [-0.95, -0.07]**

Heterogeneity: $Tau^2 = 0.18$; $Chi^2 = 14.96$, $df = 4$ ($P = 0.005$); $I^2 = 73\%$
Test for overall effect: $Z = 2.25$ ($P = 0.02$)

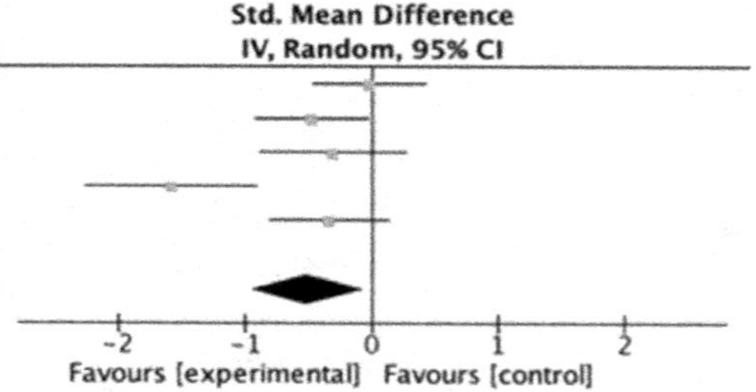

Figure 8.4 Meta-analysis of BMI.

Study or Subgroup	Experimental Mean	Experimental SD	Experimental Total	Control Mean	Control SD	Control Total	Weight	Std. Mean Difference IV, Random, 95% CI	A	B	C	D	E	F	G
Bøhn et al. 2014	24.94	3.22	37	25.02	3.25	39	28.3%	-0.02 [-0.47, 0.43]	+	+	+	+	+	+	+
Chu et al., 2011	26.86	3.17	59	28.49	3.74	30	28.8%	-0.48 [-0.92, -0.03]	+	?	?	?	?	?	+
Fujita et al. (a) 2008	22.7	1.5	25	23.4	2.81	22	17.2%	-0.31 [-0.89, 0.27]	?	-	?	?	+	?	+
Neyestani et al. 2010	29.2	1	23	30.9	1.1	23	0.0%	-1.59 [-2.26, -0.92]	?	-	-	-	+	?	-
Yang et al. 2014	-0.47	1.51	35	-0.09	0.39	35	25.7%	-0.34 [-0.81, 0.13]	+	+	+	+	+	?	?
Total (95% CI)			**156**			**126**	**100.0%**	**-0.29 [-0.53, -0.05]**							

Heterogeneity: $Tau^2 = 0.00$; $Chi^2 = 2.08$, $df = 3$ ($P = 0.56$); $I^2 = 0\%$
Test for overall effect: $Z = 2.35$ ($P = 0.02$)

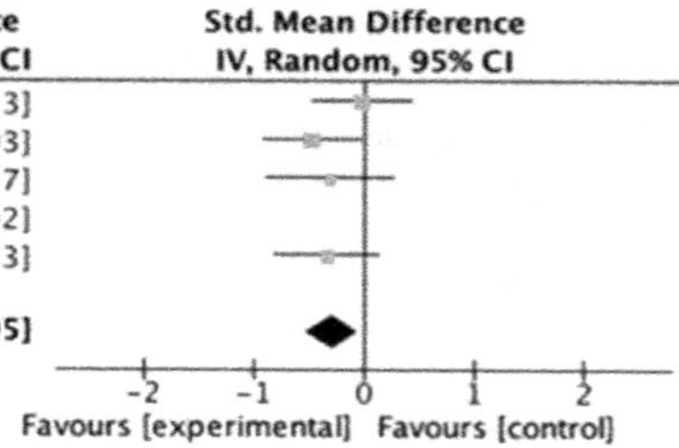

Risk of bias legend
(A) Random sequence generation (selection bias)
(B) Allocation concealment (selection bias)
(C) Blinding of participants and personnel (performance bias)
(D) Blinding of outcome assessment (detection bias)
(E) Incomplete outcome data (attrition bias)
(F) Selective reporting (reporting bias)
(G) Other bias

Figure 8.5 Sensitivity analysis for BMI.

Meta-analysis of three studies found that the overall effect of PET is not significant (p-value = 0.33) in reducing waist circumference (SMD = −0.45, 95% CI: −1.43, 0.45) (Figure 8.6). As heterogeneity was significant (I^2 = 86%), subgroup analysis and sensitivity analysis were conducted. Subgroup analysis was unable to explain heterogeneity while sensitivity analysis had an overall effect size of SMD = 0.03 (95% CI: −0.35, 0.40) with no heterogeneity (I^2 = 0%). The overall effect of PET reducing waist circumference compared to placebo was non-significant in the sensitivity analysis (p-value = 0.89) (Figure 8.7).

A meta-analysis of two studies on the effect of PET on waist-hip ratio found that the overall effect (SMD = −0.18, 95% CI: −0.50, 0.13) was not significant (p-value = 0.26) (Figure 8.8).

8.3.9.3 *Body Fat*

Body fat percentage was examined by Aizawa *et al.* which found statistical significance in the body fat percentage reduction with 0.05 g and 0.1 g BTE containing theaflavin at eight weeks onwards. Jensen *et al.* [40] found that within the intervention group treated with 3 g PET, weight reduction due to the decrease in total body fat percentage at 20 weeks compared to baseline was statistically significant.

8.3.10 *Effect of Pu'er Tea on Blood Lipids*

8.3.10.1 *Low-Density Lipoprotein*

Two studies found that PET reduced LDL significantly compared to placebo. Doses were at 1 g/day of PET [39] and 1 g/day of BTE [6] for three months. Next, although there was no statistical significance in LDL reduction when compared with placebo, Trautwein *et al.* [45] found significant reduction in LDL with 0.0775 g/day of theaflavin when comparing within the group at baseline and at 11 weeks. Similarly, Yang *et al.* [27] also found significant reduction in LDL after three months compared to baseline within the intervention group treated with 1 g BTE daily.

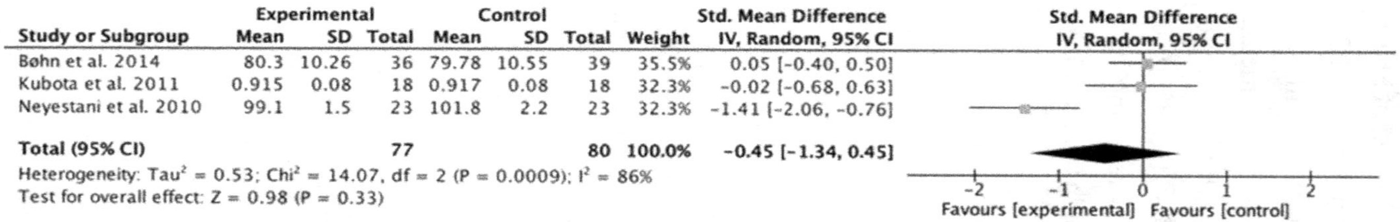

Figure 8.6 Meta-analysis of waist circumference.

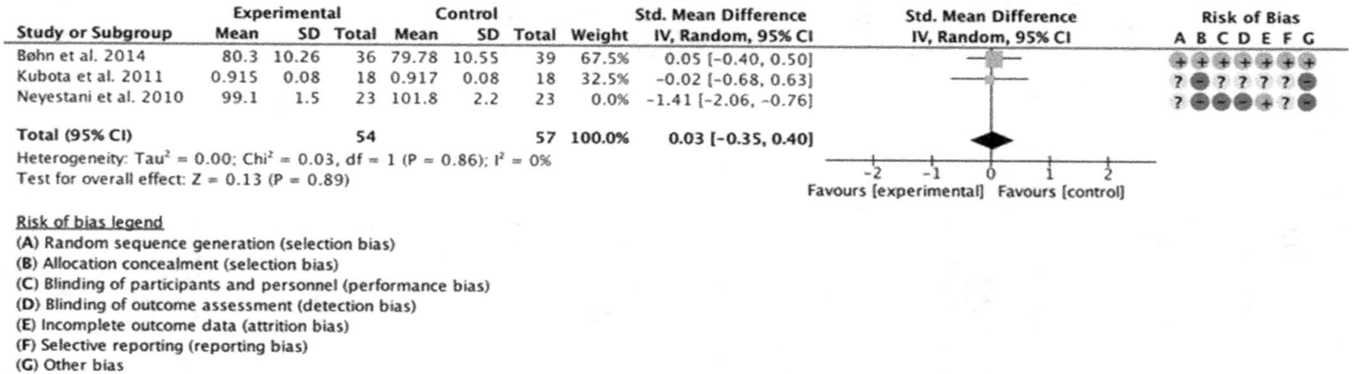

Figure 8.7 Sensitivity analysis for waist circumference.

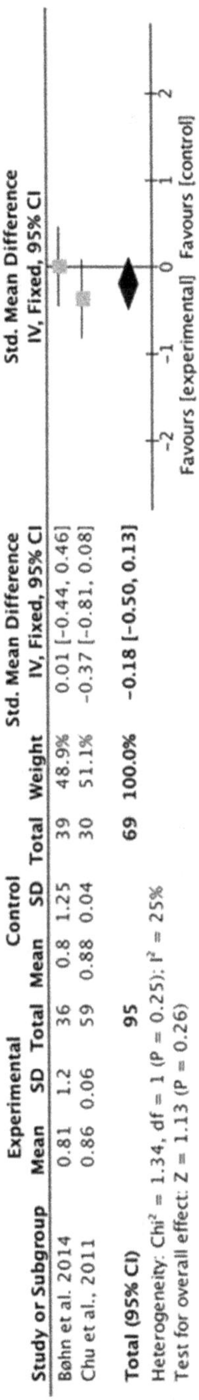

Figure 8.8 Meta-analysis of waist-hip ratio.

Meta-analysis conducted on nine studies indicated a small effect (SMD = −0.26, 95% CI: −0.68, 0.16) in favour of PET; however, it was not significant (p-value = 0.22) (Figure 8.9).

Heterogeneity was high ($I^2 = 82\%$), hence a subgroup analysis was conducted. However, the reason for heterogeneity could not be found as subgroup differences were not significant (p-value > 0.1). A sensitivity test was then conducted and the effect (SMD = −0.36, 95% CI: −0.79, 0.08) was not significant (p-value = 0.11) (Figure 8.10).

8.3.10.2 *High-Density Lipoprotein*

Statistically significant reductions in HDL were seen in two studies where 3 g BTE in 200 mL hot water three times a day [41] and 1 g of PET capsule [39] were given to the intervention group when compared to placebo. Yang *et al.* [27] found statistical significance when comparing the reduction of HDL within the intervention group treated with 1 g BTE daily at baseline and at three months.

Meta-analysis of nine studies showed that the overall effect of HDL increase in the tea group (SMD = 0.17, 95% CI: −0.18, 0.53) was not significant (p-value = 0.34). As the studies were heterogeneous ($I^2 = 74\%$), a subgroup analysis was conducted (Figure 8.11). However, no significant subgroups were found. A sensitivity analysis was conducted and the effect of increasing HDL (SMD = 0.01, 95% CI: −0.18, 0.20) was not significant (p-value = 0.93) (Figure 8.12).

8.3.10.3 *Triglycerides*

Four studies found significant reduction in triglycerides when compared to placebo. Intervention group was given 3 g BTE in 200 mL hot water three times a day [41] and 1 g PET daily [6, 39] for three months, and 3 g PET daily for five months [40].

Meta-analysis on nine studies found some effect of triglyceride reduction (SMD = −0.27, 95% CI: −0.74, 0.20) in the tea group when compared to the placebo group, but effect was not significant (p-value =

Study or Subgroup	Experimental Mean	Experimental SD	Experimental Total	Control Mean	Control SD	Control Total	Weight	Std. Mean Difference IV, Random, 95% CI
Bahorun et al. 2012	107.4094	33.3715	53	115.0842	26.1989	19	11.4%	-0.24 [-0.77, 0.29]
Bøhn et al. 2014	3.18	0.73	37	3.29	0.75	39	11.9%	-0.15 [-0.60, 0.30]
Chu et al., 2011	2.65	0.65	59	3.69	0.75	30	11.6%	-1.51 [-2.00, -1.01]
Fujita et al. (a) 2008	3.81	0.65	25	4.36	0.75	22	10.8%	-0.77 [-1.37, -0.18]
Kubota et al. 2011	3.56	0.59	18	3.38	0.76	18	10.3%	0.26 [-0.40, 0.92]
Mukamal et. al 2007	-13	37.4166	14	2	18.7083	14	9.6%	-0.49 [-1.25, 0.26]
Neyestani et al. 2010	3.2	0.2	23	3.1	0.2	23	10.9%	0.49 [-0.10, 1.08]
Trautwein et al. 2010	3.72	0.73	36	3.92	0.46	35	11.8%	-0.32 [-0.79, 0.15]
Yang et al. 2014	-0.2	19.61	35	-8.06	21.2	35	11.8%	0.38 [-0.09, 0.85]
Total (95% CI)			**300**			**235**	**100.0%**	**-0.26 [-0.68, 0.16]**

Heterogeneity: $Tau^2 = 0.34$; $Chi^2 = 43.64$, df = 8 ($P < 0.00001$); $I^2 = 82\%$

Test for overall effect: Z = 1.22 (P = 0.22)

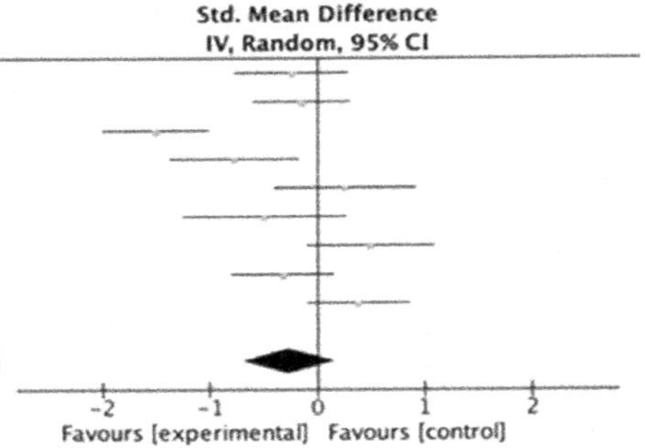

Figure 8.9 Meta-analysis of LDL.

Study or Subgroup	Experimental Mean	Experimental SD	Experimental Total	Control Mean	Control SD	Control Total	Weight	Std. Mean Difference IV, Random, 95% CI
Bahorun et al. 2012	107.4094	33.3715	53	115.0842	26.1989	19	12.8%	-0.24 [-0.77, 0.29]
Bøhn et al. 2014	3.18	0.73	37	3.29	0.75	39	13.4%	-0.15 [-0.60, 0.30]
Chu et al., 2011	2.65	0.65	59	3.69	0.75	30	13.0%	-1.51 [-2.00, -1.01]
Fujita et al. (a) 2008	3.81	0.65	25	4.36	0.75	22	12.1%	-0.77 [-1.37, -0.18]
Kubota et al. 2011	3.56	0.59	18	3.38	0.76	18	11.5%	0.26 [-0.40, 0.92]
Mukamal et. al 2007	-13	37.4166	14	2	18.7083	14	10.6%	-0.49 [-1.25, 0.26]
Neyestani et al. 2010	3.2	0.2	23	3.1	0.2	23	0.0%	0.49 [-0.10, 1.08]
Trautwein et al. 2010	3.72	0.73	36	3.92	0.46	35	13.3%	-0.32 [-0.79, 0.15]
Yang et al. 2014	-0.2	19.61	35	-8.06	21.2	35	13.2%	0.38 [-0.09, 0.85]
Total (95% CI)			**277**			**212**	**100.0%**	**-0.36 [-0.79, 0.08]**

Heterogeneity: $Tau^2 = 0.31$; $Chi^2 = 36.50$, df = 7 ($P < 0.00001$); $I^2 = 81\%$

Test for overall effect: Z = 1.61 (P = 0.11)

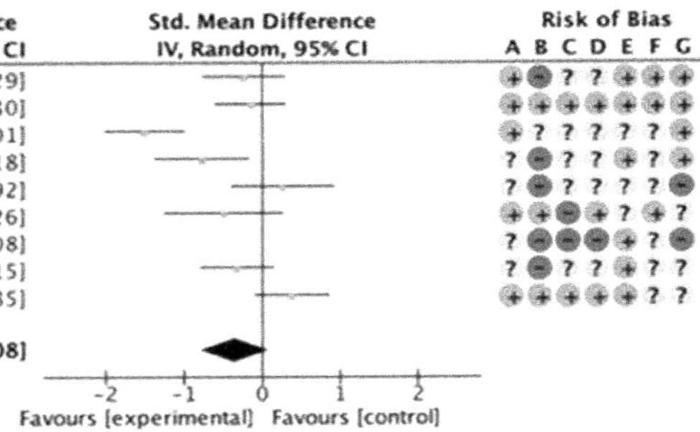

Risk of bias legend
(A) Random sequence generation (selection bias)
(B) Allocation concealment (selection bias)
(C) Blinding of participants and personnel (performance bias)
(D) Blinding of outcome assessment (detection bias)
(E) Incomplete outcome data (attrition bias)
(F) Selective reporting (reporting bias)
(G) Other bias

Figure 8.10 Sensitivity analysis for LDL.

Study or Subgroup	Experimental Mean	Experimental SD	Experimental Total	Control Mean	Control SD	Control Total	Weight	Std. Mean Difference IV, Random, 95% CI
Bahorun et al. 2012	51.7549	9.3832	51	54.32	8.6696	20	11.5%	-0.28 [-0.80, 0.24]
Bøhn et al. 2014	1.46	0.3	37	1.47	0.31	39	12.3%	-0.03 [-0.48, 0.42]
Chu et al., 2011	1.24	0.48	59	1.01	0.3	30	12.3%	0.53 [0.09, 0.98]
Fujita et al. (a) 2008	1.59	0.35	25	1.59	0.33	22	10.9%	0.00 [-0.57, 0.57]
Kubota et al. 2011	1.51	0.3	18	1.48	0.3	18	10.1%	0.10 [-0.56, 0.75]
Mukamal et. al 2007	-0.5	7.4833	14	0.1	12.7216	14	9.2%	-0.06 [-0.80, 0.69]
Neyestani et al. 2010	1	0.05	23	0.9	0.06	23	9.7%	1.78 [1.09, 2.47]
Trautwein et al. 2010	1.36	0.42	36	1.38	0.36	35	12.1%	-0.05 [-0.52, 0.41]
Yang et al. 2014	-2.46	5.29	35	-0.91	7.47	35	12.0%	-0.24 [-0.71, 0.23]
Total (95% CI)			**298**			**236**	**100.0%**	**0.17 [-0.18, 0.53]**

Heterogeneity: $Tau^2 = 0.21$; $Chi^2 = 31.16$, df = 8 (P = 0.0001); $I^2 = 74\%$
Test for overall effect: Z = 0.95 (P = 0.34)

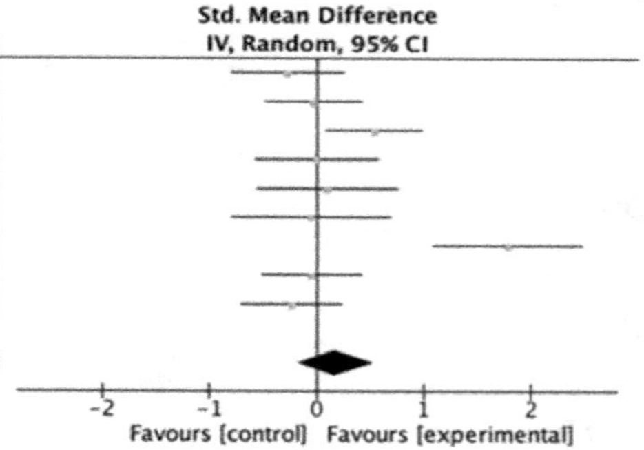

Figure 8.11 Meta-analysis of HDL.

Study or Subgroup	Experimental Mean	Experimental SD	Experimental Total	Control Mean	Control SD	Control Total	Weight	Std. Mean Difference IV, Random, 95% CI	Risk of Bias A B C D E F G
Bahorun et al. 2012	51.7549	9.3832	51	54.32	8.6696	20	12.5%	-0.28 [-0.80, 0.24]	+ - ? ? + + +
Bøhn et al. 2014	1.46	0.3	37	1.47	0.31	39	16.1%	-0.03 [-0.48, 0.42]	+ + + + + + +
Chu et al., 2011	1.24	0.48	59	1.01	0.3	30	16.3%	0.53 [0.09, 0.98]	+ ? ? ? ? ? +
Fujita et al. (a) 2008	1.59	0.35	25	1.59	0.33	22	10.4%	0.00 [-0.57, 0.57]	? - ? ? + ? +
Kubota et al. 2011	1.51	0.3	18	1.48	0.3	18	8.1%	0.10 [-0.56, 0.75]	? - ? ? ? ? -
Mukamal et. al 2007	-0.5	7.4833	14	0.1	12.7216	14	6.4%	-0.06 [-0.80, 0.69]	+ + - + ? + ?
Neyestani et al. 2010	1	0.05	23	0.9	0.06	23	0.0%	1.78 [1.09, 2.47]	? - - - + ? -
Trautwein et al. 2010	1.36	0.42	36	1.38	0.36	35	15.2%	-0.05 [-0.52, 0.41]	? - ? ? + ? ?
Yang et al. 2014	-2.46	5.29	35	-0.91	7.47	35	14.9%	-0.24 [-0.71, 0.23]	+ + + + + ? ?
Total (95% CI)			**275**			**213**	**100.0%**	**0.01 [-0.18, 0.20]**	

Heterogeneity: $Tau^2 = 0.01$; $Chi^2 = 7.67$, df = 7 (P = 0.36); $I^2 = 9\%$
Test for overall effect: Z = 0.09 (P = 0.93)

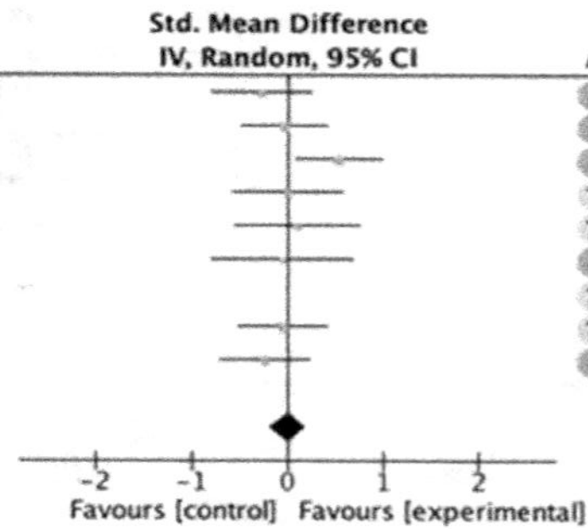

Risk of bias legend
(A) Random sequence generation (selection bias)
(B) Allocation concealment (selection bias)
(C) Blinding of participants and personnel (performance bias)
(D) Blinding of outcome assessment (detection bias)
(E) Incomplete outcome data (attrition bias)
(F) Selective reporting (reporting bias)
(G) Other bias

Figure 8.12 Sensitivity analysis for HDL.

0.26) (Figure 8.13). There was considerable heterogeneity ($I^2 = 85\%$) and subgroup differences of Asians and non-Asians were significant (p-value = 0.04). From the subgroup analysis, the effect of triglyceride reduction (SMD = −0.66, 95% CI: −1.43, 0.11) in Asians under the PET group was significant (p-value = 0.09) (Figure 8.14). Additionally, a sensitivity analysis found that by removing one study with high risk of bias, the effect of triglyceride reduction (SMD = −0.04, 95% CI: −0.35, 0.27) was also not significant (p-value = 0.80) (Figure 8.15).

8.3.10.4 *Total Cholesterol*

Chu *et al.* [39] and Fujita and Yamagami [6] found significant decrease in total cholesterol with 1 g PET and 1 g BTE, respectively, consumed daily for three months when compared to placebo. Furthermore, two studies found significant reduction in total cholesterol within the intervention group treated with 3 g BTE in 200 mL hot water three times a day [41] and 3 g PET daily [40] when comparing baseline and post-intervention total cholesterol.

Meta-analysis of eight studies found that the overall effect of total cholesterol reduction in the PET group (SMD = −0.27, 95% CI: −0.62, 0.08) compared to placebo group was not significant (p-value = 0.14) (Figure 8.16). Heterogeneity was high ($I^2 = 73\%$), but subgroup analysis did not find a significant subgroup effect. Then, a sensitivity analysis that excluded one high risk of bias study found that the overall effect of total cholesterol reduction in the remaining eight studies (SMD = −0.31, 95% CI: −0.70, 0.08) was non-significant (p-value = 0.11) (Figure 8.17).

8.3.11 *Effect of Pu'er Tea on Blood Pressure*

One study found a significant decrease in both SBP and DBP when comparing the intervention group treated with 4.317 g black tea solids daily for six months [43]. Meta-analysis was done on four studies to investigate

Study or Subgroup	Experimental Mean	Experimental SD	Experimental Total	Control Mean	Control SD	Control Total	Weight	Std. Mean Difference IV, Random, 95% CI
Bahorun et al. 2012	90.8833	63.3769	54	69.06	35.6235	20	11.5%	0.38 [-0.14, 0.89]
Bøhn et al. 2014	1.11	0.55	37	1.12	0.56	39	11.9%	-0.02 [-0.47, 0.43]
Chu et al., 2011	2.25	0.88	59	3.67	2.33	30	11.8%	-0.92 [-1.38, -0.46]
Fujita et al. (a) 2008	1.31	1.65	25	1.51	0.42	22	11.1%	-0.16 [-0.73, 0.42]
Kubota et al. 2011	1.32	0.55	18	1.29	0.38	18	10.6%	0.06 [-0.59, 0.72]
Mukamal et. al 2007	-32	19	14	-35	28	14	10.0%	0.12 [-0.62, 0.86]
Neyestani et al. 2010	2.2	0.2	23	3.5	0.7	23	9.7%	-2.48 [-3.27, -1.70]
Trautwein et al. 2010	2.09	1.55	36	1.73	0.85	35	11.8%	0.28 [-0.18, 0.75]
Yang et al. 2014	-0.46	57.81	35	-1.94	52.58	35	11.7%	0.03 [-0.44, 0.50]
Total (95% CI)			**301**			**236**	**100.0%**	**-0.27 [-0.74, 0.20]**

Heterogeneity: $Tau^2 = 0.43$; $Chi^2 = 53.71$, $df = 8$ ($P < 0.00001$); $I^2 = 85\%$
Test for overall effect: $Z = 1.13$ ($P = 0.26$)

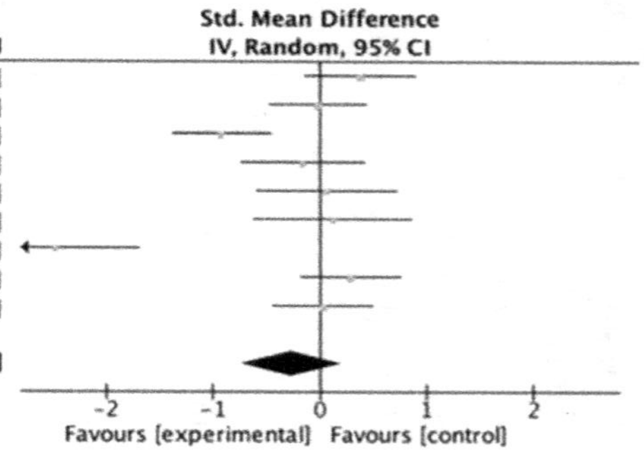

Figure 8.13 Meta-analysis of triglycerides.

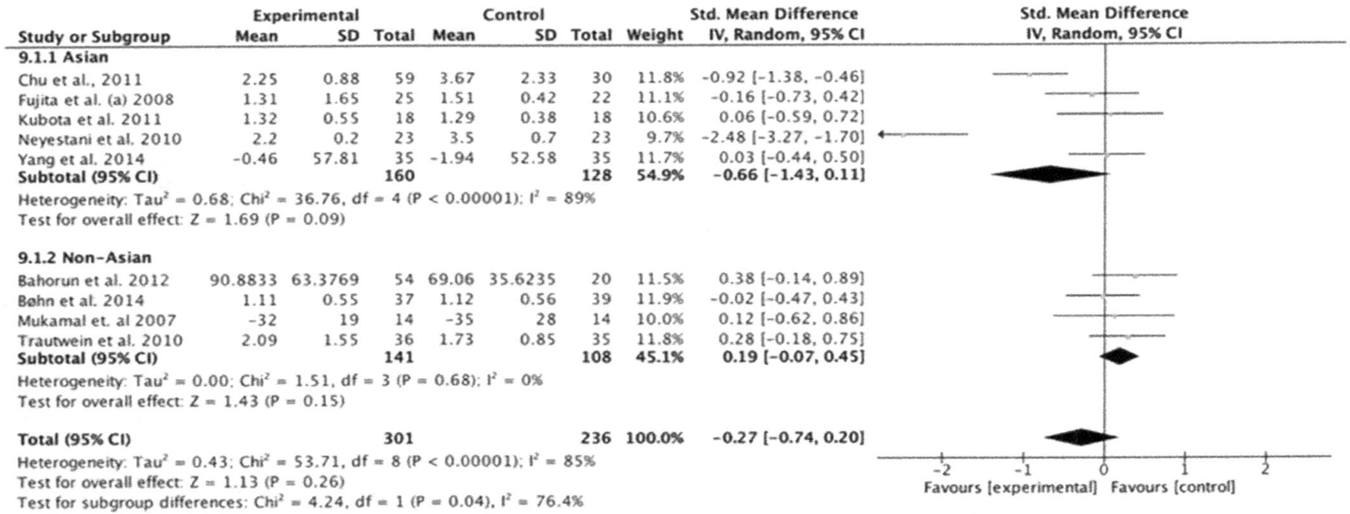

Figure 8.14 Subgroup analysis of triglycerides (Asian vs non-Asian).

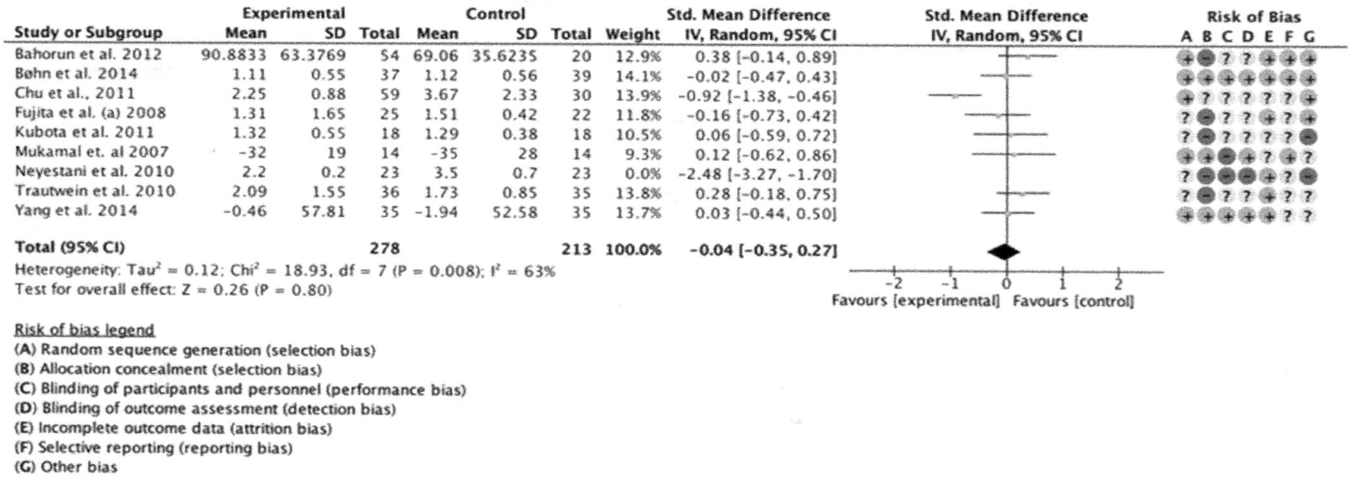

Figure 8.15 Sensitivity analysis for triglycerides.

Study or Subgroup	Experimental Mean	Experimental SD	Experimental Total	Control Mean	Control SD	Control Total	Weight	Std. Mean Difference IV, Random, 95% CI
Bahorun et al. 2012	172.6154	39.9536	52	172.68	32.2873	20	12.6%	-0.00 [-0.52, 0.51]
Bøhn et al. 2014	5.15	0.79	37	5.28	0.81	39	13.5%	-0.16 [-0.61, 0.29]
Chu et al., 2011	4.91	0.94	59	6.37	1.37	30	13.1%	-1.31 [-1.80, -0.83]
Fujita et al. (a) 2008	5.62	0.66	25	6.15	0.8	22	11.6%	-0.72 [-1.31, -0.12]
Kubota et al. 2011	5.51	0.64	18	5.47	0.72	18	10.9%	0.06 [-0.60, 0.71]
Neyestani et al. 2010	5.52	0.2	23	5.5	0.3	23	11.8%	0.08 [-0.50, 0.66]
Trautwein et al. 2010	5.55	0.86	36	5.59	0.56	35	13.3%	-0.05 [-0.52, 0.41]
Yang et al. 2014	-6.46	29.55	35	-6.64	30.91	35	13.2%	0.01 [-0.46, 0.47]
Total (95% CI)			**285**			**222**	**100.0%**	**-0.27 [-0.62, 0.08]**

Heterogeneity: $Tau^2 = 0.19$; $Chi^2 = 25.95$, df = 7 (P = 0.0005); $I^2 = 73\%$
Test for overall effect: Z = 1.49 (P = 0.14)

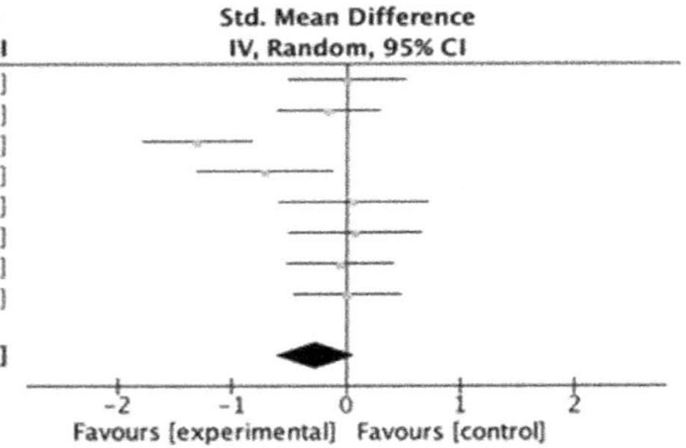

Figure 8.16 Meta-analysis of total cholesterol.

Study or Subgroup	Experimental Mean	Experimental SD	Experimental Total	Control Mean	Control SD	Control Total	Weight	Std. Mean Difference IV, Random, 95% CI	Risk of Bias A	B	C	D	E	F	G
Bahorun et al. 2012	172.6154	39.9536	52	172.68	32.2873	20	14.3%	-0.00 [-0.52, 0.51]	+	−	?	?	+	+	+
Bøhn et al. 2014	5.15	0.79	37	5.28	0.81	39	15.2%	-0.16 [-0.61, 0.29]	+	+	+	+	+	+	+
Chu et al., 2011	4.91	0.94	59	6.37	1.37	30	14.8%	-1.31 [-1.80, -0.83]	+	?	?	?	?	?	+
Fujita et al. (a) 2008	5.62	0.66	25	6.15	0.8	22	13.2%	-0.72 [-1.31, -0.12]	?	−	?	?	+	?	+
Kubota et al. 2011	5.51	0.64	18	5.47	0.72	18	12.4%	0.06 [-0.60, 0.71]	?	−	?	?	?	?	−
Neyestani et al. 2010	5.52	0.2	23	5.5	0.3	23	0.0%	0.08 [-0.50, 0.66]	?	−	−	−	+	?	−
Trautwein et al. 2010	5.55	0.86	36	5.59	0.56	35	15.0%	-0.05 [-0.52, 0.41]	?	−	?	?	+	?	?
Yang et al. 2014	-6.46	29.55	35	-6.64	30.91	35	15.0%	0.01 [-0.46, 0.47]	+	+	+	+	+	?	?
Total (95% CI)			**262**			**199**	**100.0%**	**-0.31 [-0.70, 0.08]**							

Heterogeneity: $Tau^2 = 0.21$; $Chi^2 = 24.37$, df = 6 (P = 0.0004); $I^2 = 75\%$
Test for overall effect: Z = 1.58 (P = 0.11)

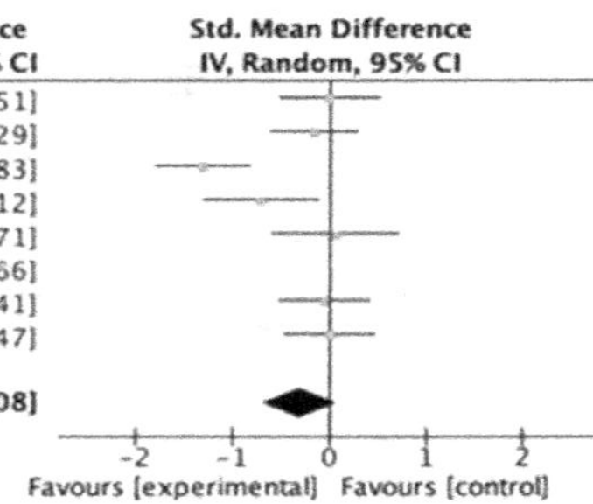

Risk of bias legend
(A) Random sequence generation (selection bias)
(B) Allocation concealment (selection bias)
(C) Blinding of participants and personnel (performance bias)
(D) Blinding of outcome assessment (detection bias)
(E) Incomplete outcome data (attrition bias)
(F) Selective reporting (reporting bias)
(G) Other bias

Figure 8.17 Sensitivity analysis for total cholesterol.

the overall effect of BP reduction in the PET group as compared to placebo (Figure 8.18). SBP decreased in the PET group (SMD = −0.25, 95% CI: −0.88, 0.37) but the difference was non-significant (p-value = 0.43). Similarly, DBP was reduced in the PET group (SMD = 0.53, 95% CI: −1.50, 0.44) when compared to the placebo group, but the effect was non-significant (p-value = 0.28) (Figure 8.19).

8.3.12 *Effect of Pu'er Tea on Blood Glucose*

Significant reduction in blood glucose was seen in two studies giving 1 g PET daily [39] and 3 tea bags daily [34] in the intervention group compared to placebo group. Additionally, Chu *et al.* [39] also reported significant reduction in blood glucose within the intervention group when comparing baseline and third month. Lastly, Mahmoud *et al.* [35] comparing high intake (3 cups/day) and low intake (1 cup/day) of BTE found a significant decrease in blood glucose in the high intake group.

Eight studies were included in a meta-analysis on the overall effect of blood glucose reduction. Results found no significant (p-value = 0.89) reduction in the PET group when compared to the placebo group (SMD = −0.03, 95% CI: −0.39, 0.34) (Figure 8.20). Heterogeneity was high (I^2 = 76%).

Subgroup analysis found significant subgroup differences for types of tea (p-value = 0.03), ethnicity (p-value = 0.06) and length of study (p-value = 0.06). However, heterogeneity within the subgroups suggests they may not represent well-defined or meaningful groupings (Figures 8.21–8.23).

A sensitivity analysis was conducted on all of the eight studies. The overall effect of blood glucose reduction of SMD = −0.04 (95% CI: −0.46, 0.37) in the tea group compared to the placebo group was non-significant (p-value = 0.84) (Figure 8.24).

8.3.13 *Effect of Pu'er Tea on Appetite*

A study found that the self-reported appetite of the PET group had a lower appetite after four weeks of intervention compared to placebo [40]. This

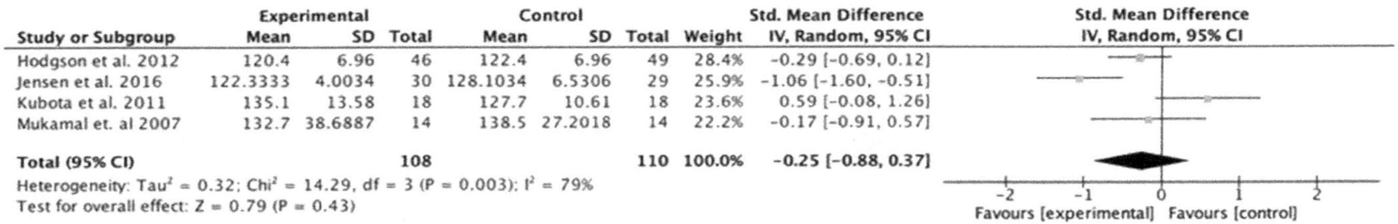

Figure 8.18 Meta-analysis for SBP.

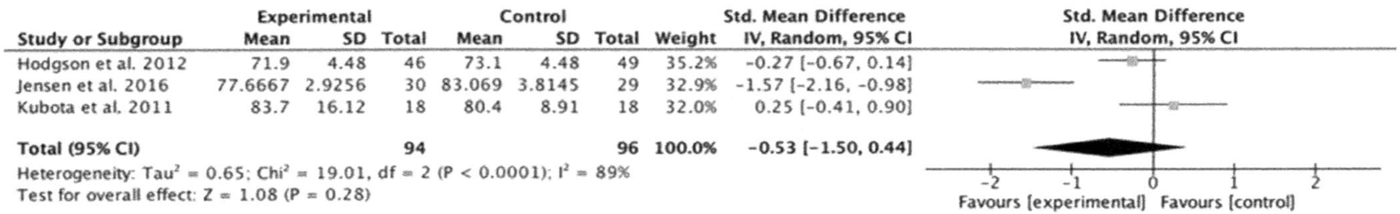

Figure 8.19 Meta-analysis for DBP.

Study or Subgroup	Experimental Mean	Experimental SD	Experimental Total	Control Mean	Control SD	Control Total	Weight	Std. Mean Difference IV, Random, 95% CI
Bahorun et al. 2012	102.5	42.3397	55	102.35	43.1595	22	13.1%	0.00 [-0.49, 0.50]
Bøhn et al. 2014	5.24	0.55	37	5.09	0.56	39	13.7%	0.27 [-0.18, 0.72]
Chu et al., 2011	7.835	2.2299	118	9.315	2.6492	60	15.2%	-0.62 [-0.94, -0.30]
Fujita et al. (a) 2008	5.58	0.4	25	6.03	0.7	22	11.9%	-0.79 [-1.39, -0.19]
Kubota et al. 2011	5.57	0.34	18	5.67	0.72	18	11.2%	-0.17 [-0.83, 0.48]
Mukamal et. al 2007	7	4	14	1	6	14	9.4%	1.14 [0.33, 1.95]
Neyestani et al. 2010	9.5	0.8	23	9.4	0.8	23	12.1%	0.12 [-0.46, 0.70]
Yang et al. 2014	0.06	0.53	35	-0.05	0.76	35	13.4%	0.17 [-0.30, 0.64]
Total (95% CI)			**325**			**233**	**100.0%**	**-0.03 [-0.39, 0.34]**

Heterogeneity: $Tau^2 = 0.21$; $Chi^2 = 28.87$, df = 7 (P = 0.0002); $I^2 = 76\%$
Test for overall effect: Z = 0.14 (P = 0.89)

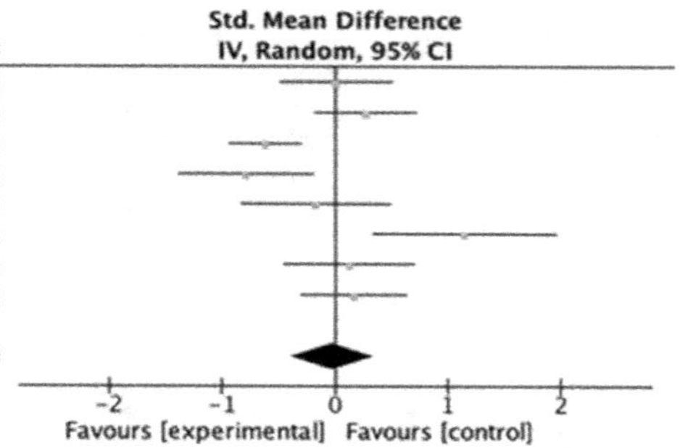

Figure 8.20 Meta-analysis of blood glucose.

Study or Subgroup	Experimental Mean	Experimental SD	Experimental Total	Control Mean	Control SD	Control Total	Weight	Std. Mean Difference IV, Random, 95% CI
13.1.1 Pu'er								
Chu et al., 2011	7.835	2.2299	118	9.315	2.6492	60	15.2%	-0.62 [-0.94, -0.30]
Fujita et al. (a) 2008	5.58	0.4	25	6.03	0.7	22	11.9%	-0.79 [-1.39, -0.19]
Kubota et al. 2011	5.57	0.34	18	5.67	0.72	18	11.2%	-0.17 [-0.83, 0.48]
Yang et al. 2014	0.06	0.53	35	-0.05	0.76	35	13.4%	0.17 [-0.30, 0.64]
Subtotal (95% CI)			**196**			**135**	**51.7%**	**-0.36 [-0.80, 0.08]**
Heterogeneity: Tau² = 0.13; Chi² = 9.51, df = 3 (P = 0.02); I² = 68%								
Test for overall effect: Z = 1.62 (P = 0.11)								
13.1.2 Non-Pu'er								
Bahorun et al. 2012	102.5	42.3397	55	102.35	43.1595	22	13.1%	0.00 [-0.49, 0.50]
Bøhn et al. 2014	5.24	0.55	37	5.09	0.56	39	13.7%	0.27 [-0.18, 0.72]
Mukamal et. al 2007	7	4	14	1	6	14	9.4%	1.14 [0.33, 1.95]
Neyestani et al. 2010	9.5	0.8	23	9.4	0.8	23	12.1%	0.12 [-0.46, 0.70]
Subtotal (95% CI)			**129**			**98**	**48.3%**	**0.30 [-0.09, 0.69]**
Heterogeneity: Tau² = 0.08; Chi² = 5.83, df = 3 (P = 0.12); I² = 49%								
Test for overall effect: Z = 1.49 (P = 0.13)								
Total (95% CI)			**325**			**233**	**100.0%**	**-0.03 [-0.39, 0.34]**
Heterogeneity: Tau² = 0.21; Chi² = 28.87, df = 7 (P = 0.0002); I² = 76%								
Test for overall effect: Z = 0.14 (P = 0.89)								
Test for subgroup differences: Chi² = 4.85, df = 1 (P = 0.03), I² = 79.4%								

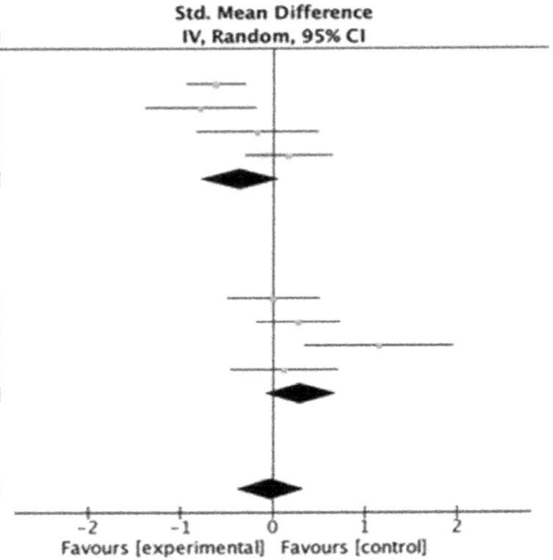

Figure 8.21 Subgroup analysis of blood glucose (PET vs BTE).

Study or Subgroup	Experimental Mean	Experimental SD	Experimental Total	Control Mean	Control SD	Control Total	Weight	Std. Mean Difference IV, Random, 95% CI
13.1.1 New Subgroup								
Bahorun et al. 2012	102.5	42.3397	55	102.35	43.1595	22	13.1%	0.00 [-0.49, 0.50]
Bøhn et al. 2014	5.24	0.55	37	5.09	0.56	39	13.7%	0.27 [-0.18, 0.72]
Mukamal et. al 2007	7	4	14	1	6	14	9.4%	1.14 [0.33, 1.95]
Subtotal (95% CI)			**106**			**75**	**36.2%**	**0.38 [-0.16, 0.93]**
Heterogeneity: $Tau^2 = 0.14$; $Chi^2 = 5.57$, df = 2 (P = 0.06); $I^2 = 64\%$								
Test for overall effect: Z = 1.38 (P = 0.17)								
13.1.2 grp 2								
Chu et al., 2011	7.835	2.2299	118	9.315	2.6492	60	15.2%	-0.62 [-0.94, -0.30]
Fujita et al. (a) 2008	5.58	0.4	25	6.03	0.7	22	11.9%	-0.79 [-1.39, -0.19]
Kubota et al. 2011	5.57	0.34	18	5.67	0.72	18	11.2%	-0.17 [-0.83, 0.48]
Neyestani et al. 2010	9.5	0.8	23	9.4	0.8	23	12.1%	0.12 [-0.46, 0.70]
Yang et al. 2014	0.06	0.53	35	-0.05	0.76	35	13.4%	0.17 [-0.30, 0.64]
Subtotal (95% CI)			**219**			**158**	**63.8%**	**-0.27 [-0.67, 0.12]**
Heterogeneity: $Tau^2 = 0.13$; $Chi^2 = 12.33$, df = 4 (P = 0.02); $I^2 = 68\%$								
Test for overall effect: Z = 1.35 (P = 0.18)								
Total (95% CI)			**325**			**233**	**100.0%**	**-0.03 [-0.39, 0.34]**
Heterogeneity: $Tau^2 = 0.21$; $Chi^2 = 28.87$, df = 7 (P = 0.0002); $I^2 = 76\%$								
Test for overall effect: Z = 0.14 (P = 0.89)								
Test for subgroup differences: $Chi^2 = 3.65$, df = 1 (P = 0.06), $I^2 = 72.6\%$								

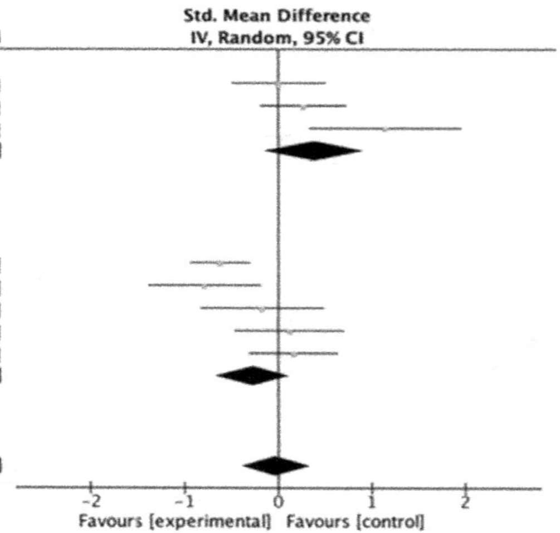

Figure 8.22 Subgroup analysis of blood glucose (Asian vs non-Asian).

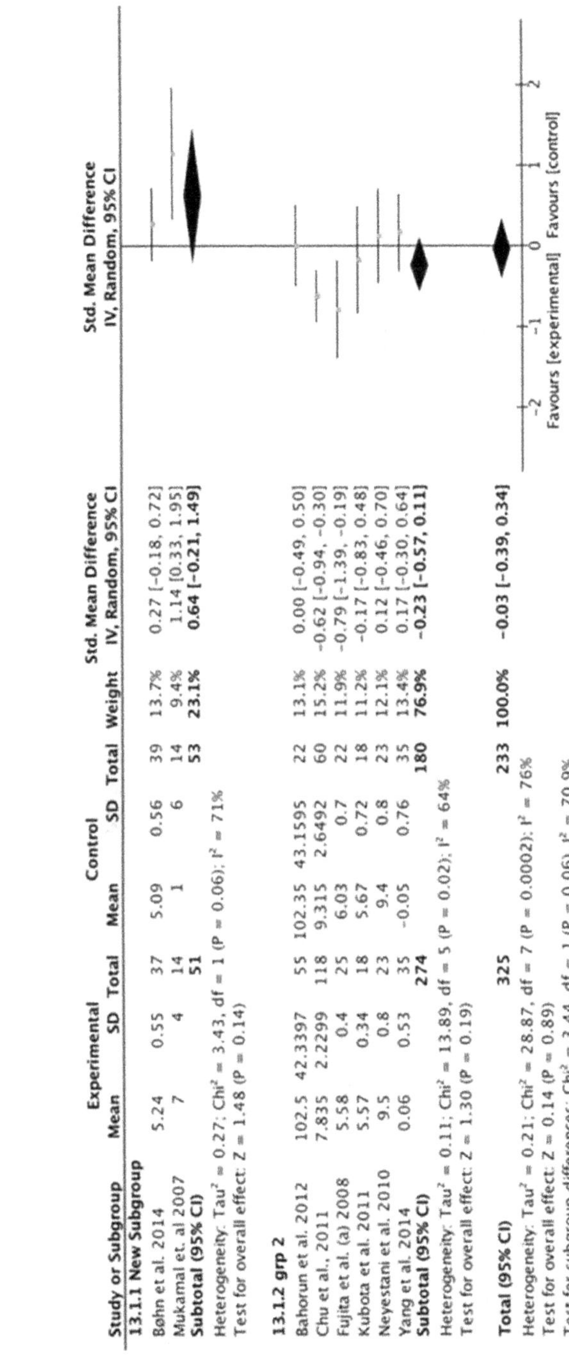

Figure 8.23 Subgroup analysis of blood glucose (length of study).

Study or Subgroup	Experimental Mean	Experimental SD	Experimental Total	Control Mean	Control SD	Control Total	Weight	Std. Mean Difference IV, Random, 95% CI	A	B	C	D	E	F	G
Bahorun et al. 2012	102.5	42.3397	55	102.35	43.1595	22	14.9%	0.00 [−0.49, 0.50]	+	−	?	?	+	+	+
Bøhn et al. 2014	5.24	0.55	37	5.09	0.56	39	15.4%	0.27 [−0.18, 0.72]	+	+	+	+	+	+	+
Chu et al., 2011	7.835	2.2299	118	9.315	2.6492	60	17.0%	−0.62 [−0.94, −0.30]	+	?	?	?	?	?	+
Fujita et al. (a) 2008	5.58	0.4	25	6.03	0.7	22	13.6%	−0.79 [−1.39, −0.19]	?	−	?	?	+	?	+
Kubota et al. 2011	5.57	0.34	18	5.67	0.72	18	12.8%	−0.17 [−0.83, 0.48]	?	−	?	?	?	?	−
Mukamal et. al 2007	7	4	14	1	6	14	11.0%	1.14 [0.33, 1.95]	+	+	−	+	?	+	?
Neyestani et al. 2010	9.5	0.8	23	9.4	0.8	23	0.0%	0.12 [−0.46, 0.70]	?	−	−	−	+	?	−
Yang et al. 2014	0.06	0.53	35	−0.05	0.76	35	15.2%	0.17 [−0.30, 0.64]	+	+	+	+	+	?	?
Total (95% CI)			**302**			**210**	**100.0%**	**−0.04 [−0.46, 0.37]**							

Heterogeneity: $Tau^2 = 0.24$; $Chi^2 = 28.01$, df = 6 ($P < 0.0001$); $I^2 = 79\%$
Test for overall effect: $Z = 0.20$ ($P = 0.84$)

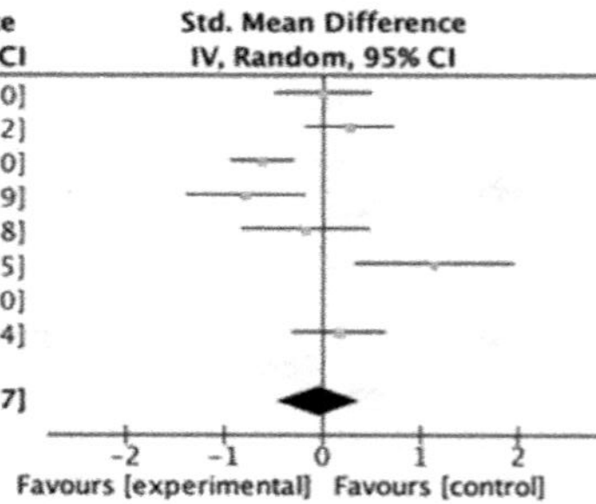

Risk of bias legend
(A) Random sequence generation (selection bias)
(B) Allocation concealment (selection bias)
(C) Blinding of participants and personnel (performance bias)
(D) Blinding of outcome assessment (detection bias)
(E) Incomplete outcome data (attrition bias)
(F) Selective reporting (reporting bias)
(G) Other bias

Figure 8.24 Sensitivity analysis of blood glucose monitoring.

trend was statistically significant at week 8. On the contrary, Bahorun *et al.* [41] reported that diet scores remained relatively constant for both tea and control groups.

8.3.14 *Adverse Effects*

Adverse events in the tea group were reported in four studies, including mild allergic-like reaction [36], diarrhoea [39], chest pain caused by lemon intake [44], tooth staining from concurrent intake with stannous fluoride [44], stomach discomfort [45] and others (common cold, throat pain, headache, whole body discomfort, gynaecological issues) [45]. On the other hand, two studies reported no adverse effects were found [27, 42].

8.3.15 *Quality of Included Studies*

Quality assessment was performed in accordance with the GRADE approach.

8.4 Discussion

14 articles were included in this review which aimed to investigate the efficacy of PET in reducing the cardiometabolic risks of metabolic syndrome and promoting weight loss. Majority of the articles suggested that PET is effective in improving body anthropometric, blood lipids and blood glucose.

Additionally, meta-analysis has been conducted on outcomes with two or more studies to estimate the overall effect size. Outcomes assessed were body anthropometric, blood lipids and blood glucose. The overall effect size for all the outcomes pointed towards the same conclusion that PET is effective in reducing cardiometabolic risks of metabolic syndrome and promoting weight loss. From the meta-analysis, BMI was found to be statistically lowered by PET when compared to placebo, while the rest of the overall effect size was non-significant.

Subgroup analysis was also performed to determine if the type of tea, ethnicity, length of study and characteristics of the population will influence the overall effect on the outcomes. First, when studies under each outcome were subdivided by the type of tea, studies included in the meta-analysis for blood glucose showed a significant subgroup difference. Second, when outcomes were segregated by ethnicity, significant differences between the subgroups were seen in triglycerides and blood glucose. Third, studies in each outcome were subgrouped into length of intervention. Blood glucose showed significant differences between its subgroups. Fourth, when studies in each outcome were subgrouped by health characteristics of the population, none of the outcomes showed significant differences in the subgroups.

Sensitivity analysis conducted showed no change in the overall effect measures when studies with high risk of bias [34] were excluded from the meta-analysis. Therefore, included studies with high risk of bias were unlikely to affect the findings of meta-analysis in this review.

8.4.1 *Limitations*

This study has several limitations. First, a limited number of studies were included as most studies were done on animals rather than humans. Second, this review allowed bioactive components of PET such as theaflavins and non-specific black tea to be included. Only five of the included studies used PET, of which three were from Yunnan and two others did not specify the origin of the PET leaves. It is to note that studies underwent subgroup analyses according to PET and non-PET categories, and the differences between subgroups were non-significant. Third, only English articles were included in this study. Tea, being a popular drink in Asia, has many studies published in languages like Mandarin and Japanese. Fourth, high heterogeneity was seen across studies.

8.4.2 *Implications*

To date, the mechanism and effect of PET to treat metabolic syndrome and obesity has not yet been determined. Findings from this study can advance the research of using PET as a safer, effective, complementary and alternative treatment for the rising number of patients with metabolic syndrome and obesity globally. Numerous animal studies were done on PET and only a few human trials were conducted. There is a need for future research to study the effect of PET on metabolic syndrome and obesity in a larger population. The specific PET doses reported in this study may be beneficial for the pharmaceutical industry and policy makers to study the natural bioactive products of PET in order to find a concoction with higher efficacy. The findings may also benefit hospitals considering introducing PET to bariatric units as part of their meal to complement the anti-obesity treatment. Health promotion programs may also refer to PET as a health beverage and recommend it as part of a healthy diet.

8.5 Summary

In conclusion, PET has numerous benefits for human health including reducing risk of metabolic syndrome and promoting weight loss. However, more human trials with longer intervention duration, and varying dosages and limitations on diet and exercise regimes are needed to identify the exact ingredients at work, optimal intervention concentration, duration, mechanism and interaction with other biomarkers.

References

1. Oliveira A, Guimarães A, Oliveira Junior R, Quintans J, Medeiros F, Barbosa Filho J, *et al.* Camellia sinensis (L.) Kuntze: a review of chemical and nutraceutical properties. 2016;44.
2. Brody H. Tea. Nature. 2019;566(Suppl 1):S1.

3. Wu CD, Wei GX. Tea as a functional food for oral health. Nutrition. 2002;18(5):443–4.
4. Cabrera C, Artacho R, Giménez R. Beneficial effects of green tea — a review. J Am Coll Nutr. 2006;25(2):79–99.
5. Zou XJ, Ding YH, Liang B. [The mechanisms of weight-cutting effect and bioactive components in Pu-erh tea]. Dong Wu Xue Yan Jiu. 2012;33(4):421–6.
6. Fujita H, Yamagami T. Antihypercholesterolemic effect of Chinese black tea extract in human subjects with borderline hypercholesterolemia. Nutr Res. 2008;28(7):450–6.
7. Du WH, Peng SM, Liu ZH, Shi L, Tan LF, Zou XQ. Hypoglycemic effect of the water extract of Pu-erh tea. J Agric Food Chem. 2012;60(40):10126–32.
8. Wang YC, McPherson K, Marsh T, Gortmaker SL, Brown M. Health and economic burden of the projected obesity trends in the USA and the UK. Lancet. 2011;378(9793):815–25.
9. Engin A. The definition and prevalence of obesity and metabolic syndrome. In: Engin AB, Engin A, editors. Obesity and Lipotoxicity. Springer; 2017. p. 1–17.
10. Cerulli J, Lomaestro BM, Malone M. Update on the pharmacotherapy of obesity. Ann Pharmacother. 2007;41(9):1505–17.
11. Pilitsi E, Farr OM, Polyzos SA, Perakakis N, Nolen-Doerr E, Papathanasiou AE, *et al.* Pharmacotherapy of obesity: available medications and drugs under investigation. Metabolism. 2019;92:170–92.
12. Li JJ, Huang CJ, Xie D. Anti-obesity effects of conjugated linoleic acid, docosahexaenoic acid, and eicosapentaenoic acid. Mol Nutr Food Res. 2008;52(6):631–45.
13. Trigueros L, Peña S, Ugidos AV, Sayas-Barberá E, Pérez-Álvarez JA, Sendra E. Food ingredients as anti-obesity agents: a review. Crit Rev Food Sci Nutr. 2013;53(9):929–42.
14. Xu J, Li M, Zhang Y, Chu S, Huo Y, Zhao J, *et al.* Huangjinya black tea alleviates obesity and insulin resistance via modulating fecal metabolome in high-fat diet-fed mice. Mol Nutr Food Res. 2020;64(22):e2000353.
15. Gurka MJ, Guo Y, Filipp SL, DeBoer MD. Metabolic syndrome severity is significantly associated with future coronary heart disease in type 2 diabetes. Cardiovasc Diabetol. 2018;17(1):17.
16. Chen L, Chen Q, Zhang Z, Wan X. A novel colorimetric determination of free amino acids content in tea infusions with 2,4-dinitrofluorobenzene. J Food Compos Anal. 2009;22(2):137–41.
17. Horžić D, Jambrak AR, Belščak-Cvitanović A, Komes D, Lelas V. Comparison of conventional and ultrasound assisted extraction techniques of yellow tea

and bioactive composition of obtained extracts. Food Bioprocess Technol. 2012;5(7):2858–70.

18. Zhang L, Zhang ZZ, Zhou YB, Ling TJ, Wan XC. Chinese dark teas: postfermentation, chemistry and biological activities. Food Res Int. 2013;53(2):600–7.
19. Chaturvedula VSP, Prakash I. The aroma, taste, color and bioactive constituents of tea. J Med Plants Res. 2011;5(11):2110–24.
20. Hursel R, Westerterp-Plantenga MS. Green tea catechin plus caffeine supplementation to a high-protein diet has no additional effect on body weight maintenance after weight loss. Am J Clin Nutr. 2009;89(3):822–30.
21. Wolfram S, Wang Y, Thielecke F. Anti-obesity effects of green tea: from bedside to bench. Mol Nutr Food Res. 2006;50(2):176–87.
22. Ho CT, Lin JK, Shahidi F. Tea and tea products: chemistry and health-promoting properties. Boca Raton: CRC Press; 2008.
23. Popkin BM, Armstrong LE, Bray GM, Caballero B, Frei B, Willett WC. A new proposed guidance system for beverage consumption in the United States. Am J Clin Nutr. 2006;83(3):529–42.
24. Kuo KL, Weng MS, Chiang CT, Tsai YJ, Lin-Shiau SY, Lin JK. Comparative studies on the hypolipidemic and growth suppressive effects of oolong, black, pu-erh, and green tea leaves in rats. J Agric Food Chem. 2005;53(2):480–9.
25. Sano M, Takenaka Y, Kojima R, Saito SI, Tomita I, Katou M, *et al.* Effects of pu-erh tea on lipid metabolism in rats. Chem Pharm Bull (Tokyo). 1986;34(1):221–8.
26. Mahdavi-Roshan M, Salari A, Ghorbani Z, Ashouri A. The effects of regular consumption of green or black tea beverage on blood pressure in those with elevated blood pressure or hypertension: a systematic review and meta-analysis. Complement Ther Med. 2020;51:102430.
27. Yang CY, Yen YY, Hung KC, Hsu SW, Lan SJ, Lin HC. Inhibitory effects of pu-erh tea on alpha glucosidase and alpha amylase: a systematic review. Nutr Diabetes. 2019;9(1):23.
28. Kris-Etherton PM, Hecker KD, Bonanome A, Coval SM, Binkoski AE, Hilpert KF, *et al.* Bioactive compounds in foods: their role in the prevention of cardiovascular disease and cancer. Am J Med. 2002;113(Suppl 9B):71S–88S.
29. Peters U, Poole C, Arab L. Does tea affect cardiovascular disease? A meta-analysis. Am J Epidemiol. 2001;154(6):495–503.
30. Higgins JPT, Thomas J, Chandler J, Cumpston M, Li T, Page MJ, Welch VA, editors. Cochrane handbook for systematic reviews of interventions. Version 6.3. Cochrane; 2022. Available from: https://www.training.cochrane.org/handbook.

31. WebPlotDigitizer [Internet]. Automeris; cited 2025 May 14. Available from: https://apps.automeris.io/wpd/.
32. Page MJ, Higgins JPT, Sterne JAC. Chapter 13: Assessing risk of bias due to missing results in a synthesis. In: Higgins JPT, Thomas J, Chandler J, Cumpston M, Li T, Page MJ, Welch VA, editors. Cochrane handbook for systematic reviews of interventions. Version 6.3. Cochrane; 2022. Available from: https://www.training.cochrane.org/handbook.
33. GRADEpro Guideline Development Tool [Internet]. McMaster University and Evidence Prime; 2021. Cited 2025 May 14. Available from: https://gradepro.org.
34. Neyestani TR, Shariatzade N, Kalayi A, Gharavi A, Khalaji N, Dadkhah M, *et al.* Regular daily intake of black tea improves oxidative stress biomarkers and decreases serum C-reactive protein levels in type 2 diabetic patients. Ann Nutr Metab. 2010;57(1):40–9.
35. Mahmoud F, Haines D, Al-Ozairi E, Dashti A. Effect of black tea consumption on intracellular cytokines, regulatory T cells and metabolic biomarkers in type 2 diabetes patients. Phytother Res. 2016;30(3):454–62.
36. Aizawa T, Yamamoto A, Ueno T. Effect of oral theaflavin administration on body weight, fat, and muscle in healthy subjects: a randomized pilot study. Biosci Biotechnol Biochem. 2017;81(2):311–5.
37. Oi Y, Fujita H. Body weight and body mass index (BMI) in pre-obese and overweight Japanese adults treated with black Chinese tea water extract (BTE) using a more appropriate statistical analysis method. Int J Food Prop. 2015;18(6):1345–9.
38. Bøhn SK, Croft KD, Burrows S, Puddey IB, Mulder TP, Fuchs D, *et al.* Effects of black tea on body composition and metabolic outcomes related to cardiovascular disease risk: a randomized controlled trial. Food Funct. 2014;5(7):1613–20.
39. Chu SL, Fu H, Yang JX, Liu GX, Dou P, Zhang L, *et al.* A randomized double-blind placebo-controlled study of Pu'er tea extract on the regulation of metabolic syndrome. Chin J Integr Med. 2011;17(7):492–8.
40. Jensen GS, Beaman JL, He Y, Guo Z, Sun H. Reduction of body fat and improved lipid profile associated with daily consumption of a Puer tea extract in a hyperlipidemic population: a randomized placebo-controlled trial. Clin Interv Aging. 2016;11:367–76.
41. Bahorun T, Luximon-Ramma A, Neergheen-Bhujun VS, Gunness TK, Googoolye K, Auger C, *et al.* The effect of black tea on risk factors of cardiovascular disease in a normal population. Prev Med. 2012;54(Suppl):S98–102.
42. Kubota K, Sumi S, Tojo H, Sumi-Inoue Y, Ichikawa H, Oi Y, *et al.* Improvements of mean body mass index and body weight in pre-obese and overweight Japanese

adults with black Chinese tea (Pu-Erh) water extract. Nutr Res. 2011;31(6): 421–8.

43. Hodgson JM, Puddey IB, Woodman RJ, Mulder TPJ, Fuchs D, Scott K, *et al.* Effects of black tea on blood pressure: a randomized controlled trial. Arch Intern Med. 2012;172(2):186–8.
44. Mukamal KJ, MacDermott K, Vinson JA, Oyama N, Manning WJ, Mittleman MA. A 6-month randomized pilot study of black tea and cardiovascular risk factors. Am Heart J. 2007;154(4):724.e21–6.
45. Trautwein EA, Du Y, Meynen E, Yan X, Wen Y, Wang H, *et al.* Purified black tea theaflavins and theaflavins/catechin supplements did not affect serum lipids in healthy individuals with mildly to moderately elevated cholesterol concentrations. Eur J Nutr. 2010;49(1):27–35.

https://doi.org/10.1142/9789819817320_0009

Chapter 9*

Effectiveness of Food Fortification in Preventing Malnutrition in Community-Dwelling Older Adults: A Systematic Review and Meta-Analysis

Xue Kee Lau[1], Min Chua[2], and Jeanette Ignacio[3,*]

[1]*Mount Alvernia Hospital, 820 Thomson Rd, Singapore 574623*

[2]*Fusionopolis Link, #03-08, Nexus @ one-north, Singapore 138543*

[3]*Alice Lee Centre for Nursing Studies, Yong Loo Lin School of Medicine, National University of Singapore, 10 Medical Drive, Singapore 117597*

**Corresponding author: nurimjj@nus.edu.sg*

9.1 Background

Adequate amounts of food and nutrients are usually required by one's body to ensure the good functionality of the various systems for physiological and metabolic processes [1]. As individuals age, physiological changes occur, altering the body's need for energy, protein, and fluids. During this process, the metabolic rate decreases and the consumption of nutrients declines, resulting in nutritional deficiency, also known as malnutrition [2]. Malnutrition is generally defined as an underconsumption or overconsumption of essential nutrients [3].

9.1.1 *Malnutrition in Older Adults*

Malnutrition is prevalent worldwide among older adults (generally defined as people aged 60 years and above) [4]. It can stem from a myriad

* Appendices to this chapter are available for download at https://www.worldscientific.com/worldscibooks/10.1142/14420#t=suppl.

of factors, ranging from inadequate nutrition intake to chronic illnesses, decreased appetite, or functional disabilities that result in chewing and swallowing problems [5, 6]. Moreover, many older adults lack a source of income and have limited social interaction, which can affect their psychosocial health and contribute to malnutrition due to decreased intake of nutrients [2]. This is similar to the local scene in Singapore, where a significant number of community-dwelling older adults live in isolation, exposing them to malnutrition risk factors [7].

In Singapore, the prevalence of older adults in the community suffering from malnourishment is 3.9%, while 31.4% are at risk [8]. Despite the relatively low percentages, it is still urgent to address the issue of malnutrition as it can increase the risk of falling and disability, impairment of immunological function, and disrupt wound healing [9–11]. An accumulation of these factors can significantly impact the overall well-being of older adults, thus making it important to prevent malnutrition in this population.

9.1.2 *Existing Strategies to Improve Malnutrition*

Some common interventions to curb malnutrition in older adults include nutritional strategies such as oral nutritional supplements (ONS), food fortification or enrichment, dietary education and dietary counselling [6, 12]. While interventions such as ONS have seen effectiveness in treating malnutrition by improving body weight and other clinical outcomes among malnourished older adults, they pose a challenge due to their poor acceptability and tolerance. ONS can result in palatability issues due to their taste and texture. In the long run, this may cause taste fatigue, which may lead to a rejection of the consumption of ONS, as often observed in clinical and residential care settings [13, 14].

Much research has been conducted to determine the efficacy of these nutritional interventions, such as nutrition education and ONS [15]. Yet, few systematic reviews have generated convincing results on fortified food being an effective strategy for preventing malnutrition in older adults. Hence, this systematic review focused on food fortification as an intervention.

9.1.3 *Food Fortification and Its Advantages in Curbing Malnutrition*

According to the World Health Organization [16], food fortification is the process of adding vitamins and minerals to increase the nutritional value of commonly consumed food [17]. Fortificants are usually micronutrients that come in various forms, such as powdered modules, cream, and oil [18]. While mandatory fortification in iodised salt and fortified flour is widespread, it may not address the full spectrum of malnutrition [19]. Studies have shown that fortification with iodine, folic acid, vitamin A and iron can significantly reduce serious diseases, proving the value of food fortification [20]. This method is advantageous as it allows the adjustment of food to suit the dietary preferences of older adults. Older adults tend to prefer familiar food and may be hesitant to try new dietary recommendations, so fortifying commonly consumed food may encourage them to consume more nutritious food [21].

9.1.4 *Measuring Outcomes for Malnutrition*

Currently, there is no universal malnutrition screening and assessment tool. Common measures used to assess malnutrition in older adults across various settings include nutritional intake, nutritional assessment tools, anthropometric measurements, and biological biomarkers.

Nutritional intake, such as calorie and energy intake [22], and the Mini-Nutritional Assessment (MNA) tool [23] are widely used to determine and evaluate the risk of malnutrition. Anthropometric measurements, such as Body Mass Index (BMI), are used to determine if an individual is obese or underweight to assess nutritional status [24]. Some biological biomarkers, such as albumin, prealbumin, haemoglobin, total protein, and total cholesterol, are found to be good indicators of malnutrition. However, other health factors like inflammation may impede the accuracy of using certain blood biomarkers as nutrition assessment tools [25].

9.1.5 *Gaps Identified in the Existing Literature*

Six existing reviews found food fortification an effective strategy for improving nutritional intake. However, the heterogeneity among included studies makes it unclear whether it is a valid intervention to improve nutritional status. This was seen in reviews conducted by Morilla-Herrera *et al.* [26] and Sossen *et al.* [27], where heterogeneity was attributed to the differences in study designs and participant characteristics. These differences were congruent with other studies as well. Also, all these reviews included primary studies from multiple settings consisting of hospitals, residential care, and the community [26–31]. No systematic review focused solely on older adults in the community setting.

Most reviews utilised primary studies dating as far back as two decades ago in which the knowledge and findings may have been outdated. Hence, the results may not be as credible as studies conducted in recent years [32]. Additionally, only two of the reviews explored the outcomes of the acceptability and cost-effectiveness of fortified food [27, 30]. As high heterogeneity exists, further research is needed to contribute to the limited existing knowledge to determine the feasibility of implementing food fortification.

9.1.6 *Rationale for Conducting the Current Systematic Review*

The literature search found that none of the existing systematic reviews included primary studies based solely in the community setting. Additionally, only a few reviews have covered the acceptability of fortified food. Hence, this review sought to close the gap highlighted by previous studies, focusing specifically on the community-dwelling older adult population and including the acceptability of fortified food in the outcome. Randomised controlled trials (RCTs) were included whenever possible to offer the highest level of evidence [33]. This allowed for a more in-depth evidence-based practice using nutritional strategies to prevent malnutrition, thus providing a foundation for future studies and potential adoption in Singapore's ageing population. This systematic review aimed to identify the best available evidence to evaluate the effectiveness of food fortification in preventing malnutrition in community-dwelling older adults. The following review questions were addressed: (1) What kind of food fortification is used to address malnutrition in older adults? (2) Is food fortification an effective strategy in preventing malnutrition and improving nutritional outcomes in older adults? (3) How is the acceptability of food fortification in older adults?

9.2 Methods

This systematic review was written following the Preferred Reporting Items for Systematic Reviews and Meta-Analyses (PRISMA) checklist [34].

9.2.1 *Eligibility Criteria*

Types of studies. RCTs and crossover trials were included in this systematic review. Restrictions on the date of publication were applied such that only studies published within the last ten years, from 2012 to 2022, were included. Due to the unavailability of translation resources, only studies written in the English language were considered for inclusion.

Types of participants. Studies focusing on older adults aged 60 years and older who were relatively independent and living in the community were included. Older adults with nutritional status at risk of undernutrition were also included.

Types of interventions. Studies with any nutritional intervention that specifically used food-based fortification or food enrichment as dietary interventions were included in this systematic review. Interventions on nutritional support by means of artificial and parenteral feedings were excluded from this study.

Comparators. Studies using any comparator of food-based intervention were included, such as studies comparing fortified food with standard food. Studies without a comparator were also included.

Types of outcome measures. The primary outcome measures were: (1) the nutrition intake of older adults (e.g., protein and energy intake), and (2) the nutritional status (e.g., MNA, BMI, blood tests [albumin and prealbumin concentration]). The secondary outcome measure was acceptability of food fortification strategies in older adults.

9.2.2 *Information Resources and Search Strategy*

Six bibliographic databases were searched for relevant studies. They included PubMed, Embase, CINAHL, Scopus, Cochrane Central Register of Controlled Trials, and Web of Science. Search for unpublished studies and grey literature was conducted on Google Scholar, ProQuest and ClinicalTrials.gov. Manual screening of reference lists of selected primary studies and systematic reviews were also performed.

The search strategy was structured based on the PICO concepts, with free-text terms and corresponding subject headings for each concept identified whenever applicable [35]. To ensure that relevant search terms and techniques were used, a medical librarian was consulted. A peer review of the search strategy and search process were also conducted and guided using the Peer Review of Electronic Search Strategies evidence-based checklist [36].

9.2.3 *Selection Process*

Search results were managed by the EndNote 20 software. Duplicate publications could result in substantial biases, as such it was crucial to identify and remove multiple reports from the same study [37]. After which, two reviewers independently reviewed the remaining studies from the databases searched. Based on the eligibility criteria, reviewers screened in stages based on the titles and abstracts. Full-text screening of the remaining studies followed. Studies that did not meet the eligibility criteria were excluded. Any discrepancies regarding the selection process were resolved by a third reviewer.

9.2.4 *Data Extraction*

Data extraction was done by two reviewers independently using an adapted data extraction form from the Cochrane Collaboration. Pilot testing was done on three studies. Data extracted included general information, characteristics of the study (methods, participants, intervention groups, outcomes), data and analysis. A third reviewer was consulted when disagreements arose. Study investigators were also contacted for clarification of existing data, and requests of missing or additional data when further information required was not found in the published study. For studies with multiple arms, only data from groups receiving fortified food and control groups were extracted.

9.2.5 *Risk of Bias*

Two reviewers undertook the risk of bias assessment in included studies independently, guided by the Cochrane risk-of-bias tool for randomised trials (RoB 1) in RevMan 5.4 [38]. The following domains were taken into consideration:

— Selection bias
— Performance bias
— Detection bias
— Attrition bias
— Reporting bias
— Other bias

Each of the domains was described based on the data reported in the studies and assigned one of the three levels of risk-of-bias judgement:

'low risk', 'unclear risk', or 'high risk'. Differing opinions were resolved through consultation with a third reviewer.

9.2.6 *Assessing the Certainty of the Evidence*

The Grading of Recommendations, Assessment, Development and Evaluation (GRADE) approach using the GRADEpro Guideline Developmental Tool [39] was used to rate the overall quality of evidence.

9.2.7 *Data Analysis and Synthesis*

Meta-analyses were undertaken to pool data with common outcomes using RevMan 5.4 software [38] under the random-effects model. For continuous data reported, effect measures were expressed as mean differences (MD) and standardised mean differences (SMD) with 95% confidence intervals (CI) under the inverse-variance method. MD was used for three of the outcome measures as the meta-analyses combined outcomes from both post-intervention and change-from-baseline measurements [40]. Z-statistics was used to assess the overall effect of the intervention with $P < 0.05$. Manual calculations were performed to retrieve missing values in mean and standard deviation.

Heterogeneity was examined statistically using the I^2 statistic and Cochran's Q χ^2 test, and through visually inspecting the forest plots. According to the Cochrane Handbook for Systematic Reviews of Interventions [40], an I^2 value above 50% and χ^2 greater than the degrees of freedom with a significance level set at $P < 0.10$ may indicate significant heterogeneity.

Studies with outcome data pooled using post-intervention measurements and changes-from-baseline were placed in separate subgroups respectively, for easier visualisation of the forest plots. Sensitivity analyses were performed to assess the strength and validity of the findings, with outliers removed whenever applicable [41]. The effects of studies which were excluded from meta-analyses were examined and summarised narratively.

9.3 Results

9.3.1 *Study Selection*

A total of 1,652 articles were identified from the six databases, as listed in the PRISMA flowchart in Figure 9.1. After duplicates were eliminated and titles and abstracts were screened, 29 articles were left for the screening of full texts, of which seven articles met the eligibility criteria of this systematic review. 204 records were also identified from other sources, and after the retrieval of full texts, four studies met the eligibility criteria. Overall, 11 studies were included in the current review.

9.3.2 *Study Characteristics*

Appendix A summarises the characteristics of the 11 included studies. Of the 11 studies, nine were RCTs and two were crossover trials. These studies were conducted across seven different countries, including four studies from the Netherlands [42–45], two studies from Thailand [46, 47], and one each from Australia [48], the United Kingdom [49], Finland [50], Indonesia [51], and France [52]. The mean age of participants ranged from 67.8 to 90.9 years. Nine studies were conducted in community settings, while two others were from nursing homes and rehabilitation centres [43, 49], respectively. The older adults were relatively independent, and those in the rehabilitation centres were prepared to be discharged into the community. There were a total of 656 participants, with sample sizes of the studies ranging between 8 and 98. The percentages of females were between 53.7% and 87.8%, while the percentages of males were between 12.2% and 46.3%.

9.3.3 *Assessment of the Risk of Bias*

All 11 included studies were assessed for risk of bias using the Cochrane risk-of-bias tool, as shown in the risk of bias summary. The GRADE approach was used to assess the overall quality of evidence. All the

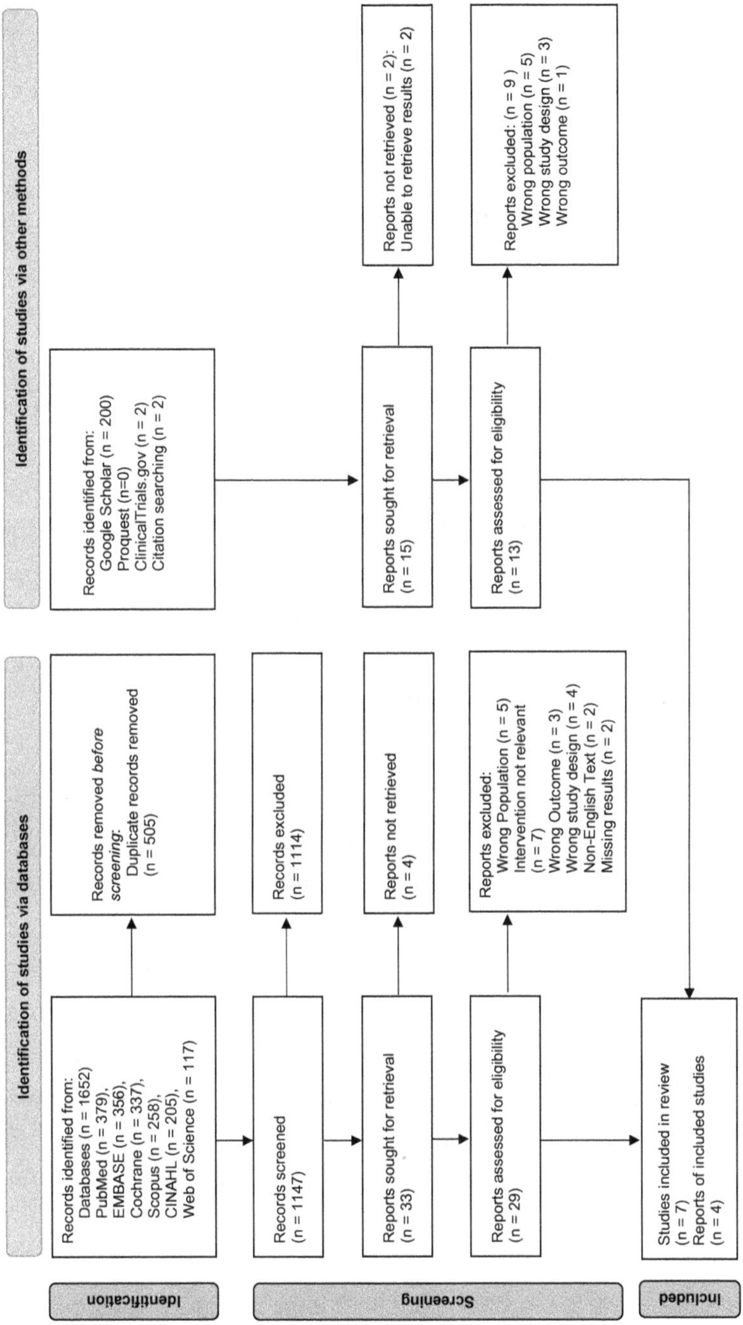

Figure 9.1 PRISMA flow diagram.

presented outcomes were reported using continuous data. Energy intake and lipid intake were rated as very low quality. Protein intake and change in MNA score were rated as low quality. Change in body weight and change in BMI were rated as moderate quality.

9.3.4 *Description of Food Fortification Interventions*

The interventions utilised in these studies consist of a variety of fortified food interventions. Of the 11 included studies, two studies provided a combination of enriched meals and snacks or dairy products [42, 46]. Three studies provided solely enriched meal interventions [44, 48, 49]. Two studies provided enriched snacks with dairy products or energy-enriched berry purées [47, 50]. The study conducted by Fatmah [51] provided only fortified snacks in the form of cookies. Additionally, three studies provided enriched bread with or without enriched meals or enriched yoghurt as interventions [43, 45, 52]. Food was generally fortified by adding skim milk powder, cream, custard, butter, rice bran oil, cheese and other ingredients into the food served.

9.3.5 *Meta-Analysis Results*

Energy intake. A meta-analysis of nine studies in Figure 9.2 showed a statistically significant difference in energy intake ($Z = 3.63$, $p = 0.0003$), with MD of 220.11 kcal (95% CI: 101.21 to 339.02). Substantial heterogeneity was observed initially ($I^2 = 73\%$, $p = 0.0003$). Upon separating the pooled results of post-intervention and change-from-baseline measurements into separate subgroups, the heterogeneity was evidently reduced in each subgroup. Sensitivity analysis done in Figure 9.3 revealed a more statistically significant difference, as seen from the higher Z-value ($Z = 4.11$, $p < 0.0001$), with MD of 278.37 kcal (95% CI: 145.70 to 411.04) after excluding the outliers.

Protein intake. A meta-analysis of eight studies in Figure 9.4 showed a statistically significant difference in protein intake ($Z = 2.28$, $p = 0.02$), with

Study or Subgroup	Fortified Food Mean	Fortified Food SD	Fortified Food Total	Standard Food Mean	Standard Food SD	Standard Food Total	Weight	Mean Difference IV, Random, 95% CI
1.1.1 Studies								
Arjuna 2018	467.97	555.35	14	151.77	935.95	16	3.7%	316.20 [-226.89, 859.29]
Borkent 2019	1,865.96	322.8	47	1,794.93	291.2	42	14.0%	71.03 [-56.53, 198.59]
Chanwikrai 2021	1,511	190	8	1,312	153	8	12.5%	199.00 [29.96, 368.04]
Chanwikrai 2022	1,565	145	15	1,303	216	16	14.0%	262.00 [133.21, 390.79]
Fatmah 2021	1,255.5	232.6	24	1,232.6	292.9	24	13.2%	22.90 [-126.74, 172.54]
Leslie 2013	556	372	16	-151	351	16	9.6%	707.00 [456.39, 957.61]
Van Til 2015	1,937	414	17	1,638	298	17	9.9%	299.00 [56.52, 541.48]
Van Wymelbeke 2016	1,394.08	312.1	29	1,135.38	264.2	22	12.9%	258.70 [100.30, 417.10]
Ziylan 2017	1,761.2	391.2	22	1,732.8	391.2	20	10.1%	28.40 [-208.49, 265.29]
Subtotal (95% CI)			**192**			**181**	**100.0%**	**220.11 [101.21, 339.02]**
Heterogeneity: Tau² = 21964.73; Chi² = 29.19, df = 8 (P = 0.0003); I² = 73%								
Test for overall effect: Z = 3.63 (P = 0.0003)								
Total (95% CI)			**192**			**181**	**100.0%**	**220.11 [101.21, 339.02]**
Heterogeneity: Tau² = 21964.73; Chi² = 29.19, df = 8 (P = 0.0003); I² = 73%								
Test for overall effect: Z = 3.63 (P = 0.0003)								
Test for subgroup differences: Not applicable								

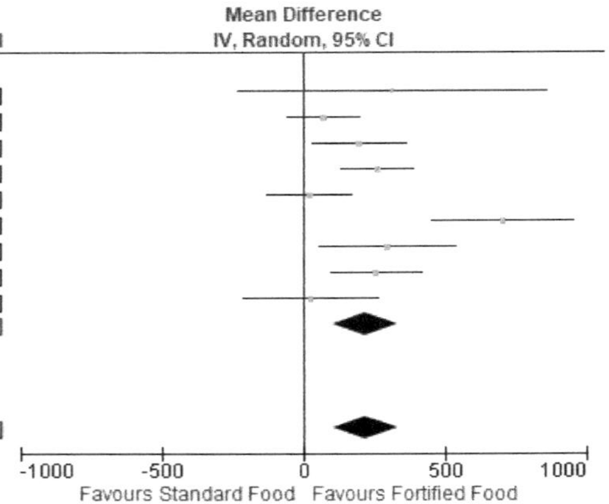

Figure 9.2 Forest plot of mean differences (95% CI) in energy intake.

Study or Subgroup	Fortified Food Mean	Fortified Food SD	Fortified Food Total	Standard Food Mean	Standard Food SD	Standard Food Total	Weight	Mean Difference IV, Random, 95% CI
1.1.1 Post-intervention readings								
Borkent 2019	1,865.96	322.8	47	1,794.93	291.2	42	18.5%	71.03 [-56.53, 198.59]
Chanwikrai 2021	1,511	190	8	1,312	153	8	16.4%	199.00 [29.96, 368.04]
Chanwikrai 2022	1,565	145	15	1,303	216	16	18.4%	262.00 [133.21, 390.79]
Fatmah 2021	1,255.5	232.6	24	1,232.6	292.9	24	0.0%	22.90 [-126.74, 172.54]
Van Til 2015	1,937	414	17	1,638	298	17	12.8%	299.00 [56.52, 541.48]
Van Wymelbeke 2016	1,394.08	312.1	29	1,135.38	264.2	22	16.9%	258.70 [100.30, 417.10]
Ziylan 2017	1,761.2	391.2	22	1,732.8	391.2	20	0.0%	28.40 [-208.49, 265.29]
Subtotal (95% CI)			**116**			**105**	**82.9%**	**204.16 [118.35, 289.97]**
Heterogeneity: Tau² = 3142.28; Chi² = 5.98, df = 4 (P = 0.20); I² = 33%								
Test for overall effect: Z = 4.66 (P < 0.00001)								
1.1.2 Change-from-baseline readings								
Arjuna 2018	467.97	555.35	14	151.77	935.95	16	4.7%	316.20 [-226.89, 859.29]
Leslie 2013	556	372	16	-151	351	16	12.4%	707.00 [456.39, 957.61]
Subtotal (95% CI)			**30**			**32**	**17.1%**	**588.92 [237.20, 940.64]**
Heterogeneity: Tau² = 29797.94; Chi² = 1.64, df = 1 (P = 0.20); I² = 39%								
Test for overall effect: Z = 3.28 (P = 0.001)								
Total (95% CI)			**146**			**137**	**100.0%**	**278.37 [145.70, 411.04]**
Heterogeneity: Tau² = 20581.47; Chi² = 20.76, df = 6 (P = 0.002); I² = 71%								
Test for overall effect: Z = 4.11 (P < 0.0001)								
Test for subgroup differences: Chi² = 4.34, df = 1 (P = 0.04), I² = 77.0%								

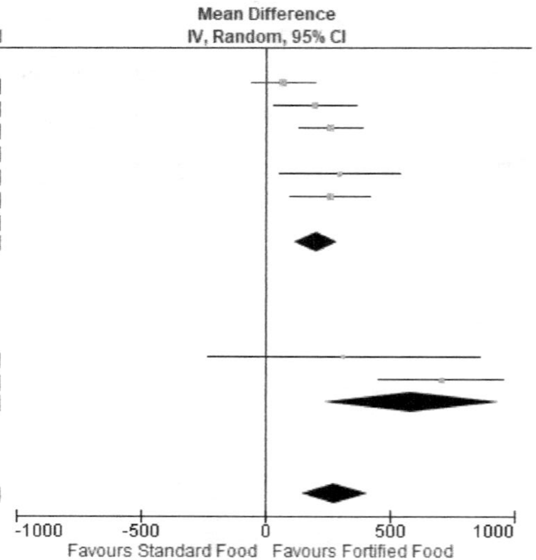

Figure 9.3 Forest plot of mean differences (95% CI) in energy intake, excluding Refs. [45] and [51].

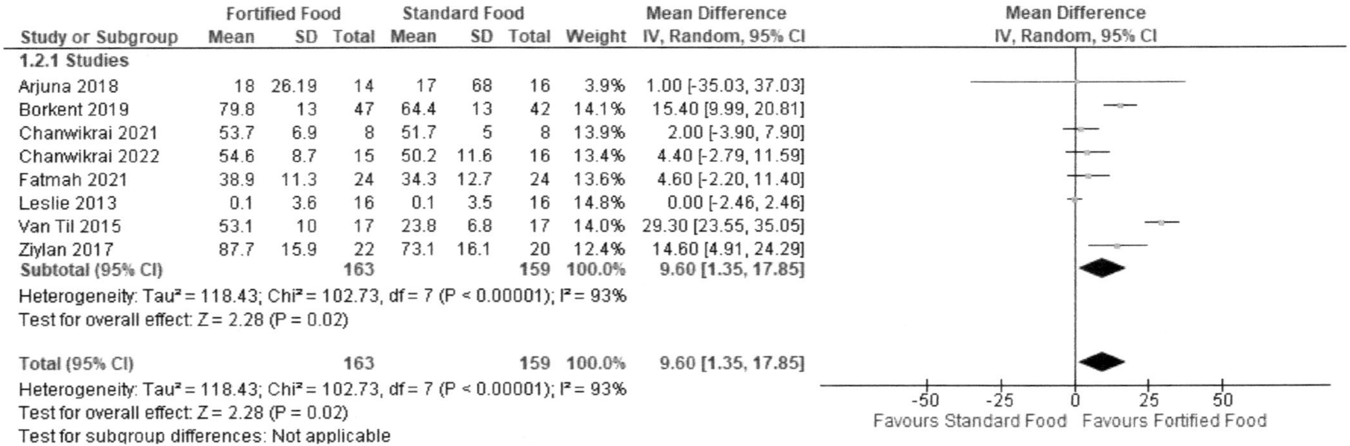

Figure 9.4 Forest plot of mean differences (95% CI) in protein intake.

MD of 9.60 g (95% CI: 1.35 to 17.85). A substantial level of heterogeneity was observed ($I^2 = 93\%$, $p < 0.00001$). Upon separating the pooled results of post-intervention and change-from-baseline measurements into separate subgroups, the heterogeneity was still present ($I^2 = 91\%$). Additionally, the overall effect for the two studies under the change-from-baseline subgroup found no significant difference in protein intake ($Z = 0$, $p = 1.00$). After sensitivity analysis was conducted where the outlier was excluded (Figure 9.5), the results revealed further statistical insignificance ($Z = 2.21$, $p = 0.03$), with MD of 6.28 g (95% CI: 0.72 to 11.84).

Lipid intake. A meta-analysis of five studies in Figure 9.6 showed a statistically significant difference in lipid intake ($Z = 3.58$, $p = 0.0003$), with MD of 11.42 g (95% CI: 5.16 to 17.67). A moderate level of heterogeneity was observed initially ($I^2 = 68\%$, $p = 0.01$). However, heterogeneity was reduced significantly after the post-intervention and change-from-baseline measurements were placed in separate subgroups, resulting in I^2 values of 20% and 0% respectively.

Change in body weight. A meta-analysis of four studies in Figure 9.7 showed no statistically significant difference in the change in body weight ($Z = 0.73$, $p = 0.46$), with SMD of 0.12 kg (95% CI: −0.21 to 0.46).

Change in BMI. A meta-analysis of five studies in Figure 9.8 showed no statistically significant difference in the change in BMI ($Z = 1.05$, $p = 0.29$), with SMD of 0.31 kg/m^2 (95% CI: −0.26 to 0.88). Substantial heterogeneity was observed ($I^2 = 73\%$, $p = 0.005$). Sensitivity analysis done where the outlier was removed resulted in a lower heterogeneity ($I^2 = 0\%$, $p = 0.88$). Consequently, the overall effect was further reduced ($Z = 0.09$, $p = 0.93$), with SMD of 0.01 kg/m^2 (95% CI: −0.30 to 0.33) (Figure 9.9).

Change in MNA scores. A meta-analysis of two studies in Figure 9.10 showed no statistically significant difference in the change in MNA scores ($Z = 0.21$, $p = 0.84$), with SMD of −0.05 (95% CI: −0.49 to 0.39).

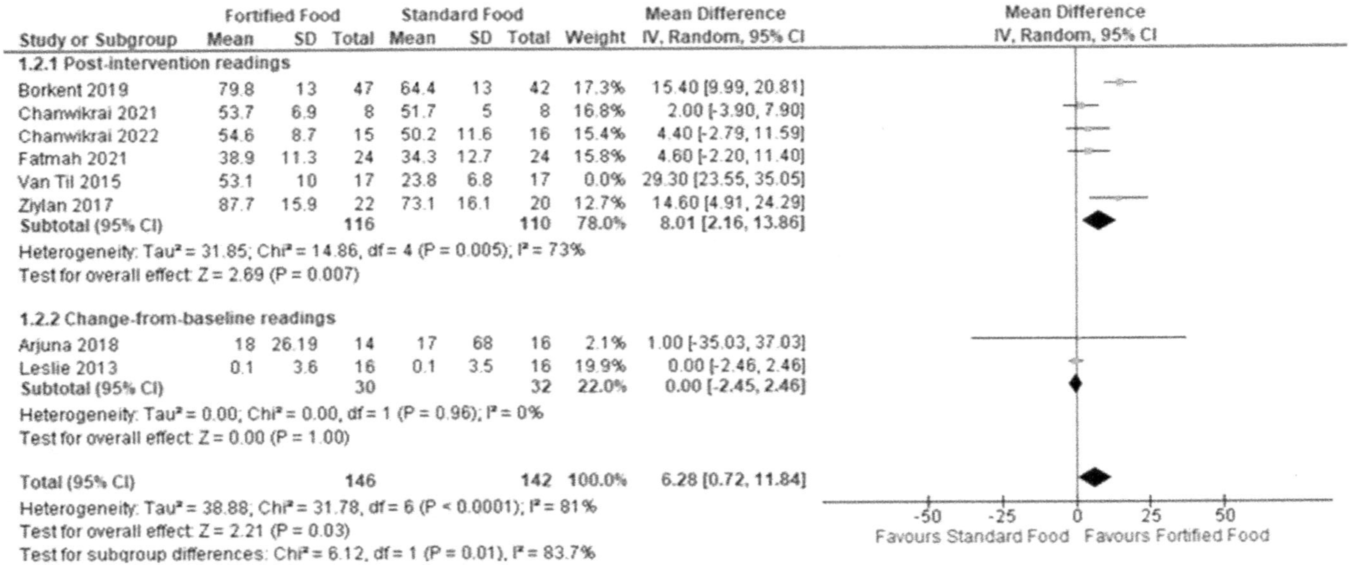

Figure 9.5 Forest plot of mean differences (95% CI) in protein intake, excluding Ref. [43].

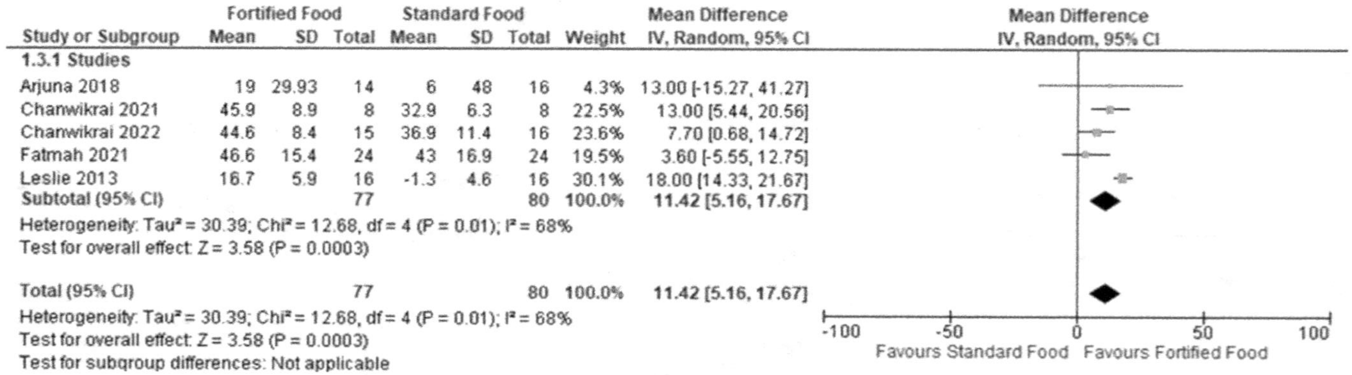

Figure 9.6 Forest plot of mean differences (95% CI) in lipid intake.

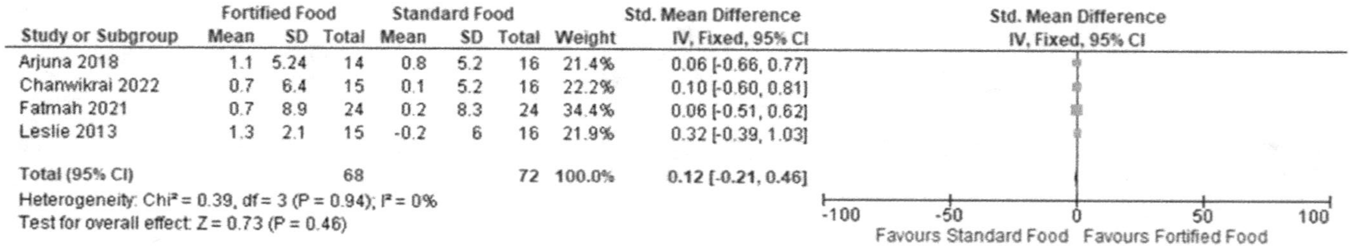

Figure 9.7 Forest plot of standardised mean differences (95% CI) in change in body weight.

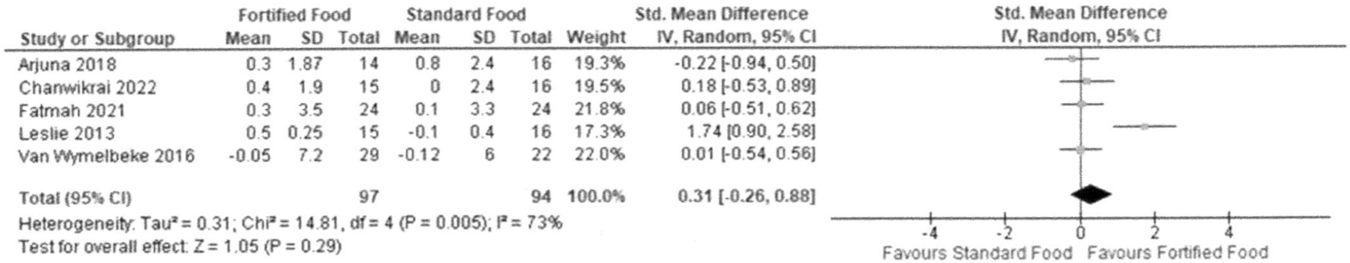

Figure 9.8 Forest plot of standardised mean differences (95% CI) in change in BMI.

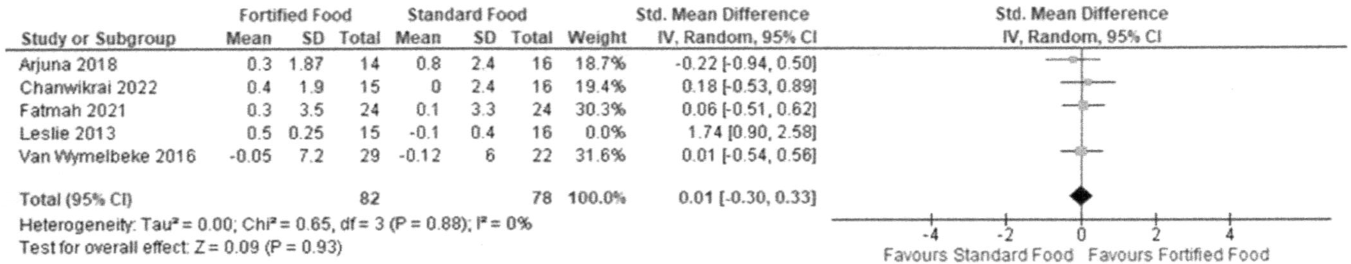

Figure 9.9 Forest plot of standardised mean differences (95% CI) in change in BMI, excluding Ref. [49].

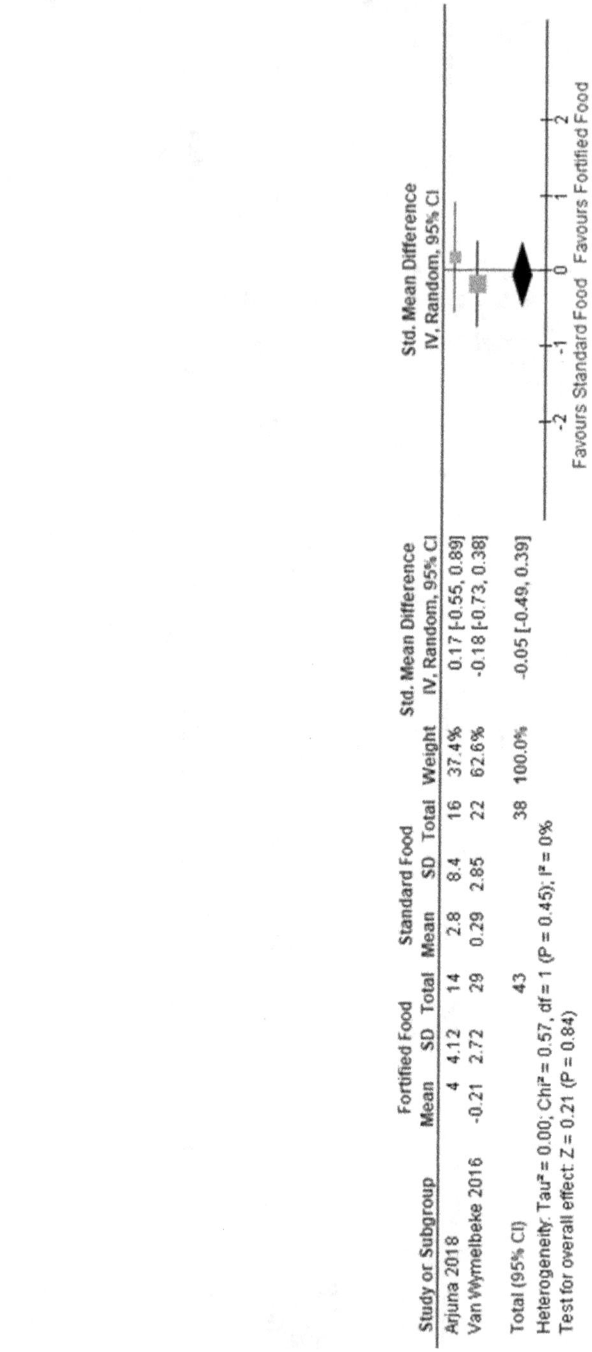

Figure 9.10 Forest plot of standardised mean differences (95% CI) in change in MNA scores.

9.3.6 *Narrative Synthesis*

Studies excluded from meta-analyses. Two studies were excluded from meta-analyses due to missing values [44, 50]. Ziylan *et al.* [44] observed a significant increase in both energy intake and protein intake when the intervention meals were enriched with energy and protein. Conversely, Nykänen *et al.* [50] reported a substantial increase in MNA scores in the intervention group and a slight decrease in MNA scores in the control group.

Plasma albumin and plasma prealbumin concentrations. Only two studies reported results for plasma albumin and plasma prealbumin concentrations [50, 52]. Both studies observed higher plasma albumin and plasma prealbumin concentrations in their intervention groups compared to their control groups.

Acceptability of fortified food. Six studies assessed the acceptability of the food provided to participants during their study. Most participants in both intervention and control groups rated high scores for the respective food consumed. It was found that there was no significant difference in acceptability scores between the two groups. Feedback from participants found that they were more inclined to consume these fortified foods if they were affordable and convenient to obtain [45, 48].

9.4 Discussion

9.4.1 *Summary of Findings*

The evidence from this systematic review suggested that food fortification may effectively prevent malnutrition in community-dwelling older adults, where a significant increase in energy and nutrient intake was observed in the intervention groups. However, there were no differences in findings in the change in body weight, BMI, and MNA scores between both intervention and control groups. Despite having a small effect size, the findings of this review were generally consistent with existing reviews, where food fortification interventions showed improvements in outcomes measured.

9.4.2 *Nutrition Intake*

Results from meta-analyses and narrative synthesis showed higher energy, protein, and lipid intake in participants consuming fortified food than standard food. The findings are in line with previous reviews by Morilla-Herrera *et al.* [26] and Mills *et al.* [30], where both reported a distinct rise in energy intake among the intervention groups. However, while Morilla-Herrera *et al.* [26] noted an increase in protein intake among the intervention group, Mills *et al.* [30] did not observe any notable difference between the intervention and control groups.

After excluding the outliers in the meta-analysis of energy intake, the overall results further improved the mean difference in the energy intake in intervention groups. Fatmah [51] did not report similar findings as other studies due to its intervention providing solely fortified cookies rather than proper meals. Hence, this could have resulted in a less significant increase in energy intake compared to other studies which utilised fortified meals.

Additionally, the high heterogeneity observed in the analysis of protein intake could be explained by the methodological differences present in each of the included studies provided. Each study intervention provided various forms of fortified foods, including meals, bread, snacks, and dairy products. The significant differences in the amount of protein present in each type of food thus could have resulted in the lack of homogeneity. As such, while the overall pooled results presented significant findings in protein intake, these results should still be taken with caution.

Lipids are known to be important energy sources, and they lower the risks of diseases [53]. Although lipid intake is not as frequently examined in studies investigating food fortification and malnutrition, it is still a crucial factor to include lipids in the prevention of malnutrition, considering its benefits. The meta-analysis in this review demonstrated a positive outcome, in which a higher intake of lipids was observed in the intervention groups.

Fortified food is designed to contain higher quantities of energy and nutrients in comparison to standard food of the same portion size [19]. This is particularly crucial in addressing malnutrition in older adults, who are more susceptible to loss of appetite [5]. The use of energy-dense fortified food allows older adults to consume smaller portions of food with greater nutrient content. As such, measuring energy and nutrient intake is an essential approach to evaluating the effectiveness of food fortification, as it determines whether older adults are consuming an adequate amount of energy and nutrients. The studies included in this review demonstrated that participants who received fortified food had higher energy and nutrient intake, indicating that food fortification is likely an effective strategy for addressing malnutrition in older adults within the community.

9.4.3 *Nutritional Status*

Meta-analyses undertaken revealed that there was no difference in findings in the body weight, BMI, and MNA scores between participants consuming fortified food and standard food. An existing review conducted by Douglas *et al.* [29], which was based in hospital and nursing home settings, found that the body weight and BMI of participants consuming fortified food did not differ much from those consuming standard food. This finding was consistent with the meta-analyses conducted in the current review. In another review conducted by Sossen *et al.* [27], while an increase in weight was observed, the BMI and MNA between intervention and control groups from aged residential care saw little differences as well.

Although most studies in the meta-analysis of MNA scores did not reveal notable findings, Nykänen *et al.* [50] found a substantial increase in MNA scores among the intervention groups, as reported in the narrative synthesis earlier. This difference in effect could be attributed to the differences in the study duration and frequencies among the three studies which measured MNA scores as outcomes [48, 50, 52].

From the narrative synthesis, both Nykänen *et al.* [50] and Van Wymelbeke *et al.* [52] also reported higher plasma albumin and prealbumin concentrations in the intervention groups than control groups. No previous systematic reviews have reported outcome measures on these biomarkers. However, it would be insightful to explore these biomarkers as studies have presented findings related to them being useful indicators in assessing nutritional status [54]. Low levels of plasma prealbumin and albumin concentrations are observed in people with malnutrition, and they have been associated with a higher risk of morbidity and mortality in older adults [55]. Hence, it would be value-adding to include them as outcome measures in studies examining malnutrition.

9.4.4 *Acceptability of Food Fortification Strategies*

Narrative synthesis in this review found that while participants in both intervention and control groups rated high scores for the respective food received, there were no differences in findings as the acceptability scores of foods between the two groups were similar. This outcome is consistent with a review previously conducted by Mills *et al.* [30], where the acceptability of fortified food and standard food was similar, thus no meaningful finding could be drawn.

Acceptability of food is important in influencing the decision of older adults to adopt fortified food into mealtimes. By providing nutritious and appealing food, older adults are more likely to consume them regularly, promoting improved health outcomes [21]. Furthermore, two of the six studies which assessed the acceptability of food examined the factors that might influence participants' acceptance or rejection of fortified food. These studies employed readymade meals or meals-on-wheels services. Arjuna *et al.* [48] reported that participants were unlikely to accept meals-on-wheels if their families prepared the meals. Ziylan *et al.* [45] found that some participants would only utilise readymade meals if they preferred to cook for themselves. Overall, the affordability and convenience of these interventions are likely to influence participants' willingness to adopt them. However, since the intervention food and standard food in each study have high similarities, it is difficult to gauge if the acceptability of food is a considerable factor in influencing older adults' uptake of fortified food.

9.4.5 *Strengths and Limitations*

As of current knowledge, no studies conducted previously have investigated the effectiveness of food fortifications in preventing malnutrition in community-dwelling older adults. Previous systematic reviews had only conducted narrative synthesis, whereas this review also included meta-analyses which more comprehensively assessed the research questions.

This review also strived to include only RCTs to ensure the highest level of evidence to increase overall confidence in the results [33]. However, the limited number of available RCTs posed a challenge to meeting this goal. Nonetheless, the reviewers addressed this issue by including as many RCTs as possible, with only two of the included studies utilising a crossover design, while the remaining studies used an RCT design.

Furthermore, there were several other limitations present. Firstly, only English language studies were included due to the lack of translation resources and time constraints for translation. Such language bias can result in a biased summary of the evidence, leading to an overestimation or an underestimation of treatment effects, affecting the generalisability of the review's findings [56]. Secondly, the high heterogeneity present was likely attributed to the methodological differences between each study, including differences in intervention duration and types of intervention food. This can make it challenging to determine the true effect of food fortification when the studies are too distinct from each other [57]. Thirdly, the limited number of primary studies on this topic led to meta-analyses consisting of a small number of studies, potentially impacting the reliability and quality of the outcomes [58]. Lastly, there was no follow-up indicated in any of the studies, and the lack of continuation may limit the ability to assess long-term effects of food fortification [59].

9.4.6 *Recommendations for Future Practice and Research*

As the ageing population increases in many countries, including Singapore, food fortification may provide a viable means for older adults to enhance their nutritional status. Given Singapore's significant number of community-dwelling older adults, effective and practical strategies can be adopted through affordable and accessible methods such as meals-on-wheel services or readymade fortified foods. This was demonstrated in some of the primary studies included in this review. However, the presence of heterogeneity in the studies raises concerns regarding the true effect of food fortification, thus caution must be taken during implementation. Future research should aim to include more RCTs with larger sample sizes, as well as having follow-up measures to provide more robust evidence and to encourage continuous assessment of long-term outcomes. Furthermore, future studies could focus on providing a more standardised intervention food to avoid inconsistencies in findings.

9.4.7 *Summary*

Overall, this systematic review and meta-analysis have provided insightful findings on the effectiveness of food fortification in preventing malnutrition in community-dwelling older adults. The review showed a significant improvement in energy and nutrient intakes, highlighting the effectiveness of this approach. However, the quality of future research could be improved to reduce heterogeneity between studies. This would further strengthen the evidence for recommending fortified food adoption among older adults in the community to prevent malnutrition.

References

1. Chen Y, Michalak M, Agellon LB. Importance of nutrients and nutrient metabolism on human health. Yale J Biol Med. 2018;91(2):95–103.
2. DiMaria-Ghalili RA, Amella E. Nutrition in older adults: intervention and assessment can help curb the growing threat of malnutrition. Am J Nurs. 2005;105(3):40–50.
3. World Health Organization. Malnutrition [Internet]. Geneva: World Health Organization; 2021 Jun 9 [cited 2025 May 14]. Available from: https://www.who.int/news-room/fact-sheets/detail/malnutrition
4. United Nations High Commissioner for Refugees. Older persons [Internet]. Geneva: UNHCR; [cited 2025 May 14]. Available from: https://emergency.unhcr.org/entry/43935/olderpersons
5. Fávaro-Moreira NC, Krausch-Hofmann S, Matthys C, Vereecken C, Vanhauwaert E, Declercq A, *et al.* Risk factors for malnutrition in older adults: a systematic review of the literature based on longitudinal data. Adv Nutr. 2016;7(3):507–22.
6. Volkert D. Malnutrition in older adults — urgent need for action: a plea for improving the nutritional situation of older adults. Gerontology. 2013;59(4):328–33.
7. Li J, Theng YL, Foo S. Depression and psychosocial risk factors among community-dwelling older adults in Singapore. J Cross Cult Gerontol. 2015;30(4):409–22.
8. Wei K, Nyunt MSZ, Gao Q, Wee SL, Yap KB, Ng TP. Association of frailty and malnutrition with long-term functional and mortality outcomes among community-dwelling older adults. JAMA Netw Open. 2018;1(3):e180650.
9. Amarya S, Singh K, Sabharwal M. Changes during aging and their association with malnutrition. J Clin Gerontol Geriatr. 2015;6(3):78–84.
10. Norman K, Haß U, Pirlich M. Malnutrition in older adults — recent advances and remaining challenges. Nutrients. 2021;13(8):2764.
11. Posthauer ME. The role of nutrition in wound care. Adv Skin Wound Care. 2012;25(2):62–3.
12. Khor PY, Vearing RM, Charlton KE. The effectiveness of nutrition interventions in improving frailty and its associated constructs related to malnutrition and

functional decline among community-dwelling older adults: a systematic review. J Hum Nutr Diet. 2021;35(3):566–82.

13. Lester S, Kleijn M, Cornacchia L, Hewson L, Taylor MA, Fisk I. Factors affecting adherence, intake, and perceived palatability of oral nutritional supplements: a literature review. J Nutr Health Aging. 2022;26(7):663–74.
14. Nieuwenhuizen WF, Weenen H, Rigby P, Hetherington MM. Older adults and patients in need of nutritional support: review of current treatment options and factors influencing nutritional intake. Clin Nutr. 2010;29(2):160–9.
15. Poscia A, Milovanovic S, La Milia DI, Duplaga M, Grysztar M, Landi F, *et al.* Effectiveness of nutritional interventions addressed to elderly persons: umbrella systematic review with meta-analysis. Eur J Public Health. 2017;28(2):275–83.
16. World Health Organization. Food fortification [Internet]. Geneva: World Health Organization; [cited 2025 May 14]. Available from: https://www.who.int/health-topics/food-fortification#tab=tab_1
17. Aa M. The role of fortification and supplementation in mitigating the 'hidden hunger.' J Nutr Food Sci. 2016;6(1).
18. Chadare FJ, Idohou R, Nago E, Affonfere M, Agossadou J, Fassinou TK, *et al.* Conventional and food-to-food fortification: an appraisal of past practices and lessons learned. Food Sci Nutr. 2019;7(9):2781–95.
19. Olson R, Gavin-Smith B, Ferraboschi C, Kraemer K. Food fortification: the advantages, disadvantages and lessons from Sight and Life programs. Nutrients. 2021;13(4):1118.
20. Mkambula P, Mbuya MN, Rowe LA, Sablah M, Friesen VM, Chadha M, *et al.* The unfinished agenda for food fortification in low- and middle-income countries: quantifying progress, gaps and potential opportunities. Nutrients. 2020;12(2):354.
21. van der Zanden LDT, van Kleef E, de Wijk RA, van Trijp HCM. Knowledge, perceptions and preferences of elderly regarding protein-enriched functional food. Appetite. 2014;80:16–22.
22. Mathewson SL, Azevedo PS, Gordon AL, Phillips BE, Greig CA. Overcoming protein-energy malnutrition in older adults in the residential care setting: a narrative review of causes and interventions. Ageing Res Rev. 2021;70:101401.
23. Kaiser MJ, Bauer JM, Ramsch C, Uter W, Guigoz Y, Cederholm T, *et al.* Validation of the Mini Nutritional Assessment Short-form (MNA®-SF): a practical tool for identification of nutritional status. J Nutr Health Aging. 2009;13(9):782–8.
24. Sánchez-García S, García-Peña C, Duque-López MX, Juárez-Cedillo T, Cortés-Núñez AR, Reyes-Beaman S. Anthropometric measures and nutritional status in a healthy elderly population. BMC Public Health. 2007;7:2.

25. Zhang Z, Pereira S, Luo M, Matheson E. Evaluation of blood biomarkers associated with risk of malnutrition in older adults: a systematic review and meta-analysis. Nutrients. 2017;9(8):829.
26. Morilla-Herrera JC, Martín-Santos FJ, Caro-Bautista J, Saucedo-Figueredo C, García-Mayor S, Morales-Asencio JM. Effectiveness of food-based fortification in older people: a systematic review and meta-analysis. J Nutr Health Aging. 2015;20(2):178–84.
27. Sossen L, Bonham M, Porter J. Can fortified, nutrient-dense and enriched foods and drink-based nutrition interventions increase energy and protein intake in residential aged care residents? A systematic review with meta-analyses. Int J Nurs Stud. 2021;124:104088.
28. Cave DP, Abbey KL, Capra SM. Can foodservices in aged care homes deliver sustainable food fortification strategies? A review. Int J Food Sci Nutr. 2019;71(3):267–75.
29. Douglas JW, Lawrence JC, Knowlden AP. The use of fortified foods to treat malnutrition among older adults: a systematic review. Qual Ageing Older Adults. 2017;18(2):104–19.
30. Mills SR, Wilcox CR, Ibrahim K, Roberts HC. Can fortified foods and snacks increase the energy and protein intake of hospitalised older patients? A systematic review. J Hum Nutr Diet. 2018;31(3):379–89.
31. Trabal J, Farran-Codina A. Effects of dietary enrichment with conventional foods on energy and protein intake in older adults: a systematic review. Nutr Rev. 2015;73(9):624–33.
32. Patsopoulos NA, Ioannidis JPA. The use of older studies in meta-analyses of medical interventions: a survey. Open Med. 2009;3(2):62–8.
33. Glasofer A, Townsend AB. Determining the level of evidence. Nurs Crit Care. 2019;14(6):22–5.
34. Page MJ, McKenzie JE, Bossuyt PM, Boutron I, Hoffmann TC, Mulrow CD, *et al.* The PRISMA 2020 statement: an updated guideline for reporting systematic reviews. Int J Surg. 2021;88:105906.
35. Aromataris E, Riitano D. Constructing a search strategy and searching for evidence. Am J Nurs. 2014;114(5):49–56.
36. McGowan J, Sampson M, Salzwedel DM, Cogo E, Foerster V, Lefebvre C. PRESS peer review of electronic search strategies: 2015 guideline statement. J Clin Epidemiol. 2016;75:40–6.
37. Lefebvre C, Glanville J, Briscoe S, Littlewood A, Marshall C, Metzendorf MI, *et al.* Searching for and selecting studies. In: Higgins JPT, Thomas J, Chandler J, Cumpston M, Li T, Page MJ, *et al.*, editors. Cochrane Handbook for Systematic

Reviews of Interventions. Version 6.0. Chichester (UK): John Wiley & Sons; 2019. p. 67–107.

38. Review Manager (RevMan) [Computer program]. Version 5.4. Copenhagen: The Cochrane Collaboration; 2020.
39. GRADEpro Guideline Development Tool [Internet]. McMaster University and Evidence Prime; 2022 [cited 2025 May 14]. Available from: https://gradepro.org
40. Deeks JJ, Higgins JPT, Altman DG. Analysing data and undertaking meta-analyses. In: Higgins JPT, Thomas J, Chandler J, Cumpston M, Li T, Page MJ, *et al.*, editors. Cochrane Handbook for Systematic Reviews of Interventions. Version 6.0. Chichester (UK): John Wiley & Sons; 2019. p. 241–84.
41. Thabane L, Mbuagbaw L, Zhang S, Samaan Z, Marcucci M, Ye C, *et al.* A tutorial on sensitivity analyses in clinical trials: the what, why, when and how. BMC Med Res Methodol. 2013;13(1):92.
42. Borkent JW, Beelen J, Linschooten JO, Roodenburg AJ, de van der Schueren MA. The CONSUMEER study: a randomised trial towards the effectiveness of protein-rich ready-made meals and protein-rich dairy products in increasing protein intake of community-dwelling older adults after switching from self-prepared meals towards ready-made meals. J Nutr Sci. 2019;8:e27.
43. Van Til AJ, Naumann E, Cox-Claessens IJ, Kremer S, Boelsma E, de van der Schueren MA. Effects of the daily consumption of protein enriched bread and protein enriched drinking yoghurt on the total protein intake in older adults in a rehabilitation centre: a single blind randomised controlled trial. J Nutr Health Aging. 2015;19(5):525–30.
44. Ziylan C, Kremer S, Eerens J, Haveman-Nies A, de Groot LCPGM. Effect of meal size reduction and protein enrichment on intake and satiety in vital community-dwelling older adults. Appetite. 2016;105:242–8.
45. Ziylan C, Haveman-Nies A, Kremer S, de Groot LCPGM. Protein-enriched bread and readymade meals increase community-dwelling older adults' protein intake in a double-blind randomized controlled trial. J Am Med Dir Assoc. 2017;18(2):145–51.
46. Chanwikrai Y, Wangrath J, Techangam S, Pachotikarn C, Yamamoto S. Energy rich snacks may be preferable to lunch with high lipid to increase energy intakes in older adults at risk of malnutrition, Northern Thailand. Asian J Diet. 2021;3(2):49–54.
47. Chanwikrai Y, Wungrath J, Techangam S, Pachotikarn C, Yamamoto S. Frequent snacks improved energy intake and nutritional status in community-dwelling older adults at risk of malnutrition, Chiang Mai, Thailand. J Educ Community Health. 2022;9(1):11–7.

48. Arjuna T, Miller M, Ueno T, Visvanathan R, Lange K, Soenen S, *et al.* Food services using energy- and protein-fortified meals to assist vulnerable community-residing older adults meet their dietary requirements and maintain good health and quality of life: findings from a pilot study. Geriatrics. 2018;3(3):60.
49. Leslie WS, Woodward M, Lean ME, Theobald H, Watson L, Hankey CR. Improving the dietary intake of undernourished older people in residential care homes using an energy-enriching food approach: a cluster randomised controlled study. J Hum Nutr Diet. 2012;26(4):387–94.
50. Nykänen I, Törrönen R, Schwab U. Dairy-based and energy-enriched berry-based snacks improve or maintain nutritional and functional status in older people in home care. J Nutr Health Aging. 2018;22(10):1205–10.
51. Fatmah. The effect of potato almond orange cookies on their weight, BMI, hemoglobin, and lymphocyte status of undernourished older people during COVID-19 pandemic. Curr Nutr Food Sci. 2021;17(7):753–63.
52. Van Wymelbeke V, Brondel L, Bon F, Martin-Pfitzenmeyer I, Manckoundia P. An innovative brioche enriched in protein and energy improves the nutritional status of malnourished nursing home residents compared to oral nutritional supplement and usual breakfast: Farine+ project. Clin Nutr ESPEN. 2016;15: 93–100.
53. Alabdulkarim B, Bakeet ZA, Arzoo S. Role of some functional lipids in preventing diseases and promoting health. J King Saud Univ Sci. 2012;24(4):319–29.
54. Keller U. Nutritional laboratory markers in malnutrition. J Clin Med. 2019;8(6):775.
55. Cabrerizo S, Cuadras D, Gomez-Busto F, Artaza-Artabe I, Marín-Ciancas F, Malafarina V. Serum albumin and health in older people: review and meta-analysis. Maturitas. 2015;81(1):17–27.
56. Jackson JL, Kuriyama A. How often do systematic reviews exclude articles not published in English? J Gen Intern Med. 2019;34(8):1388–9.
57. Melsen WG, Bootsma MCJ, Rovers MM, Bonten MJM. The effects of clinical and statistical heterogeneity on the predictive values of results from meta-analyses. Clin Microbiol Infect. 2014;20(2):123–9.
58. Møller AM, Myles PS. What makes a good systematic review and meta-analysis? Br J Anaesth. 2016;117(4):428–30.
59. Cuzick J. The importance of long-term follow up of participants in clinical trials. Br J Cancer. 2022;128(3):432–8.

https://doi.org/10.1142/9789819817320_0010

Chapter 10*

Efficacy of a Symptom Self-Management Program Delivered Via Virtual Reality Headset and Face-to-Face on Inpatients Post-Acute Myocardial Infarction: A Pilot Randomised Controlled Trial

Piyanee Klainin-Yobas[1,*], Lian Kwang Tang[2], Karen Wei Ling Koh[3], Anand Adinath Ambhore[3], Ping Chai[3], and Ying Lau[1]

[1]*Alice Lee Centre for Nursing Studies, Yong Loo Lin School of Medicine, National University of Singapore, Level 5, Centre of Translational Medicine, Block MD6, 14 Medical Drive, Singapore 117599*

[2]*Raffles Hospital, 585 North Bridge Road, Singapore 188770*

[3]*National University Hospital, 5 Lower Kent Ridge Road, Main Building 1, CCU, Singapore 119074*

**Corresponding author: nurpk@nus.edu.sg*

10.1 Introduction

More than 17 million people worldwide experience cardiovascular disease each year [1]. The Western Pacific region (such as Australia and New Zealand) has the highest mortality from cardiovascular disease, followed by European, Eastern Mediterranean, America, Africa, and Southeast Asia [2]. Cardiovascular disease has various forms such as ischemic heart disease (insufficient blood supply to the heart muscle due to narrowed or obstructed coronary arteries), cerebrovascular disease (insufficient

* Appendices to this chapter are available for download at https://www.worldscientific.com/worldscibooks/10.1142/14420#t=suppl.

blood supply to the brain due to blockage or rupture of a blood vessel), congestive heart failure (inability of the heart to produce sufficient blood supply to the body), among others [3]. Of which, the top cause of death is ischemic heart disease resulting in acute myocardial infarction (AMI or heart attack) [4]. In Singapore, ischemic heart disease is the third leading cause of hospitalisation and mortality (18.8%) in 2019. The incidence of AMI has significantly increased from 6,817 cases in 2007 (the crude incidence rate of 234.7 per 100,000 population) to 11,887 cases in 2018 (349.3 per 100,000 population) [4].

AMI reflects irreversible damages to the heart muscle resulting from diminished blood supply to the heart [5]. AMI would be diagnosed if at least two of the following criteria are present: (a) ischemic symptom, (b) electrocardiographic ST segment changes, (c) pathological Q wave on the electrocardiogram, and (d) abnormality of the regional wall motion [5]. People experiencing AMI report severe and diffuse chest pain, which may radiate to arms, jaws and back [6]. Such pain is not mitigated by pain medications. Patients may report associating symptoms, encompassing eructation, retrosternal burning, vomiting, sweating and breathlessness [6]. Evidence suggests that stressful life, diabetes, hypertension, hypercholesterolemia, smoking, and alcohol consumption increase the risk of developing AMI [7]. Studies show that patients post-AMI reported the lowest quality of life in the first week after an AMI episode [8]. Subsequently, all quality of life domains (physical, psychological and social) improved over time [7]. Low quality of life is linked with many variables including the feeling of shock after receiving the AMI diagnosis, fatigue [9], loss of job [10], loss of income [10], and changes in social and family life [9].

Stress refers to non-specific physiological or psychological responses of the body to noxious stimuli from the environment [11]. A vicious cycle between stress and AMI is observed. On the one hand, stress may contribute to the development of AMI [12], medical complications (such as obesity, hypertension and diabetes), harmful lifestyle (such as smoking) and psychological symptoms (such as depression) [12]. Financial stress is linked with worse AMI symptoms at baseline, worse clinical outcomes during a recovery period, higher risk of rehospitalisation at one-year post-discharge, and higher mortality risk at four years [13]. Furthermore, extreme stress such as natural disasters could trigger the occurrence of AMI. Research in New Zealand suggests a significant increase in hospital admissions of AMI cases in the first two weeks following the Christchurch earthquakes [14]. On the other hand, AMI may traumatise the patients with life-threatening and unpredictable conditions, and thus increase their stress levels. Evidence shows that post-AMI patients with moderate/high perceived stress had increased risks of mortality and poorer health outcomes, including increased angina, more physical limitations due to angina, lower quality of life, and poorer mental health status [12]. Gender difference was observed whereby women reported significantly higher perceived stress during a 12-month period post-AMI than their male counterpart [15]. Moreover, post-AMI stress is linked with other psychological symptoms including depression and anxiety [16].

Depression is characterised by persistent depressed mood, anhedonia, changes in body weight, sleep problems, fatigue, poor concentration, feeling of guilt and suicidal ideation [17]. Anxiety is manifested by persistent and excessive worry about various things accompanied by such physical symptoms as restlessness, fatigue, poor concentration, muscle aches and sleep problems [17]. AMI may play a major role in the occurrence of depression and anxiety. Research shows the prevalence of depression as 26% during hospitalisation, and that number becomes 38% and 37% at four months and 12 months respectively [16]. The risk of suicidal thought was increased during the first month of AMI conditions [18]. Furthermore, the prevalence of anxiety is in the range of 24–31% among patients post-AMI [16]. Additionally, anxiety may trigger the next episode of AMI. Specifically, anxiety is linked with decreased vagal tone and increased sympathetic activity, which lead to diminished heart rate variability. Anxiety is also associated with imbalanced platelet activity, which may trigger thrombus foundation and another AMI attack [16]. There is a need to help patients post-AMI manage their stress, depression and anxiety more effectively.

Symptom self-management refers to an individual's ability to use their cognitive and behavioural efforts to regulate symptoms resulting from AMI such as chest pain, stress and anxiety [19]. To our knowledge, there are limited studies examining symptom self-management interventions for people post-AMI. However, a systematic review involving 18 studies suggested that face-to-face psychosocial interventions improved stress and anxiety among people with cardiovascular diseases [20]. Additionally, a pilot randomised controlled trial was conducted on inpatients with ischemic heart disease in Singapore [21]. In this study, a control group (n = 13) received only standard care while an intervention group (n = 12) received standard care and the psychoeducation program delivered through a face-to-face method. Each intervention session contained psychoeducation (stress, anxiety and depression) and relaxation therapy (guided by a 20-minute relaxation CD). Results suggested that the face-to-face psychosocial intervention had the potential to improve anxiety, depression and perceived relaxation [21]. Nevertheless, such a small sample size impeded the generalisability of the findings.

Virtual reality (VR) is a set of technologies comprising graphical presentations, sounds, and synthesised forces/sensations that generate a convincing interface where an individual is immersed in an interactive virtual world [22]. VR has two major components: immersion and presence. The former signifies how the technical aspects (such as visual, audio and tactile sensations) are offered to generate illusions of reality [22]. The latter reflects a subjective psychological state and indicates how the users are absorbed in the virtual world and respond physically and emotionally to it like being in the actual place [22]. VR technology that can generate immersive virtual environments encompasses VR cave (multiple projection screens creating 360-degree VR reality), head-mounted display (HMD: images projected directly to users' eyes), sensors (motion-tracking device), and haptics (creating a sense of touch) [22]. Thus far, the applications of VR are observed in gaming, training, basic science, healthcare, and e-commerce (such as online shopping) [18].

The first immersive HMD for VR (HMD-VR) was invented in 1968 [23]. The device was later modified and it has become more portable, affordable and desirable [23]. A scoping review involving 21 studies suggested that HMD-VR can be used to deliver interventions for patients with stroke, spinal cord injuries, and congenital limb deficiency [24]. Furthermore, the HMD-VR was used for the assessment for Parkinson's disease vestibular impairment and balance, and cervical range of motion [24]. It is concluded that the HMD-VR increased participants' motivation, concentration and engagement during the intervention periods [24]. Another systematic review involving 27 studies indicated that HMD-VR were effective in delivering education for healthcare providers, including medical students [25]. The HMD-VR appeared to be salient, motivating, engaging, and non-inferior to a face-to-face traditional method of teaching [24]. Nevertheless, it is unclear if the non-immersive HMD will produce similar positive effects for the assessment, intervention and education domains.

Thus far, there is limited evidence on the effectiveness of face-to-face symptom self-management programs for people post-AMI. Furthermore, it is unknown if non-immersive HMD (such as SONY Headset) can be used to deliver self-management programs for people post-AMI. Moreover, it is inconclusive if self-management programs would reduce psychological symptoms (stress, anxiety, and depression) associated with the occurrence of AMI. Consequently, we developed a two-session symptom self-management program that can be delivered via a VR screen (IManage-HSet) and traditional face-to-face method (IManage-FF). Contents of the interventions were adapted from the previous systematic review concerning other psychosocial interventions [19] and pilot RCT conducted in Singapore [21]. Both IManage-HSet and IManage-FF had the same education contents with two sessions: (a) stress and stress management and (b) emotion and emotion management. This study aimed to evaluate the two programs on people post-AMI. Research questions are:

1. In comparison with a control group, will the symptom self-management program delivered via SONY headset (IManage-HSet) enhance participants' knowledge, perceived relaxation and satisfaction, while reducing objective stress, subjective stress, anxiety and depression?
2. In relation to the control group, will the symptom self-management program delivered face-to-face (IManage-FF) increase participants' knowledge, perceived relaxation and satisfaction, while decreasing objective stress, subjective stress, anxiety and depression?

10.2 Methods

10.2.1 *Research Design*

This study was a single-centre, randomised controlled trial using three arms in a 1:1:1 ratio. Participants were randomly allocated to one of these groups: (a) IManage-HSet (intervention), (b) IManage-FF (intervention), and (c) control group (Figure 10.1). A random allocation list was generated using Microsoft Excel. The allocation list was concealed from other researchers until the recruited participants completed baseline measurements. All participants were assigned a unique ID sequentially according to order of entry to the study. After the baseline assessment, they were allocated to the group that contained the number that matched their ID.

The randomisation and allocation concealment were used to prevent selection bias [26]. Participants were aware of the group allocation. However, we asked them not to reveal any research information with other patients. Note that all patients were in a private room and they were less likely to communicate with each other. All healthcare providers in the hospital were blinded to the group allocation. However, research

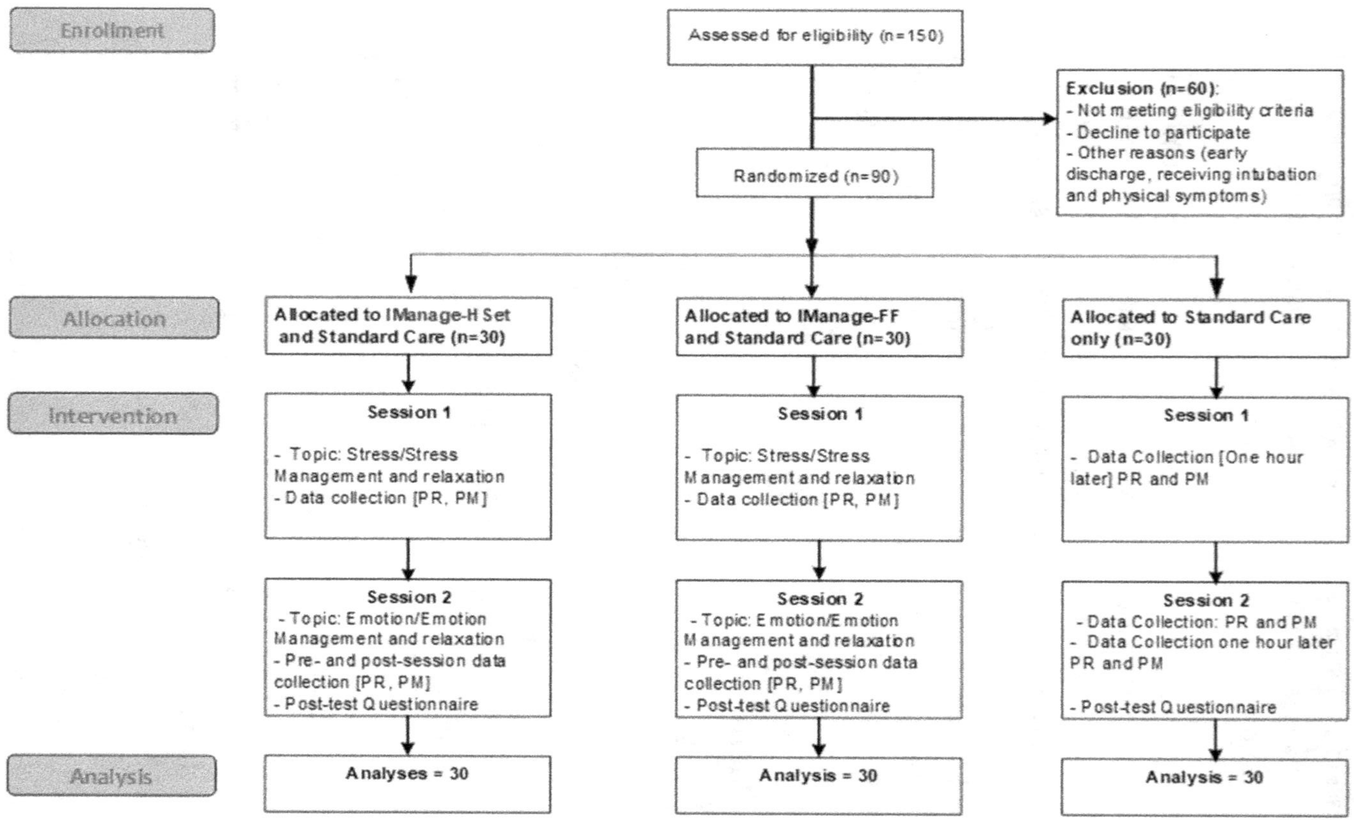

Figure 10.1 Modified CONSORT diagram.

Note: PR: perceived relaxation scale; PM: physiological measures of objective stress (blood pressure, heart rate, skin temperature).

staff were not blinded as they had to coordinate with hospital staff and deliver the interventions.

10.2.2 *Participants*

A target population included adults post-AMI who were hospitalised at a cardiac care unit in a tertiary hospital in Singapore. A convenience sample was used to recruit potential participants. Eligibility criteria encompassed adult inpatients who: (a) were aged 21–65 years, (b) had a diagnosis of AMI by their physician, and (c) were able to communicate in English. Participants were excluded if they had severe complications such as congestive heart failure, unstable angina, uncontrolled arrhythmia, and severe hypertension with blood pressure more than 200/120 mmHg. Those with a confirmed diagnosis of mental disorders such as schizophrenia and mood disorders were also excluded. These conditions were excluded as they might affect study outcomes or add more stress to the participants.

Power analysis for repeated measure of variance was used to estimate a sample size for this study [27]. The following elements were required: correlations among study variables ranging from 0.50 to 0.75, type-I error (α) = 0.05, type II error (β) = 0.2, the number of pre-measurement measures = 7, and the number of post-measurement measures = 7. Taken all together, an adequate sample size for each group would be at least 20 [27]. However, to account for possible attrition, 30 participants were recruited for each group, making a total sample size of 90.

10.2.3 *Intervention*

Participants in the intervention groups received standard care plus IManage-VR or IManage-FF programs. The control group received only standard care.

The IManage-HSet program entailed two one-hour individual-based symptom self-management sessions delivered on two consecutive

Table 10.1 Outline of the IManage-HSet program (two daily sessions).

Session	Topics	Activities
0 (One hour)	**Standard Care** — Education about AMI and management of AMI (such as including medication adherence, healthy diet, and exercise)	— A single-session, individual-based, one-hour education session
1 (One hour)	**The IManage-HSet programme: Stress and Stress Management** — Education component — Practice of relaxation techniques	— Education video #1: Stress-Demolishing Room — Relaxation video #1: Escape–A Fantastic Journey to Relaxation
2 (One hour)	**The IManage-HSet programme: Emotion and Emotion Management** — Education component — Practice of relaxation techniques	— Education video #2: Emotion Wellness Room — Relaxation video #2: Escape–A Fantastic Journey to Relaxation

days (Table 10.1). This program, delivered via a headset device, comprised an educational component and practice of relaxation techniques. Participants sat or lied down in a comfortable position while wearing the headset, SONY HMZ-T2 [28].

The SONY HMZ-T2 is a light device with an adjustable headband with attaching earbuds. With this headset, a user can watch 3D movies with a big-screen cinematic experience, play 3D games and hear sound effects produced by the virtual-phone technology [28]. Conventionally, the headset is used for entertainment purposes. In this study, we utilised the headset as a delivery method for the symptom self-management intervention and expected that the device would enhance learning experiences. Although a non-interactive mode was used in our study, this headset offered a high-definition screen (1280 × 720) and allowed vivid video experiences with virtual surround sound [26]. It was also expected that participants would engage in pleasant learning experiences without environmental distractions.

During the Stress and Stress Management session (session 1), participants viewed an education video, **Stress Demolishing Room**, via the headset SONY HMZ-T2. To make the education more interesting, the video was presented as a story, where a student nurse spoke to a viewer and described information regarding AMI, its treatments, stress and available strategies to manage stress. Case scenarios, stories, images and video clips were also presented. Subsequently, the participants viewed two relaxation videos (A Fantastic Journey to Relaxation, Tracks A and B) to guide their practice on abdominal breathing and muscle relaxation. The abdominal breathing track contained beach-themed images while the muscle relaxation track showed meadow, mountain and rain forest images. A soothing female narrator was also presented with calming music.

During the Emotion and Emotion Management education (session 2), participants watched an education video, **Emotional Wellness Room**. This video was presented as a scenario where a nurse and a patient with post-AMI have a conversation about emotions, emotional problems (anxiety and depression) and possible strategies to manage the emotional problems. Case scenarios, images and video clips were also used to maximise the learning process. Subsequently, participants watched three short videos (via the headset) to guide relaxation practice. The videos encompassed abdominal breathing, A Fantastic Trip to Japan (images concerning vibrant flowers and colourful gardens), and A Relaxation Trip to Bhutan: A Land of Happiness (images about nature, mountain landscape, and river valley). Note that we created the relaxation videos (a fantastic journey to relaxation) to use for this research (Supplementary file: Appendix B). Some images of the education videos are illustrated in Supplementary file: Appendix A.

The IManage-FF Program is a two one-hour individual-based symptom self-management intervention delivered on two consecutive

Table 10.2 Outline of the IManage-FF program (two daily sessions).

Session	Topics	Activities
0 (One hour)	**Standard Care** — Education about AMI and management of AMI (such as including medication adherence, healthy diet, and exercise)	— A single-session, individual-based, one-hour education session
1 (One hour)	**The IManage-FF programme: Stress and Stress Management** — Education component — Practice of relaxation techniques	— Conventional face-to-face discussion — Audio relaxation CD
2 (One hour)	**The IManage-FF programme: Emotion and Emotion Management** — Education component — Practice of relaxation techniques	— Conventional face-to-face discussion — Audio relaxation CD

days. It contained two major components: education and the practice of relaxation techniques (Table 10.2). However, this program was delivered using a conventional face-to-face method. The first session delivered knowledge concerning stress and stress management. Then, participants practiced abdominal breathing and muscle relaxation guided by audio-tape instruction (relaxation CD). The second session covered information regarding emotion and emotion management. Depression and anxiety were included. Similar to session 1, participants practiced abdominal breathing and muscle relaxations using a relaxation CD.

Both IManage-HSet and IManage-FF interventions were delivered in a private room in the cardiac care unit by two researchers (a student nurse and registered nurse). Before delivering the interventions, both researchers received two training sessions conducted by the first author to ensure standardisation of the intervention procedures. Participants in both groups received an education booklet (containing knowledge imparted during the programs) (Appendix C). This booklet might help maximise outcomes as participants would be able to review materials at their convenience.

Standard care included usual evidence-based treatments and services provided by the study hospital. All patients in the cardiac care unit also received a single-session, individual-based, one-hour patient education. This session taught patients about AMI and management of AMI (such as healthy diet and exercise). Clinical staff at the cardiac care unit delivered the patient education and they were blinded to participants' group allocation.

10.2.4 *Measurements*

Objective stress was measured by bio-physiological instruments. Heart rate was assessed in beats/min and blood pressure was measured in mmHg. Skin temperature was measured by Stress Thermometer TM #SC911 [29], in which lower skin temperature reflects a higher level of objective stress. An electrode of the stress thermometer was placed at the participant's fingertip for one minute. Validity of the stress thermometer was established among inpatients in Singapore [30].

Subjective stress, anxiety, and depression were measured with corresponding subscales of the Depression, Anxiety, and Stress scale [31]. Each subscale has seven items with four response categories ranging from 0 (did not apply to me at all) to 3 (applied to me most of the time). Possible scores of each subscale are in the range of 0–21 with higher scores indicating higher stress (anxiety or depression) levels. Cronbach's alphas of the stress (0.86–0.90), anxiety subscale (0.86–0.90), and depression (0.82–0.90) are in acceptable ranges [32].

Perceived relaxation was measured by the perceived relaxation scale [33]. Participants rated their relaxation level on a single-item Numeric Rating Scale: a 10-centimeter continuum line starting from "0" (very tensed) to "10" (very relaxed). Validity of the perceived relaxation scale was established in previous research on people with cardiovascular disease in Singapore [33].

Knowledge was measured by the six-item IManage knowledge scale developed by the researchers. Two sets of items (three items each) were determined by contents taught in the IManage programs. The first set tested knowledge concerning stress and stress management strategies and it was administered before and after intervention session one. Another set, addressing knowledge about emotion and emotion management, was administered before and after intervention session two. Respondents answered 1 (True) or 0 (False) and a total score would add to 3 for each set of items.

Patient satisfaction was measured by the four-item satisfaction with the IManage program scale developed by the researchers. The scale captures how respondents were satisfied with the overall programs, contents, education materials and relaxation practice. They responded on five categories from 1 (very dissatisfied) to 5 (very satisfied) and they also provided qualitative feedback for the programs.

10.2.5 *Statistical Analysis*

We entered all research data into IBM SPSS Statistics 26.0 and then verified the accuracy of data entry by two researchers. The intent-to-treat principles were used to guide the data analyses and all of them were two-tailed with a significance level at $\alpha = 0.05$. Univariate analyses were performed to explore study variables and respondents' characteristics. Chi-square (χ^2) tests were used to test if there were significant differences in the respondent characteristics across the three groups. Efficacy of the interventions was evaluated by using changes of variable scores from baseline to each post-intervention assessment. Descriptive statistics was used to analyse patient satisfaction and content analyses were used to summarise qualitative data. Analysis of variance was used to compare changed scores of subjective stress, depression, anxiety, and knowledge across the three groups. Repeated measure analysis of variance was to analyse perceived relaxation, skin temperature, heart rate, and blood pressure. Partial eta square (Partial η^2) was used to determine an effect size of the interventions. The value of Partial η^2

0.01, 0.06, and 0.14 would be interpreted as small, medium and large effect size respectively [34].

10.2.6 *Ethical Considerations*

This research received ethical approval from the Domain Specific Review Board of the study hospital (Ref: 00801, RCB No: 200002150H). The researchers approached eligible patients at their bedside, provided details of this research, distributed a patient information sheet, answered questions that they might have and requested their participation. The researchers also emphasised that participation in this study would be voluntary and their information would be kept strictly confidential. All interested participants were asked to sign a written consent form before partaking in this study.

10.3 Results

10.3.1 *Participant Characteristics*

In total, 150 inpatients were assessed for eligibility, 90 of which fulfilled the inclusion criteria and were randomly assigned to IManage-HSet (n = 30), IMnange-FF (n = 30), and control group (n = 30) (Figure 10.1). Participants' age ranged from 21 to 65 years with an average of 51 years (standard deviation (SD) = 8.68). They were predominantly male, Singaporean citizens, and married (Table 10.3). A significant difference in marital status was observed ($\chi^2 = 12.77$, $p < 0.01$) where there were more singles in the IManage-HSet group and more divorcees in the IManage-FF group. Nevertheless, there were no significant differences in gender, education, nationality, ethnic groups, and religions across the three groups.

10.3.2 *Efficacy of the IManage Interventions*

10.3.2.1 *Knowledge*

Knowledge was measured twice at the end of intervention sessions 1 and 2. Mean scores and SD for knowledge are displayed in Table 10.4.

Table 10.3 Demographic information of study participants.

Variables	IManage-HSet n(%)	IManage-FF n(%)	Control group n(%)	Chi-square (df)
Gender				
— Male	29(96.70)	28(93.30)	29(96.7)	0.52 (2)
— Female	1(3.30)	2(6.70)	1(3.30)	
Education				
— Primary school	5(16.70)	7(23.30)	8(26.70)	4.38 (12)
— Secondary school	10(33.30)	13(43.30)	13(43.30)	
— Junior college	1(3.30)	1(3.30)	1(3.30)	
— Polytechnic	5(16.70)	3(10.00)	4(13.30)	
— University	3(10.00)	4(13.30)	3(10.00)	
— Postgraduate	2(6.70)	1(3.30)	—	
— Others	4(13.30)	1(3.30)	1(3.30)	
Nationality				
— Singaporean	23(76.70)	24(80.00)	26(86.70)	0.49 (2)
— Others	7(23.30)	6(20.00)	4(13.30)	
Ethnic group				
— Chinese	10(33.30)	12(40.00)	14(46.70)	3.14 (6)
— Malay	10(33.30)	9(30.00)	8(26.70)	
— Indian	8(26.70)	9(30.00)	7(23.30)	
— Others	2(6.70)	—	1(3.30)	
Marital status				
— Married	23(76.70)	26(86.70)	28(93.30)	12.77 (4)**
— Divorced	—	4(13.30)	1(3.30)	
— Single	5(16.70)	—	1(3.30)	
— Missing	2(6.70)	—	—	
Religion				
— Buddhism	4(13.30)	11(36.70)	9(30.00)	5.82 (8)
— Christianity	2(6.70)	1(3.30)	2(6.70)	
— Hinduism	7(23.30)	7(23.30)	6(20.00)	
— Islam	11(36.70)	10(33.30)	11(36.70)	
— Others	6(20.00)	1(3.30)	2(6.70)	

Note: ** = Significance at 0.01 level.

Knowledge scores concerning stress and stress management (session 1) for the IManage-HSet (Mean = 3.00, SD = 0.00) and IManage-FF (Mean = 2.90, SD = 0.40) were significantly higher than those in the control group (Mean = 1.90, SD = 0.55) with a large effect size (Partial $\eta^2 = 0.62$). Furthermore, knowledge scores regarding emotion and emotion management (session 2) for the IManage-HSet (Mean = 3.00, SD = 0.00) and IManage-FF (Mean = 3.00, SD = 0.00) were significantly higher than those in the control group (Mean = 0.67, SD = 1.12) with a large effect size (Partial $\eta^2 = 0.75$).

10.3.2.2 *Subjective Stress, Depression and Anxiety*

Subjective stress, depression and anxiety were measured twice at baseline and the end of intervention session 2. Changed scores are displayed in Table 10.4. The IManage-HSet group had higher changed scores on all three variables than the IManage-FF and control groups. Nonetheless, the changes did not achieve statistical significance. Effect sizes were small for subjective stress (Partial $\eta^2 = 0.04$), depression (Partial $\eta^2 = 0.01$), and anxiety (Partial $\eta^2 = 0.03$).

10.3.2.3 *Objective Stress*

To capture immediate changes, all measures of objective stress were measured before and after each intervention session, making a total of four assessment points (Table 10.5). At session 1, changed scores in skin temperature for the IManage-HSet (changed scores = 0.43, SD = 1.48, $p = 0.01$) and IManage-FF group (changed scores = 0.57, SD = 1.59, $p = 0.00$) were significantly higher than that of the control group (changed scores = −0.99, SD = 2.18). A strong effect size was reported (Partial $\eta^2 = 0.14$). These findings suggested that both intervention groups had lower objective stress than the control. At session 2, changed scores for the IManage-HSet (changed scores = 0.55, SD = 1.39, $p = 0.76$) and IManage-FF groups (changed scores = 1.29, SD = 2.14, $p = 0.07$) were higher than that of the control group (changed scores = 0.21, SD = 1.69). A medium effect size

Table 10.4 Comparisons of changed scores of study variables.

Variables	Session 1 (Pre-intervention)		Session 2 (Post-intervention)		Changed score (Time 1-2)		Partial η^2 (p-value)
	Mean	**SD**	**Mean**	**SD**	**Mean**	**SD**	
Subjective Stress							**0.04**
— Control	4.53	3.10	2.77	3.04	1.77	3.05	—
— IManage-FF	5.40	3.92	2.23	3.63	3.17	3.07	(0.33)
— IManage-HSet	5.60	3.99	2.34	3.25	3.57	3.64	(0.16)
Depression							**0.01**
— Control	2.87	2.74	1.23	1.85	1.63	2.06	—
— IManage-FF	2.43	2.93	1.23	3.06	1.20	2.02	(0.87)
— IManage-HSet	4.16	4.47	2.07	3.49	2.10	4.57	(0.85)
Anxiety							**0.03**
— Control	3.10	3.49	2.26	3.11	0.83	2.35	—
— IManage-FF	3.87	3.43	2.13	3.57	1.73	2.80	(0.55)
— IManage-HSet	4.23	4.03	1.97	3.17	2.27	4.14	(0.23)
					Mean	**SD**	**Partial η^2 (p-value)**
Knowledge Time 1							**0.62**
— Control	—	—	—	—	1.90	0.55	**(0.000)**
— IManage-FF	—	—	—	—	2.90	0.40	
— IManage-HSet	—	—	—	—	3.00	0.00	
Knowledge Time 2							**0.75**
— Control	—	—	—	—	0.67	1.12	**(0.000)**
— IManage-FF	—	—	—	—	3.00	0.00	
— IManage-HSet	—	—	—	—	3.00	0.00	

Note: The Post-Hoc test used the control group as a reference group.

Table 10.5 Comparisons of changed scores of study variables.

Variables	Session 1 Pre-test		Session 1 Post-test		Changed score		Partial η^2 (p-value)	Session 2 Pre-test		Session 2 Post-test		Changed score		Partial η^2 (p-value)
	Mean	SD	Mean	SD	Mean	SD		Mean	SD	Mean	SD	Mean	SD	
Perceived Relaxation							**0.11**							**0.12**
— Control	3.53	3.94	6.53	3.47	3.00	3.85	—	3.70	4.13	6.33	3.93	2.63	3.76	—
— IManage-FF	3.77	4.19	9.10	1.27	5.33	4.23	0.08	4.07	4.25	9.58	0.67	5.52	4.20	0.02**
— IManage-HSet	3.03	3.62	9.13	1.07	6.10	3.64	0.01**	4.00	3.88	9.65	0.73	5.65	3.78	0.02**
Skin Temperature							**0.14**							**0.06**
— Control	28.89	3.75	27.90	3.22	−0.99	2.18	—	28.50	3.18	28.71	3.46	0.21	1.69	—
— IManage-FF	29.64	3.39	30.22	3.19	0.57	1.59	0.00**	28.83	3.94	30.12	3.54	1.29	2.14	0.07
— IManage-HSet	29.23	3.59	29.66	3.24	0.43	1.48	0.01**	29.64	3.50	30.19	3.24	0.55	1.39	0.76
Heart Rate							**0.06**							**0.06**
— Control	75.83	11.14	76.13	9.90	−0.30	4.93	—	73.97	9.60	75.13	8.32	−1.17	3.58	—
— IManage-FF	74.40	9.98	74.47	8.62	−0.07	5.83	0.99	74.00	9.15	73.47	7.54	0.53	3.81	0.26
— IManage-HSet	77.13	12.88	74.50	10.77	2.63	5.36	0.11	75.77	11.48	74.43	10.77	1.33	4.50	0.06
Systolic blood pressure							**0.01**							**0.03**

(*Continued*)

Table 10.5 *(Continued)*

Variables	Session 1 Pre-test		Session 1 Post-test		Changed score		Partial η^2 (p-value)	Session 2 Pre-test		Session 2 Post-test		Changed score		Partial η^2 (p-value)
	Mean	SD	Mean	SD	Mean	SD		Mean	SD	Mean	SD	Mean	SD	
— Control	117.83	20.75	118.53	18.95	−0.70	5.85	—	115.77	14.20	116.20	13.39	−0.43	12.60	—
— IManage-FF	115.93	18.45	114.57	15.66	1.37	9.83	0.68	118.93	15.12	115.97	13.75	2.97	5.60	0.34
— IManage-HSet	117.47	18.99	117.43	20.21	0.03	10.64	0.95	113.17	14.14	112.83	13.39	0.33	6.90	0.95
Diastolic blood pressure							**0.03**							**0.00**
— Control	73.33	12.86	74.33	12.47	−1.00	5.48	—	73.67	8.27	72.80	8.78	0.87	7.07	—
— IManage-FF	72.93	9.36	73.37	9.46	−0.43	8.13	0.99	73.40	8.32	72.50	7.48	0.90	6.14	0.99
— IManage-HSet	77.40	19.46	73.70	13.72	3.70	20.60	0.39	70.97	9.83	69.80	11.26	1.17	6.07	0.98

Note: The Post-Hoc test used the control group as a reference group.
**Statistical significance at alpha = 0.01

was reported (Partial $\eta^2 = 0.06$) despite the fact that the changes did not achieve statistical significance. However, there were no significant differences in other measures of objective stress including heart rate, systolic blood pressure, and diastolic blood pressure across the three groups.

10.3.2.4 *Perceived Relaxation*

To capture immediate changes, perceived relaxation was assessed before and after each intervention session, adding to four assessment points (Table 10.5). At session 1, only a changed score of the IManage-HSet (changed scores = 6.10, SD = 3.64, $p = 0.01$) was significantly higher than that of the control group (changed scores = 3.00, SD = 3.85). A medium effect was observed (Partial $\eta^2 = 0.11$). At session 2, however, changed scores of the IManage-HSet (changed scores = 5.65, SD = 3.78, $p = 0.02$) and IManage-FF group (changed scores = 5.52, SD = 4.20, $p = 0.02$) were significantly higher than that of the control group (changed scores = 2.63, SD = 3.76). A medium effect size was reported (Partial $\eta^2 = 0.12$).

10.3.2.5 *Patient Satisfaction*

Patient satisfaction was assessed at the end of IManage interventions. Table 10.6 suggested that all respondents (n = 30) were either satisfied or very satisfied with the overall IManage-HSet program, its contents, educational materials and relaxation practice. Respondents provided positive comments on the use of headset and videos for patient education, which was more effective than a face-to-face approach (Table 10.6). The program contents were perceived to be very good, clear, effective, understandable, straightforward, helpful, and sufficient. Furthermore, the relaxation instructions were clear, easy, and helpful, and the practice induced focus, relaxation, happiness, and good feelings.

Similarly, those who attended the IManage-FF program (n = 30) were either satisfied or very satisfied with the overall program, contents, educational materials and relaxation practice (using audio-guided instructions) (Table 10.7). Respondents commented that the program

Table 10.6 Satisfaction with the IManage-HSet programme (n = 30).

	Very Dissatisfied n(%)	Dissatisfied n(%)	Neutral n(%)	Satisfied n(%)	Very Satisfied n(%)	Additional Comments[1]
1. Overall, how satisfied are you with the IManage-HSet programme?	0	0	0	25(83.3)	5(16.7)	"Very good" "Not bad" "Not so lengthy" "There must be buddy in guiding you"
2. How satisfied are you with the content of the programme?	0	0	0	25(83.3)	5(16.7)	"Good and clear explanation" (n = 4) "Presentation and explanation are very effective to the patient" "Straight to point and clear explanation" "Contents of the videos and booklets are sufficient" "Helpful, the contents are generally sufficient"
3. How satisfied are you with the educational materials?	0	0	0	26(86.7)	4(13.3)	"Nice gadget" "Different method (attractive)" "Interesting mode of education" "Interesting from the other mode of education" "More interesting than usual face-to-face education" "Understand more by watching video" "Clear explanation with visual presentations, interesting" "Audio very relaxing"
4. How satisfied are you with the relaxation practice?	0	0	0	26(86.7)	4(13.3)	"Easy techniques for relaxation" (n = 2) "Very relaxing: Help to relax" (n = 3) "Help the patient to focus" "Make me so happy and have a good body" "Clearer instructions on how to breathe and use techniques"

[1]Publisher's Note: This column was not copyedited for language errors to retain originality.

Table 10.7 Satisfaction with the IManage-FF programme (n = 30).

	Very Dissatisfied n(%)	Dissatisfied n(%)	Neutral n(%)	Satisfied n(%)	Very Satisfied n(%)	Additional Comments[2]
1. Overall, how satisfied are you with the IManage-FF programme?	0	0	0	27(90.0)	3(10.0)	"Good approach" "Good techniques" "Clear explanation easy to understand" "Not so lengthy, session period just nice" "It is useful and helpful" "Practical interventions"
2. How satisfied are you with the content of the programme?	0	0	1(3.3)	25(83.3)	4(13.3)	"Education on stress management" "It helps us to understand and focus on actions to take to overcome our stress/depression/anxiety" "I am able to understand the education" "More knowledgeable to stress, relax, and depression" "Very good for me, study a lot on things good on my heart" "Very informative"
3. How satisfied are you with the educational materials?	0	0	2(6.7)	25(83.3)	4(13.3)	"Contents of the booklet are enough and understandable" "Techniques are easy to follow" "Good explanation; relaxing audio" "Good explanation; easy to understand. I can refer to the booklet"
4. How satisfied are you with the relaxation practice?	0	0	0	24(80.0)	6(20.0)	"Clear explanation on the relaxation techniques" "Easy to understand the relaxion audios" "Gives time to relax" "So relaxing" "Help us relax and think positive" "Made me feel calm" "Tell people how to make themselves into a relaxed body, not having stress" "The relaxation techniques were very useful"

[2]Publisher's Note: This column was not copyedited for language errors to retain originality.

was clear, useful, helpful, understandable, and informative. The relaxation audios helped patients to relax, feel calm and think positive.

10.3.3 *Comparisons Between the IManage-HSet and IManage-FF Programmes*

To compare differences between the Imanage-HSet and Imanage-FF groups, we examined the following statistical parameters: Difference in changed scores (DC), Standard error (Se) and p-value. Findings suggested there were no significant differences between the two groups in terms of subjective stress (DC = 0.40, Se = 0.93, p = 1.00) depression (DC = 0.90, Se = 0.81, p = 0.80), anxiety (DC = 0.53, Se = 0.82, p = 1.00), knowledge Time 1 (DC = 0.10, Se = 0.10, p = 0.98) and knowledge Time 2 (DC = 0.00, Se = 0.17, p = 1.00).

Furthermore, there were no significant differences between the two groups on perceived relaxation Time 1 (DC = 0.77, Se = 1.01 , p = 1.00), perceived relaxation Time 2 (DC = 0.13, Se = 1.01, p = 1.00), skin temperature Time 1 (DC = 0.14, Se = 0.46, p = 1.00), skin temperature Time 2 (DC = 0.74, Se = 0.46, p = 0.33), heart rate Time 1 (DC = 2.70, Se = 1.39, p = 0.17), heart rate Time 2 (DC = 0.80, Se = 1.03, p = 1.00), systolic blood pressure Time 1 (DC = 1.33, Se = 2.33, p = 1.00), systolic blood pressure Time 2 (DC = 2.63, Se = 2.30, p = 0.77), diastolic blood pressure Time 1 (DC = 4.13, Se = 3.40, p = 0.68) and diastolic blood pressure Time 2 (DC = 0.27, Se = 1.67 , p = 1.00).

10.4 Discussion

This RCT evaluated the efficacy of two symptom self-management programs on inpatients post-AMI in Singapore. Findings suggested that respondents in the IManage-HSet group had improvement in knowledge (large effect size), perceived relaxation (large effect size) and periphery skin temperature (medium effect size) than those of the control group. Similarly, the IManage-FF group demonstrated improvement in knowledge score (large effect size), perceived relaxation (large effect size) and skin temperature (medium effect size). Nearly all participants were satisfied or very satisfied with both programs and positive comments were provided. However, there were no significant differences in outcomes between the IManage-HSet and IManage-FF groups.

Stress increases the risk of AMI, aggravates AMI-related complications, leads to poorer clinical outcomes and increases mortality risks at post discharge [12, 13]. Acute stress activates sympathetic nervous responses and the hypothalamus-pituitary-adrenal axis by triggering the secretion of stress-related hormones such as catecholamines and glucocorticoids [35]. People under stress would exhibit higher heart rate, blood pressure and respiration. Stress also triggers peripheral vasoconstriction, leading to a rapid drop in skin temperature [36]. On the contrary, a relaxation state generates lower heart rate, blood pressure and respiration, but higher skin temperature (peripheral vasodilation) [35, 36]. In line with this, patients in our study who attended either IManage-HSet or IManage-FF programs reported more improvement in skin temperature (lower objective stress) than the control counterparts at both intervention sessions. It may be logical to conclude that the IManage-HSet and I-Manage-FF programs helped minimise objective stress. Similarly, a previous feasibility study revealed that the eight-week virtual world program in Second Life mitigated perceived stress among healthy Americans [38].

Relaxation response reflects a physiological state that counteracts the stress responses [38]. Relaxation responses are found to mitigate stress-related illnesses such as cardiovascular diseases, hypertension, sleep problems, chronic pain, anxiety and depression [38]. Patients in our study revealed improvement in perceived relaxation (with a large effect size) after attending both symptom self-management interventions. Relaxation audios used in the IManage-FF program might induce relaxation responses among the respondents. For the IManage-HSet program, the use of the SONY headset might enhance the experiences of relaxation. Respondents practiced abdominal breathing, muscle relaxation and total body relaxation. The headset is perceived to generate deeper and faster relaxation as it concurrently offers visual presentations (e.g., peaceful and pleasant sceneries) and audio (e.g., music and voice instruction). Moreover, the headset might reduce environmental distractions. Consistent with our findings, a previous RCT examined the efficacy of a relaxing narrative program on university students in Italy [37]. It is reported that immersive VR experiences, DVD and audio tapes produced significant improvement in relaxation (measured through self-reported questionnaire) and skin conductance parameters [36].

At the end of each intervention session, participants had significantly higher knowledge and satisfaction levels than controls with a large effect size. For the IManage-FF, the intervention facilitator delivered knowledge concerning stress management and emotion management; and assisted with the relaxation practice (abdominal breathing and muscle relaxation). Such interactive individual sessions might enhance the learning process and satisfaction. Moreover, participants in the IManage-HSet viewed educational videos (stress demolishing room and emotion wellness room) through the VR device. They felt that the VR device was an attractive gadget and a more interesting mode of patient education. The videos contained useful information, case scenarios, stories, colourful images, examples of activities (such as exercise and healthy lifestyles) and interactive conversations among actors, which might enhance learning outcomes. Participants also viewed relaxation videos (A Fantastic Journey to Relaxation) via the SONY headset and concurrently practiced relaxation. An education booklet was distributed to all respondents so that they could review the learned information at their convenience. An intervention facilitator was also presented to help respondents use the headset, ensure their comfort levels, provide emotional support, answer questions regarding education videos, and assist with relaxation practice.

In comparison to controls, both interventions had higher changed scores on subjective stress, depression, anxiety and other measures of objective stress (heart rate and blood pressure) with small effect sizes. Nevertheless, such scores did not achieve statistical significance. A possible explanation could be that the IManage-HSet and IManage-FF programs might have an immediate effect on skin temperature (objective stress) but a delayed effect on subjective stress. Hence, it might take longer durations and more sessions to induce significant changes on subjective stress. Another possible explanation could be that the contents of interventions did not directly improve subjective stress, anxiety and depression. Furthermore, scores of blood pressure and heart rate were already in a normal range for participants across three groups. Therefore, there was not much room to improve the scores. Similarly, a previous RCT examined a VR-based cardiac rehabilitation program among people with coronary artery disease [39]. There were no significant differences in subjective stress, anxiety and depression (as measured by the DASS-21) between the intervention and control groups [39]. The researchers concluded that the relationships between depression and cardiovascular diseases are complex and more research is required to explore such relationships.

There were non-significant differences in study outcomes between the IManage-Hset and IManage-FF interventions. A possible explanation could be that the two programs entailed similar contents (educations on AMI, stress management and emotion management), same format (two-daily sessions) and same education booklet. The differences between two programs were the use of delivery methods and mindfulness practices. Cancer survivors in the IManage-HSet group commented that the use of SONY headset (non-immersive device) was an attractive and interesting mode of education, which enhanced understanding. Furthermore, the headset was perceived to be a good technique to enhance relaxation. Similarly, a systematic review revealed that an immersive device (HMD-VR) increased motivation, concentration and engagement during the intervention periods for people with different illnesses [24]. Additionally, HMD-VR appeared to be outstanding, motivating, and engaging, and non-inferior to a face-to-face traditional method of teaching for healthcare students [25].

10.4.1 *Limitations*

Strengths of this research were the use of a RCT to examine the effects of two interventions and the computation of sample size through power analysis. However, there are some limitations and the first is the lack of a follow-up assessment. Hence, it is unclear if the beneficial effects of the interventions would sustain over time. Secondly, the cardiac care unit used centralised air conditioning. Temperature in the patient rooms was low and could not be manually adjusted. Such low temperatures might affect the accuracy of skin temperature scores. Thirdly, due to limited manpower, we were unable to blind the outcome assessor, which might increase the risk of detection bias. However, this study also included physiological measures, which produced objective data and might help minimise the bias. Fourthly, neither researchers and participants were blinded due to the nature of interventions, which might lead to detection bias. Finally, the sample demographics might raise an issue of generalisability. Nearly all participants were male and thus the findings might not be generalisable to female patients. Furthermore, marital status was significantly different among the three groups, which might affect the findings. Future research may explore the effect of marital status on outcome variables using RCTs with a larger sample size.

10.4.2 *Future Directions*

This study has implications to future research. More RCTs with a larger sample size and multi-site arrangements may be carried out to test both IManage-HSet and IManage-FF programs. Booster sessions of the programs may be developed and offered to patients post-hospitalisation. Several objective data (such as salivary cortisol, salivary alpha amylase, periphery skin temperature, blood pressure and heart rate) and subjective data (such as subjective stress, self-efficacy, and motivation to change) may be collected. Follow-up assessments should be utilised to measure long-term effects of the interventions. A qualitative approach may be added to elicit in-depth information concerning participants' experiences of the program.

10.5 Conclusions

This is the first study to examine the symptom self-management programs on patients post-AMI at a tertiary hospital in Singapore. Apparently, it is feasible to conduct the two-session interventions at the cardiac care unit in the study hospital. Findings suggested that the program delivered via the SONY headset (IManage-HSet) and traditional face-to-face approach (IManage-FF) had the potential to improve objective stress (as measured by peripheral skin temperature), perceived relaxations, knowledge and satisfaction. Given that both programs did not produce significantly different effects on the study outcomes, they may be offered to cancer survivors in clinical settings. The delivery methods (SONY headset or face-to-face arrangement) may be selected by the patients based on their preference.

Acknowledgement

This research was supported by the Ministry of Health, Health Service Research New Investigator Grant, Singapore [Grant NO. HSR-NIG12NOV005].

References

1. World Health Organization. Cardiovascular diseases [Internet]. Geneva: World Health Organization; 2020 [cited 2025 Jul 16]. Available from: http://www.who.int/mediacentre/factsheets/fs317/en/index.html
2. World Health Organization. Global health estimates: deaths by cause, age, sex and country, 2000–2012 [Internet]. Geneva: World Health Organization; 2014 [cited 2025 Jul 16]. Available from: http://www.who.int/healthinfo/global_burden_disease/en/
3. World Health Organization. Heart: Technical package for cardiovascular disease management in primary health care. Geneva: World Health Organization; 2016.

4. Health Promotion Board. Singapore myocardial infarction registry annual report 2018 [Internet]. 2020 [cited 2025 Jul 16]. Available from: https://www.nrdo.gov.sg/docs/librariesprovider3/default-document-library/smir-web-report-2018.pdf?sfvrsn = ccde799a
5. Mechanic OJ, Grossman SA. Acute myocardial infarction. In: StatPearls [Internet]. Treasure Island (FL): StatPearls Publishing; 2020 [cited 2025 Jul 16]. Available from: https://www.ncbi.nlm.nih.gov/books/NBK459269/
6. Panday R, Gupta N, Wander G. Diagnosis of acute myocardial infarction. J Assoc Physician India. 2015;59:8–13.
7. Bahall M, Seemungal T, Legall G. Risk factors for first-time acute myocardial infarction patients in Trinidad. BMC Public Health. 2018;18(1):161.
8. Bahall M, Khan K. Quality of life of patients with first-time AMI: a descriptive study. Health Qual Life Outcomes. 2018;16(1):32.
9. Alsén P, Brink E. Fatigue after myocardial infarction — a two-year follow-up study. J Clin Nurs. 2013;22(11–12):1647–52.
10. Dreyer RP, Xu X, Zhang W, Du X, Strait KM, Bierlein M, *et al.* Return to work after acute myocardial infarction: comparison between young women and men. Circ Cardiovasc Qual Outcomes. 2016;9 Suppl 1:S45–52.
11. Selye H. The stress concept: past, present, and future. In: Cooper CL, editor. Stress research: issues for the eighties. New York: John Wiley & Sons; 1983.
12. Arnold SV, Smolderen KG, Buchanan DM, Li Y, Spertus JA. Perceived stress in myocardial infarction: long-term mortality and health status outcomes. J Am Coll Cardiol. 2012;60(18):1756–63.
13. Shah SJ, Krumholz HM, Reid KJ, Rathore SS, Mandawat A, Spertus JA, Ross JS. Financial stress and outcomes after acute myocardial infarction. PLoS One. 2012;7(10):e47420.
14. Chan C, Elliott J, Troughton R, Frampton C, Smyth D, Crozier I, Bridgman P. Acute myocardial infarction and stress cardiomyopathy following the Christchurch earthquakes. PLoS One. 2013;8(7):e68504.
15. Xu X, Bao H, Strait KM, Edmondson DE, Davidson KW, Beltrame JF, Krumholz HM. Perceived stress after acute myocardial infarction: a comparison between young and middle-aged women versus men. Psychosom Med. 2017;79(1):50–8.
16. Kumar M, Nayak PK. Psychological sequelae of myocardial infarction. Biomed Pharmacother. 2017;95:487–96.
17. American Psychiatric Association. Anxiety disorders. In: Diagnostic and Statistical Manual of Mental Disorders. 5th ed. Arlington (VA): American Psychiatric Association; 2013.

18. Klarsen KK, Agerbo E, Christensen B, Søndergaard J, Vestergaard M. Myocardial infarction and risk of suicide: a population-based case-control study. Circulation. 2010;122(23):2388–93.
19. Klainin-Yobas P, Koh KWL, Ambhore A, Chai P, Chan SWC, He HG. A study protocol of a randomised controlled trial examining the efficacy of a symptom self-management programme for people with acute myocardial infarction. J Adv Nurs. 2015;71(6):1299–309.
20. Klainin-Yobas P, Ng S, Stephen PDM, Lau Y. Efficacy of psychosocial interventions on psychological outcomes among people with cardiovascular diseases: a systematic review and meta-analyses. Patient Educ Couns. 2016;99(4):512–21.
21. Ramos P. Testing the efficacy of the psychosocial intervention with standard care on inpatients with ischemic heart disease in Singapore: a pilot randomized controlled trial. Honours research project. Alice Lee Ctr for Nursing St, Yong Loo Lin Sch of Med, Natl Univ Singapore; 2013.
22. Bohil C, Owen C, Jeong E, Alicea B, Biocca F. Virtual reality and presence [Internet]. 2009 [cited 2025 Jul 16]. Available from: https://www.researchgate.net/publication/263619590
23. Sherman WR, Craig AB. Understanding virtual reality: interface, application, and design. Burlington (MA): Morgan Kaufmann; 2002.
24. Saldana D, Neureither M, Schmiesing A, *et al.* Applications of head-mounted displays for virtual reality in adult physical rehabilitation: a scoping review. Am J Occup Ther. 2020;74(5):7405205060p1–7405205060p15.
25. Barteit S, Lanfermann L, Bärnighausen T, Neuhann F, Beiersmann C. Augmented, mixed, and virtual reality-based head-mounted devices for medical education: systematic review. JMIR Serious Games. 2021;9(3):e29080.
26. Moher D, Hopewell S, Schulz KF, Montori V, Gøtzsche PC, Devereaux PJ, Altman DG. CONSORT 2010 explanation and elaboration: updated guidelines for reporting parallel group randomised trials. BMJ. 2010;340:c869.
27. Frison L, Pocock SJ. Repeated measures in clinical trials: analysis using mean summary statistics and its implications for design. Stat Med. 1992;11(13):1685–704.
28. Sony Corporation. SONY head mounted display: reference guide [Internet]. 2012 [cited 2025 Jul 16]. Available from: https://www.sony.com/electronics/support/res/manuals/4439/44390203M.pdf
29. Stress Market. Stress thermometer SC 911 [Internet]. 2011 [cited 2025 Jul 16]. Available from: http://www.cliving.org/SC911/SC911instr.pdf

30. Klainin-Yobas P, Ignacio J, Wong PHH, La Y, He HG, Ngooi B, Koh SQD. Effects of the stress management (S-Manage) program for inpatients with mental disorders: a feasibility study. Biol Res Nurs. 2016;18(2):213–20.
31. Lovibond SH, Lovibond PF. Manual for the Depression Anxiety Stress Scales. 2nd ed. Sydney: Psychology Foundation; 1995.
32. Mahmoud JSR, Hall LA, Staten R, Pritchard M. The psychometric properties of the 21-item Depression Anxiety and Stress Scale (DASS-21) among a sample of ... [abstract]. Br J Nurs. 2009;18(7):416–9.
33. Lee SY. Developing a stress management intervention for adult patients with hypertension and ischemic heart disease: a pilot study. Unpublished honours thesis. Alice Lee Ctr for Nursing St, Natl Univ Singapore; 2010.
34. Cohen J. Statistical power analysis for the behavioral sciences. 2nd ed. Hillsdale (NJ): Lawrence Erlbaum Associates; 1988.
35. Halm MA. Relaxation: a self-care healing modality reduces harmful effects of anxiety. Am J Crit Care. 2009;18(2):169–72.
36. Herborn KA, Graves JL, Jerem P, Evans NP, Nager R, McCafferty DJ, McKeegan DE. Skin temperature reveals the intensity of acute stress. Physiol Behav. 2015;152(Pt A):225–30.
37. Villani D, Riva G. Presence and relaxation: a preliminary controlled study. PsychNology J. 2008;6(1):7–26.
38. Hoch DB, Watson AJ, Linton DA, Bello HE, Senelly M, Milik MT, Kvedar JC. The feasibility and impact of delivering a mind-body intervention in a virtual world. PLoS One. 2012;7(3):e33843.
39. Vieira A, Melo MCDA, Noites SPARS, Machado J, Gabriel MMJ. The effect of virtual reality on a home-basewd cardiac rehabilitation program on body composition, lipid profile and eating patterns. Eur J Integr Med. 2017;9:69–78.

https://doi.org/10.1142/9789819817320_0011

Chapter 11

Toward a Culturally Adapted Positive Psychological Framework for Thai Individuals with Chronic Kidney Disease: Reflections for Future Psychosocial Intervention Design

Nopporn Vongsirimas[1,*], Sirada Kesornsri[1], and Piyanee Klainin-Yobas[2]

[1]*Faculty of Nursing, Mahidol University, 999, Phuttamonthon 4 Road, Salaya, Nakhon Pathom 73170, Thailand*

[2]*Alice Lee Centre for Nursing Studies, Yong Loo Lin School of Medicine, National University of Singapore, Level 5, Centre of Translational Medicine, Block MD6, 14 Medical Drive, Singapore 117599*

**Corresponding author: nopporn.von@mahidol.ac.th*

11.1 Introduction

This chapter presents a reflective and forward-looking exploration of how psychosocial care — particularly Positive Psychological Interventions (PPIs) — may be applied to the context of chronic kidney disease (CKD) in Thailand. While some narrative elements and themes are conceptually informed by previously published research, this work does not replicate or summarise empirical findings. Instead, it synthesises existing literature, lived experience, and psychosocial theory into a proposed framework for future intervention design. It aims to serve as a conceptual guide for researchers, educators, and practitioners interested in developing culturally attuned and digitally adaptable psychosocial interventions for Thai individuals undergoing dialysis.

Future care models for individuals with CKD may benefit from acknowledging the multifaceted challenges that patients are likely to encounter — not only in terms of medical complexity, but also emotional vulnerability, social disconnection, and lifestyle disruption. In the Thai context, these psychosocial factors are often intensified by deeply rooted cultural expectations and variable access to supportive services. While medical treatment continues to advance, there is an increasing need to conceptualise care in ways that holistically support patients' psychological and social well-being alongside physical health. Patients undergoing haemodialysis face substantial lifestyle disruptions, psychological vulnerability, and diminished quality of life. In Thailand, these challenges are further complicated by cultural values, familial roles, and unequal access to psychosocial resources. While medical management has advanced, the psychosocial dimension remains underdeveloped within the continuum of CKD care.

This chapter proposes that future care models integrate the principles of positive psychology, particularly through the use of Internet-Based Positive Psychological Interventions (IPPIs). These interventions offer scalable, flexible formats suitable for patients with mobility constraints and limited access to in-person care. The following sections offer conceptual guidance for the development of such programs, informed by theoretical foundations, cultural considerations, and emerging global practices.

11.2 Chronic Kidney Disease: A Global Public Health Concern

Noncommunicable diseases constitute a significant global health challenge, contributing substantially to mortality and economic losses worldwide. These diseases disrupt national development through their impact on healthcare systems, labour productivity, and societal well-being. Globally, noncommunicable diseases account for a majority of all deaths, particularly affecting individuals aged 30 to 70 — an age group vital to economic sustainability. In the Americas, for instance, approximately 80% of all deaths are attributable to noncommunicable diseases, with 35% occurring within this economically productive age bracket [1].

Thailand bears a disproportionate burden of noncommunicable diseases relative to the global average. Current data indicate that approximately 14 million Thai citizens are living with one or more noncommunicable diseases. These conditions are the leading cause of mortality nationwide, with over 300,000 deaths recorded in 2009 alone — accounting for 73% of total mortality. The associated economic cost has been estimated at 200 billion Thai Baht annually, signalling a critical need for enhanced public health responses.

Among these diseases, CKD has emerged as a particularly urgent concern. It is currently ranked as the fifth leading cause of death in Thailand and is primarily associated with long-term complications from diabetes mellitus and hypertension. CKD prevalence is notably high among the elderly, with some studies reporting rates of up to 88.6% [2]. In cases where CKD progresses to end-stage renal disease, patients require lifelong renal replacement therapy, including modalities such as haemodialysis, peritoneal dialysis, or kidney transplantation.

The demand for renal replacement therapy in Thailand has shown a consistent upward trajectory. According to the Thai Renal Replacement Therapy Registry, the number of patients receiving haemodialysis increased from 47,410 in 2013 to 54,104 in 2015 [3]. Parallel to this trend, the implementation of the Universal Coverage Scheme in 2008 significantly expanded access to continuous ambulatory peritoneal dialysis (CAPD). The number of CAPD recipients increased from just 60 in 2007 to 16,513 in 2013 [4], marking an exponential rise in uptake.

These developments underscore the necessity of integrating psychosocial dimensions into CKD care. Beyond managing physiological symptoms, effective interventions must address emotional distress, social disruption, and the psychological adaptation required for long-term disease management. The subsequent sections of this chapter explore how PPIs can fulfil this need within the Thai healthcare context.

11.3 Psychosocial and Economic Burden of Haemodialysis Patients in Thailand

The financial and emotional toll of CKD, particularly for patients undergoing haemodialysis, presents a multifaceted challenge to both individuals and the national healthcare system. Haemodialysis, typically administered two to three times per week in specialised clinics, requires extensive time, financial resources, and strict treatment adherence. According to Phunmuangrat *et al.* [5], the direct cost per dialysis session in Thailand — excluding laboratory testing — is approximately 2,394.85 Thai Baht (≈USD 68.42), translating to over 40,000 Baht per patient per month [6]. National expenditure for renal replacement therapy has reached an estimated 3 billion Baht annually (≈USD 85.7 million) [7].

While CAPD represents a more cost-effective option and allows patients to self-administer treatment at home, the overall psychosocial burden remains substantial. Both forms of dialysis disrupt daily routines, limit physical activity, and introduce emotional stressors related to dependency, isolation, and uncertainty.

The emergence of the COVID-19 pandemic further intensified these burdens by increasing infection risk, disrupting care continuity, and heightening psychological distress. Patients reported elevated levels of anxiety, hopelessness, and emotional exhaustion. Studies have shown that depression is particularly prevalent in this population, with Thai patients undergoing haemodialysis and CAPD exhibiting depressive symptoms at rates of 46% and 42%, respectively [8, 9]. These mental health challenges contribute to reduced quality of life, non-adherence to treatment regimens, increased hospitalisation, and higher mortality.

Moreover, the psychological burden is exacerbated by the high pill burden associated with CKD treatment. On average, patients in developed healthcare systems such as the United States consume approximately 12 pills per day [10]. The complexity of medical regimens and limited psychosocial support infrastructure underscore the need for integrative approaches that prioritise emotional well-being.

Despite the high prevalence of depression among dialysis patients, access to psychiatric care remains limited. Pharmacological interventions are typically reserved for severe cases involving suicidal ideation or marked treatment refusal, due to concerns about polypharmacy. Cognitive behavioural therapy (CBT) has demonstrated efficacy in reducing depressive symptoms in this group; however, its cost and resource-intensive nature render it less feasible in resource-limited settings or during public health crises.

These findings point to the importance of exploring alternative, scalable psychosocial interventions that can address the emotional needs of CKD patients while remaining accessible and culturally appropriate. PPIs, which emphasise strength-based coping and emotional resilience, offer a promising pathway for improving mental health outcomes in this vulnerable population.

11.4 Psychological Vulnerability in Chronic Kidney Disease

In addition to its well-documented physiological consequences, CKD is strongly associated with elevated psychological vulnerability, particularly depressive symptoms. Depression is one of the most common comorbid psychiatric conditions observed in individuals with CKD, with prevalence rates ranging from 20% to 30% — significantly higher than those reported in the general population. This heightened psychological burden is multifactorial in origin, stemming from the persistent stress of living with a chronic condition, financial strain, disruptions to daily life, loss of autonomy, and neurobiological alterations associated with uraemia [11].

If left unrecognised or inadequately managed, depression in CKD patients can have far-reaching clinical implications. It may compromise patients' adherence to treatment regimens, contribute to increased rates of hospitalisation, and negatively affect overall survival outcomes [11]. These findings underscore the importance of integrating psychological assessment and evidence-based mental health interventions as core components of comprehensive CKD care.

11.5 Psychosocial Dynamics of Thai Women with Chronic Kidney Disease: A Nursing Perspective

From a psychosocial nursing perspective, understanding the subjective experiences of patients is not merely supplementary — it is central to the provision of person-centred care. In Thailand, a growing body of research has illuminated the nuanced psychosocial realities of women living with CKD, offering contextually grounded insights that are essential for culturally sensitive interventions.

Evidence suggests that depression remains a predominant factor influencing quality of life among Thai female patients receiving dialysis treatment. A study by Praha *et al.* identified depression as the most powerful predictor of diminished quality of life in Thai women undergoing haemodialysis [8]. Complementing this, Prapaiwong *et al.* found that depressive symptoms, the quality of spousal relationships, and sexual dysfunction significantly contributed to reduced well-being among women on CAPD [9].

Further comparative insight was offered by Sriyuktasuth *et al.*, who revealed that although depression levels were comparable, women receiving haemodialysis scored higher in domains related to psychosocial functioning and spousal relationships than those on CAPD. These findings point toward modality-specific psychosocial dynamics that must be addressed in care planning [12]. Adding to the depth of this evidence, Phuka, Vongsirimas, and Thanoi explored factors associated with psychological well-being in Thai haemodialysis patients. Their study demonstrated strong correlations between psychological well-being and factors such as perceived stress, resilience, and social support. These findings align closely with the theoretical principles of positive psychology, emphasising not only the mitigation of distress but also the cultivation of strengths — particularly emotional resilience — as a pathway to enhancing patients' quality of life [13].

In this context, psychosocial nursing is uniquely positioned to serve as both a clinical practice and a humanistic science — one that not only alleviates suffering but also empowers individuals to discover meaning, adaptation, and dignity within the trajectory of chronic illness.

11.6 Psychological Well-being and the Emergence of Positive Psychological Interventions

Psychological well-being is increasingly recognised as a central component of comprehensive CKD care. Defined by dimensions such as autonomy, environmental mastery, purpose in life, self-acceptance, personal growth, and positive social relationships [14, 15], psychological well-being encompasses not only the absence of psychological disorders but the presence of optimal psychological functioning. In patients with CKD, higher levels of psychological well-being have been associated with improved treatment adherence, enhanced quality of life, and lower levels of depressive symptoms [16, 17].

In recent years, PPIs have emerged as a novel and evidence-based strategy to foster psychological resilience and enhance emotional well-being. Unlike conventional therapeutic approaches that primarily focus on symptom reduction, PPIs aim to cultivate positive emotions, strengths, and meaning in life. These interventions include activities such as gratitude journaling, identifying personal strengths, practicing mindfulness, and engaging in acts of kindness [18-20].

A growing body of research supports the effectiveness of PPIs in reducing depressive symptoms across various clinical populations, including individuals with chronic illnesses such as cardiovascular disease, diabetes, and HIV [21, 22]. Meta-analyses have demonstrated outcomes comparable to those of pharmacological and traditional psychotherapeutic treatments, with the added advantage of lower cost and greater adaptability [23].

Particularly relevant in the context of CKD care is the adaptation of PPIs into digital formats — known as IPPIs. These interventions offer scalable, flexible, and socially distanced delivery methods, which are especially beneficial for dialysis patients who face mobility constraints and frequent hospital visits. Studies from high-income countries have shown that online PPIs can improve mood, increase life satisfaction, and reduce psychological distress in both general and clinical populations [24, 25].

However, there remains a significant research gap concerning the application of PPIs in patients undergoing dialysis, particularly in non-Western settings. To address this, the subsequent sections of the chapter explore culturally adapted PPI frameworks developed specifically for Thai patients with CKD, highlighting their relevance, acceptability, and potential for integration into existing care systems.

11.7 Positive Psychological Interventions in the Context of Chronic Kidney Disease Care: A Holistic Alternative

In the care of patients with CKD, addressing psychological distress remains a clinical imperative. While conventional approaches to depression — such as pharmacotherapy and CBT — demonstrate robust efficacy, their limitations must be critically acknowledged, especially in medically complex populations. For CKD patients, polypharmacy heightens the risk of adverse interactions, while the in-person nature of CBT often creates logistical and systemic barriers, particularly during public health emergencies like the COVID-19 pandemic [26].

To navigate these challenges, the field has witnessed the emergence of PPIs — an evidence-based paradigm shift that reframes psychological care from deficit correction to strength cultivation. Rather than focusing exclusively on symptom reduction, PPIs aim to enhance well-being by nurturing positive affect, personal meaning, social engagement, and psychological resilience [20, 26]. Core elements such as gratitude journaling, mindfulness, strengths identification, and prosocial behaviour form the foundation of these interventions, aligning closely with the inner resources and lived experiences of patients navigating chronic illness.

Notably, the digital transformation of healthcare has facilitated the advent of IPPIs — an innovation particularly suited to the needs of CKD populations. These interventions offer accessible, low-cost, and scalable formats that accommodate physical limitations and reduce reliance on in-person visits. In a U.S.-based initiative, CKD patients who engaged in IPPIs demonstrated improved coping mechanisms and enhanced emotional resilience [27]. Similarly, a five-week digital PPI adapted for haemodialysis patients led to measurable improvements in both mood and quality of life [28].

Systematic reviews published in journals such as *Journal of Behavioural Medicine* and *Cureus* further affirm the value of Internet-based psychological interventions and online CBT in managing psychological distress among patients with chronic conditions — including diabetes and cardiovascular diseases — offering promising translational value for the CKD context [29, 30]. In the evolving landscape of psychosocial nursing, IPPIs represent more than a technological workaround. They are an opportunity to reimagine care in ways that are empathetic, empowering, and congruent with the deeply human endeavour of healing.

11.8 Reimagining Emotional Care in Chronic Kidney Disease through Digital Positive Psychology

Within the psychosocial care continuum for patients with CKD, the urgency of rethinking psychological support cannot be overstated. Traditional treatments — whether pharmacological or psychotherapeutic — are often constrained by the practical realities of polypharmacy, patient fatigue, and limitations in clinical reach. In this light, PPIs offer not merely an alternative, but a paradigm shift.

PPIs aim to cultivate strengths such as gratitude, mindfulness, and emotional resilience, thereby supporting patients not through symptom suppression alone, but by restoring meaning and vitality. Of particular significance in today's healthcare landscape is the transformation of these interventions into IPPIs — accessible, scalable, and integrative tools for enhancing mental well-being among patients with limited mobility.

One seminal study that reinforces this direction is the work by Hernandez and colleagues [31], who piloted a five-week IPPI among haemodialysis patients with depressive symptoms. The intervention, grounded in structured online modules delivered during dialysis sessions, resulted in a statistically significant reduction in depressive symptoms, high retention rates (85.7%), and overwhelmingly positive user feedback. Patients reported enhanced coping capacity, emotional clarity, and a renewed sense of self-efficacy — hallmarks of psychological well-being that pharmacotherapy alone seldom delivers.

From a psychosocial nursing lens, such findings invite us to envision a clinical practice model that does not merely "treat" but "re-engages" the personhood of patients. By merging behavioural science with compassionate technology, IPPIs are not just feasible — they are deeply humane. As we stride into an era where emotional healing must coexist with chronic disease management, the integration of interventions like those tested by Hernandez *et al.* becomes not just advisable, but ethically imperative [31].

11.8.1 *Culturally Adapted Positive Psychological Interventions for Thai Chronic Kidney Disease Patients*

To ensure the effectiveness of PPIs in the Thai context, a culturally grounded framework must be developed that aligns with local values, spiritual beliefs, and social structures. Research conducted in Thailand — funded by the National Research Council of Thailand in the fiscal year 2024 — by the author and research team has identified five core psychosocial themes influencing the perception of individuals with CKD: emotional suppression due to cultural norms (*kreng jai*), disrupted social roles and identity, the centrality of Buddhist spirituality, family dynamics as both support and stressor, and the desire for reconnection and normalcy.

11.8.2 *Critical Reflections and Future Direction*

What remains essential is cultural translation. While evidence from the West affirms the efficacy of PPIs, the Thai context demands adaptation. Local values — such as *kreng jai*, family interconnectedness, and Buddhist-informed views of suffering — must shape how interventions are designed and delivered. Furthermore, the nurse's role must evolve from provider to partner — co-creating care pathways that honour lived experience.

As we stand at the intersection of chronic disease, emotional distress, and digital innovation, psychosocial nursing is uniquely poised to lead. Not through high-cost innovation, but through high-touch understanding. In this space, PPIs become more than interventions — they become invitations to rediscover the humanity of care.

11.8.3 *Reflection: Beyond the Screen, Towards the Soul*

The study by Hernandez *et al.* catalyses a critical insight: technology, in the context of psychosocial care, is not merely a tool — it is a bridge [31]. A bridge that leads patients toward self-discovery, self-acceptance, and emotional healing. Yet in the Thai context, the challenge lies not only in digital accessibility, but in emotional resonance. An intervention must go beyond the ability to "reach the screen" — it must be designed to "*reach the heart*".

This is why psychosocial interventions cannot remain solely clinical in intent; they must also be culturally attuned and spiritually sensitive. Thai patients live not in isolation, but within a matrix of family, faith, and community. To truly serve them, psychosocial nursing must do more than relieve distress — it must *translate suffering into a pathway for transformation.* This is the moral and professional calling of the modern psychosocial nurse: not merely to provide care, but to restore meaning, honour resilience, and walk with patients through the sacred terrain of chronic illness.

11.9 Toward Contextualised Innovation: Thai-Singaporean Research Collaboration

In light of the aforementioned reflections, a team of Thai nurse researchers from the Faculty of Nursing, Mahidol University, in collaboration with colleagues from the National University of Singapore, initiated a cross-cultural research initiative. This project, supported by national-level research funding from the National Research Council of Thailand in fiscal year 2024, aims to develop a culturally attuned PPI tailored specifically for Thai individuals living with CKD.

To ensure that the intervention is truly responsive to the lived realities of Thai patients, the research team identified the need to first gain a comprehensive understanding of the psychosocial context surrounding

CKD in Thailand. This contextual inquiry serves as the foundation for the intervention design process.

Findings from the preliminary qualitative phase have provided rich insight into the emotional, cultural, and relational landscapes of Thai CKD patients. These insights are now being integrated into the next stage of the project: the co-creation of a culturally grounded PPI that is not only evidence-based but also emotionally resonant and socially relevant. The following section outlines key findings from this initial phase of research.

11.9.1 *The Voice from Haemodialysis Patients: A Foundation for Digital Intervention Design*

To ensure that psychosocial interventions are truly responsive to the lived experiences of Thai individuals undergoing haemodialysis, in-depth interviews were conducted with a diverse group of patients. These narratives offered rich insights into the emotional, social, and practical realities of life on long-term dialysis. What emerged was not merely a list of needs, but a textured portrait of resilience, vulnerability, and cultural adaptation.

One of the most immediate challenges voiced by participants centred on the disruption of daily functioning and financial security. Haemodialysis — typically scheduled multiple times per week — imposed significant limitations on their ability to maintain employment. Some participants reported adjusting work hours or changing occupations altogether, while others were compelled to stop working entirely. Though Thailand's government healthcare schemes were acknowledged as helpful, patients often described a persistent sense of lost autonomy, financial pressure, and an increased reliance on family members for both economic and emotional support.

Emotionally, the diagnosis of CKD and the initiation of dialysis triggered a spectrum of psychological responses. Feelings of fear, helplessness, sadness, and even anger were common in the early stages of treatment. Over time, however, many patients described a gradual emotional shift — an emerging capacity to reflect, accept, and seek meaning. This form of psychological adaptation was often facilitated through cultural and spiritual frameworks, highlighting the role of internal and external resources in shaping resilience.

The role of family support surfaced as a foundational element in the patients' coping processes. Emotional and logistical assistance from spouses, children, siblings, and extended relatives were described not merely as helpful, but as essential. Family members often assumed caregiving responsibilities, provided financial assistance, and offered companionship during treatment. In many cases, patients equated the quality of their dialysis experience with the strength of their family ties, reinforcing the need to design interventions that extend beyond the individual and encompass the broader social system.

Patients also articulated a range of personal coping strategies aimed at regaining a sense of stability and control. These included strict adherence to medical regimens, cognitive reframing, and reliance on religious or spiritual practices. Many drew strength from Buddhist teachings, engaging in prayer, meditation, or listening to Dhamma talks to soothe anxiety and cultivate emotional balance. Others turned to simple pleasures — music, humorous videos, or daily routines — to reclaim a sense of normalcy amidst uncertainty.

Lifestyle adjustments, while often perceived as burdensome, were generally met with high levels of motivation when instructions were clear and contextually appropriate. Changes in diet, fluid intake, and physical activity were frequently cited, with patients expressing a desire for personalised guidance that aligned with both medical advice and cultural preferences.

When discussing the potential for digital health tools, participants expressed a surprisingly high level of openness. The majority indicated regular use of smartphones and social media platforms, and voiced interest in receiving psychosocial support via these channels. Preferences leaned toward brief, visually engaging content — such as short videos, real-life patient stories, or guided mindfulness exercises — that could be accessed on demand. Importantly, participants emphasised the need for content that was not only informative, but also inspiring and emotionally supportive.

These patient narratives provide critical insight into the psychosocial terrain of living with CKD in Thailand. They highlight the interplay of emotional vulnerability, cultural values, family interdependence, and adaptive strength. Rather than treating patients as passive recipients of care, these stories position them as active interpreters of their own lives — individuals who draw on diverse resources to navigate the demands of long-term illness. The voices documented here are not only expressions of lived reality but are also guiding beacons for the development of a culturally attuned IPPI, to be detailed in the following section.

Note: Portions of this chapter, particularly the section on voice from haemodialysis patients, draw upon findings previously reported in a peer-reviewed article by the author and colleagues. The original research provides an in-depth exploration of patients' emotional responses, coping strategies, and expectations regarding digital health interventions. As the manuscript is currently under peer review for publication in an academic journal, those wishing to access the full findings are advised to contact the corresponding author directly.

11.10 Suggested Characteristics and Structure of a Culturally Adapted Internet-Based Positive Psychological Intervention Program for Thai Patients with Chronic Kidney Disease

To support the evolving landscape of CKD care in Thailand, future psychosocial interventions may benefit from incorporating culturally sensitive, psychologically grounded approaches that address the emotional and existential dimensions of living with chronic illness. Particularly in the Thai context — where care experiences are shaped by cultural values, family roles, and spiritual traditions — there is a growing need to move beyond models focused solely on clinical management. Guided by the foundational principles of positive psychology, including psychological well-being, resilience, and mindfulness, this section introduces a preliminary conceptual framework for a five-week IPPI. While not yet implemented, the proposed structure reflects an integration of theoretical models, insights from prior literature, experiential understanding, and theoretical models, rather than from finalised empirical results for a digital IPPI model tailored to Thai CKD patients. It is presented as a forward-looking suggestion to inform the development of future psychosocial programs tailored to the needs of Thai individuals undergoing dialysis.

11.10.1 *Conceptual Foundations*

Any future IPPI program designed for Thai CKD patients should ideally integrate the following theoretical constructs:

- **Psychological Well-being:** The intervention should aim to support dimensions such as self-acceptance, autonomy, environmental mastery, positive relationships, personal growth, and purpose in life [14].
- **Resilience:** Given the ongoing psychological stressors associated with CKD, interventions should foster adaptive functioning through identification of personal strengths, emotional flexibility, and support system mobilisation.
- **Mindfulness:** The use of culturally embedded mindfulness practices may help patients develop emotional regulation and existential coherence, particularly when aligned with familiar Buddhist principles and rituals.

The development of effective psychosocial interventions for Thai individuals with CKD requires not only a sound theoretical foundation but also a deep appreciation of the cultural context that shapes patients' lived experiences. Research conducted by the authors highlighted the complex psychosocial landscape facing Thai CKD patients, including disrupted personal identity, emotional vulnerability, and the influence of cultural values such as *kreng jai*, filial obligation, and Buddhist-informed beliefs about suffering.

In light of these findings, the integration of three core constructs — psychological well-being, resilience, and mindfulness — into future IPPI programs is both theoretically grounded and culturally resonant. Each construct addresses distinct yet interconnected dimensions of patients' psychological needs:

1. Psychological Well-being: Ryff's model of psychological well-being emphasises six key dimensions: self-acceptance, autonomy, environmental mastery, positive relationships, personal growth, and purpose in life. For Thai CKD patients, whose illness often results in reduced independence, altered family roles, and emotional uncertainty, this framework offers a holistic path toward rebuilding meaning and identity. By supporting patients in discovering new forms of self-worth and purpose beyond the boundaries of illness, interventions grounded in this model can serve as a counterbalance to the loss and disruption experienced during long-term treatment [14].
2. Resilience: CKD imposes chronic and often unpredictable physical, emotional, and financial stress. Resilience — the capacity to adapt positively to adversity — plays a critical role in maintaining psychological functioning under such conditions. Interventions that cultivate resilience can help patients identify personal strengths, navigate emotional fluctuations, and mobilise support systems such as family and peers. This strength-based approach is particularly fitting for Thai patients, many of whom rely heavily on familial networks for caregiving and emotional stability. Empowering individuals to become active agents in their own coping process may counteract feelings of helplessness and dependency.

3. Mindfulness: Mindfulness is not only an evidence-based therapeutic practice but also one deeply embedded within Thai culture through its alignment with Buddhist philosophy and rituals. Thai CKD patients frequently turn to religious practices such as chanting, prayer, or listening to Dhamma talks as a means of emotional regulation. Mindfulness-based components, when presented in familiar and culturally respectful formats, can promote acceptance, reduce anxiety, and provide existential grounding. In contrast to pharmacological treatments, mindfulness practices offer a sustainable, non-invasive method for managing emotional distress while honouring the spiritual dimension of the patient experience.

In sum, the integration of psychological well-being, resilience, and mindfulness into psychosocial intervention design allows for a comprehensive response to the emotional, existential, and cultural needs of Thai CKD patients. Rather than viewing these constructs as therapeutic add-ons, they should be understood as essential building blocks for person-centred care — facilitating not only the alleviation of distress but also the cultivation of strength, meaning, and psychological growth. Such an approach aligns with the core tenets of holistic nursing and affirms the value of culturally attuned innovation in chronic illness care.

11.10.2 *Suggested Structure of a Five-Week Internet-Based Positive Psychological Intervention Program*

Building on these theoretical foundations and patient insights, the following is a proposed five-week structure for an IPPI tailored to the cultural and psychosocial context of Thai individuals with CKD.

- ***Week 1:*** *Gratitude and Emotional Awareness*
  The program could begin by introducing gratitude practices that help patients shift attention from illness-related concerns to

meaningful aspects of their daily life. Guided journaling or multimedia prompts may assist in enhancing emotional awareness and self-acceptance.

- *Suggested objectives*: Increase positive affect, foster emotional regulation, support reflective practice
- *Theoretical foundations*: Broaden-and-build theory; Ryff's self-acceptance dimension

- ***Week 2:** Strengths Identification and Empowerment*
  Future modules may focus on helping patients recognise personal strengths and sources of resilience. Activities might include narrative recall, goal setting, and reflection on personal roles within family and society.
  - *Suggested objectives*: Enhance autonomy and self-efficacy, validate inner resources
  - *Theoretical foundations*: Resilience theory; Psychological well-being — autonomy and mastery
- ***Week 3**: Kindness and Relationship Reinforcement*
  Given the relational orientation in Thai culture, a module encouraging small acts of kindness and family-based engagement could play a crucial role. This may help reduce interpersonal burden and strengthen social connectedness.
  - *Suggested objectives*: Improve relational well-being, reduce perceived burden
  - *Theoretical foundations*: Positive psychology of prosocial behaviour; Psychological well-being — positive relationships
- ***Week 4:** Mindfulness and Spiritual Integration*
  Incorporating mindfulness practices such as breathing, guided reflection, or short Dhamma-based videos could offer culturally consonant methods for enhancing psychological stability. These may be delivered via audio or video, respecting spiritual diversity and accessibility.

- *Suggested objectives*: Promote emotional regulation, cultivate inner peace
- *Theoretical foundations*: Mindfulness-based stress reduction; Spiritual resilience

- ***Week 5:*** *Hope and Future Orientation*

  The concluding week might encourage patients to envision realistic future goals and aspirations, emphasising continuity, hope, and self-directed meaning-making. Peer testimonies and visual tools could reinforce a forward-looking mindset.

  - *Suggested objectives*: Support purposeful living, encourage future-minded resilience
  - *Theoretical foundations*: Ryff's dimension of purpose in life and personal growth

11.10.3 *Additional Design Considerations*

To optimise both usability and impact, several key design considerations should be taken into account during the development of the IPPI platform.

Digital Accessibility: The program should be mobile-first, low-bandwidth compatible, and designed with visual simplicity to ensure usability across different literacy and technology levels. In the Thai healthcare landscape, especially among individuals living in rural areas or with limited mobility due to CKD, ensuring digital access is a fundamental prerequisite for intervention equity. Mobile-first and low-bandwidth-compatible platforms can overcome barriers posed by technological disparity and allow patients to access support from their homes or dialysis centres. Furthermore, simplified user interfaces and clear visual designs enhance usability for individuals with varying levels of health literacy or digital proficiency.

Personalisation: Optional features such as private journaling, modular pacing, and content choice could increase patient engagement. Given the diversity among CKD patients in terms of illness stage, cultural beliefs, caregiving contexts, and digital familiarity, personalised intervention design is essential. Offering options such as self-paced modules, topic preferences, and private journaling features allows users to tailor the experience to their own needs. This autonomy fosters greater emotional investment, enhances engagement, and supports sustained participation by recognising the individuality of each patient's journey.

Social Integration: A community storytelling space (e.g., anonymous forums or peer video clips) may help foster shared meaning and normalise lived experiences. Social support is deeply embedded in Thai cultural values, with family and community playing integral roles in coping with illness. Incorporating features that enable patients to share stories, interact anonymously in forums, or view testimonial videos from peers can normalise experiences and build a sense of shared humanity. These social mechanisms contribute to reduced feelings of isolation and enhance the psychological benefits of the intervention through connection and belonging.

As healthcare systems in Thailand and elsewhere seek more culturally responsive models of chronic illness care, future psychosocial interventions for CKD patients **should consider adopting a positive psychology-informed approach**. Programs designed along the suggested structure above may not only address emotional vulnerabilities but also enhance psychological strengths, spiritual resilience, and long-term quality of life. Importantly, such models emphasise that meaningful care begins not with instruction, but with deep listening — translating the lived narratives of patients into interventions that are both compassionate and evidence-informed.

11.11 Suggestions for Future Development of Psychosocial Interventions in Chronic Kidney Disease Care: Implications for Policy and Practice

In anticipation of future efforts to improve the quality of life among individuals living with CKD in Thailand, this section outlines key suggestions for the potential development of psychosocial care models — particularly those grounded in positive psychology and adapted for digital delivery. Drawing on synthesised evidence, theoretical foundations, and cultural considerations, these recommendations are intended to inform the design, integration, and support of future interventions that extend beyond medical symptom management to include emotional, relational, and existential well-being.

While the IPPI proposed earlier has not yet been implemented, the following points highlight key elements that may be considered in guiding its future development and practical application.

11.11.1 *Key Considerations for Future Program Design*

Drawing from both empirical insights and cultural context, the following considerations highlight essential elements for shaping effective and meaningful future interventions.

Multidimensional Psychosocial Impact: CKD presents not only biomedical challenges, but also profound psychosocial implications that affect patients' emotional stability, financial security, and sense of life purpose. Programs that address only the physical aspects of illness risk neglecting key dimensions of suffering that influence long-term engagement and health outcomes. Future psychosocial interventions should therefore adopt a whole-person approach, recognising the interconnectedness of mind, body, and social context. This requires moving beyond symptom management toward frameworks that promote emotional resilience, financial coping, and existential meaning-making as integral parts of healing. Such comprehensive designs are more likely to foster sustained patient participation and enhance overall quality of life.

Cultural Responsiveness: In the Thai context, cultural values such as *kreng jai* (consideration and emotional restraint), the influence of Buddhist teachings, and deep-rooted familial interdependence shape how patients experience illness and seek support. Effective program design must not only acknowledge these values, but actively integrate them into intervention content, communication style, and delivery methods. Culturally responsive strategies may include using local metaphors, integrating mindfulness rooted in Buddhist principles, and encouraging family involvement in therapeutic processes. These adaptations will increase the emotional resonance of the intervention, foster trust, and ensure greater acceptability and adherence among Thai participants.

Digital Accessibility and Design: With mobile technology increasingly embedded in everyday life — particularly among rural and low-income populations — digital interventions must be designed with accessibility in mind. This includes optimising content for mobile-first use, ensuring compatibility with low-bandwidth environments, and employing visually simple, user-friendly interfaces. Inclusive digital design helps overcome barriers related to health literacy, age, and education level, thereby expanding reach and equity in care delivery. Aesthetically engaging and functionally intuitive platforms can also enhance sustained use, which is critical for achieving long-term psychosocial benefits in digital health programs.

Promotion of Patient Agency: A growing body of evidence supports the importance of promoting patient agency — the capacity for individuals to make choices, set goals, and act meaningfully in their own care. In the context of CKD, where illness can often feel disempowering, interventions should intentionally create space for patient voice, reflection, and self-directed growth. Practical strategies may include values clarification exercises, guided journaling, or tools for setting and tracking personal goals. Empowering patients in this way not only enhances intrinsic motivation, but also facilitates deeper psychological transformation and resilience — outcomes that are rarely achieved through directive or top-down models of care.

11.11.2 *Suggestions for Policy Development*

In order to translate research insights into sustainable change, the following policy-oriented recommendations are proposed to support the integration of psychosocial care into Thailand's national health system.

Formal Inclusion of Psychosocial Care: Despite increasing evidence supporting the effectiveness of psychosocial interventions in improving health outcomes for individuals with chronic diseases, such care remains marginal in Thailand's formal health policy. It is therefore recommended that psychosocial interventions — particularly those grounded in positive psychology — be formally recognised as essential components of chronic disease management frameworks. This inclusion should extend to national clinical guidelines, nephrology service protocols, and continuing education programs for healthcare professionals. Recognising the psychosocial domain as a core element of care would promote a more holistic approach and validate the psychological dimensions of living with CKD.

Strategic Budgeting and Resource Allocation: Effective policy implementation requires not only conceptual acknowledgment but also dedicated financial and structural support. Policymakers should consider creating specific budget lines for the research, development, and implementation of digital psychosocial interventions within chronic disease care, particularly for nephrology services. Prioritisation should be given to pilot programs that address the needs of underserved populations, such as those in rural areas or with limited access to mental health services.

Such strategic allocation of resources would help reduce disparities in care and ensure that innovations in digital health are equitably accessible across demographic and geographic groups.

Cross-sectoral Collaboration: To ensure both cultural relevance and implementation feasibility, policy development should be driven by collaboration across multiple sectors. Academic researchers can contribute theoretical and empirical knowledge, while healthcare providers bring insights from clinical practice. Digital health innovators offer the technical infrastructure needed to reach patients effectively, and community stakeholders — such as patient groups and local health volunteers — can help ensure alignment with real-world needs. Establishing structured partnerships and knowledge-sharing platforms among these actors would facilitate co-design processes, foster innovation, and support scalability and sustainability of psychosocial interventions within the public health system.

11.11.3 *Suggestions for Clinical and Educational Practice*

To translate research findings into day-to-day practice, the following recommendations are proposed for enhancing clinical implementation and professional training in psychosocial care.

Training in Psychosocial and Digital Competencies: The evolving landscape of chronic illness care, particularly in relation to psychosocial interventions, demands an expanded skill set among healthcare providers. Nurses and frontline clinicians, who often serve as the first point of contact for patients, are uniquely positioned to deliver psychosocial support. However, many currently lack formal training in areas such as narrative-based care, mindfulness facilitation, and digital intervention delivery. It is therefore recommended that continuing education programs and clinical training curricula integrate these competencies as core modules. Equipping providers with these skills will not only enhance the therapeutic quality of care, but also ensure more confident and competent use of digital tools in clinical settings.

Integration of Family-Centred Care: In the Thai cultural context, family members play a central role in the daily care of individuals with chronic illness. They often serve as informal caregivers, assisting with treatment adherence, emotional support, and health decision-making. Yet, traditional care models tend to overlook or underutilise this vital resource. Clinical interventions should be restructured to include clearly defined and culturally respectful roles for family members. Doing so may strengthen patients' support systems, reduce the emotional burden on caregivers, and promote shared ownership of health goals. Training providers to engage families effectively and respectfully is a key component of this shift toward relationally oriented care.

Mechanisms for Feedback and Iteration: Effective and sustainable psychosocial interventions require mechanisms for continuous improvement. Building systems that collect structured feedback from patients — whether through digital surveys, user experience interviews, or clinical observations — can help ensure that content remains relevant, culturally attuned, and user-friendly. Usability testing during pilot phases should be followed by periodic content reviews and iterative refinement. Involving patients and providers in these processes promotes co-ownership, enhances trust, and increases the likelihood that interventions will be embraced in real-world clinical practice. Ultimately, integrating a feedback-driven development model ensures that psychosocial care evolves alongside patient needs and technological advancements.

11.12 Conclusion

Caring for individuals with CKD in Thailand requires more than the management of physical symptoms; it calls for an intentional re-centring of the psychosocial, cultural, and existential dimensions of illness. The burden borne by patients — intertwined with disruptions in identity, emotional strain, family dynamics, and spiritual dissonance — underscores the need for care models that see beyond the clinical to the deeply human. Within this context, the incorporation of psychosocial support is not a peripheral concern, but a central tenet of holistic, person-centred care.

This chapter has explored the possibilities of integrating IPPIs into the landscape of CKD care. While the proposed framework remains conceptual, it reflects a deliberate synthesis of empirical insights, cultural grounding, and theoretical principles relevant to the Thai context. The emphasis on psychological well-being, resilience, and mindfulness offers a pathway toward emotional healing that is not only scalable but also congruent with the values and lived realities of Thai patients.

For particularly vulnerable groups — such as women undergoing dialysis — IPPIs represent more than a digital innovation; they embody a humanising approach to care, one that affirms inner strength, nurtures meaning, and honours the social and spiritual fabric of patients' lives. As the healthcare system moves toward models that embrace whole-person care, it is essential that institutional mechanisms support the co-design, implementation, and evaluation of such interventions.

Ultimately, this chapter affirms that psychosocial care is not simply about alleviating distress — it is about restoring dignity, cultivating resilience, and walking alongside patients in their journey through chronic illness. Future efforts should continue to invest in interdisciplinary collaboration, policy integration, and cultural adaptation, ensuring that the vision of holistic care becomes a lived reality for all individuals with CKD in Thailand.

References

1. Pan American Health Organization. Noncommunicable diseases: the leading causes of death in the Americas. Washington (DC): PAHO; 2015.

2. Thanakitcharu S. Epidemiology of CKD in Thailand. Nephrol J Thailand. 2015;31(1):12–18.
3. The Nephrology Society of Thailand. Annual report of the Thai Renal Replacement Therapy Registry. Bangkok: NST; 2015.
4. National Health Security Office (NHSO). Annual report 2013. Bangkok: NHSO; 2013. Available from: https://www.nhso.go.th/images/nhsoEn/Document/Annual%20Reports/NHSO%20Annual%20Report%202013.pdf
5. Phunmuangrat S, Sathirayon P, Inpanya W, Boonyaprasop N, Ruengorn C. A cost analysis of hemodialysis treatment in end-stage renal disease patients under the universal coverage scheme in Thailand. J Med Assoc Thai. 2017;100(6):664–72.
6. Thiansaard J. Health expenditures among hemodialysis patients in Bangkok. Thai J Public Health. 2017;47(1):72–81.
7. Ministry of Public Health. Annual report: health statistics and indicators 2015. Nonthaburi: Strategy and Planning Division, Ministry of Public Health; 2015.
8. Praha S, Sriyuktasuth A, Kusuma Na Ayuthya S, Vongsirimas N. Factors predicting quality of life in women receiving hemodialysis. J Nurs Sci. 2015;33(4):27–39.
9. Prapaiwong P, Sriyuktasuth A, Kusuma Na Ayuthya S, Vongsirimas N. Depression in patients with chronic kidney disease receiving CAPD. Thai J Nurs. 2015;64(2):9–20.
10. Manley HJ, Drayer DK, McClaran ML, *et al.* Medication prescribing patterns in ambulatory hemodialysis patients: comparisons of USRDS to a large not-for-profit dialysis provider. Pharmacoepidemiol Drug Saf. 2004;13(3):177–84.
11. Palmer SC, Vecchio M, Tonelli M, *et al.* Prevalence of depression in chronic kidney disease: updated systematic review and meta-analysis. Kidney Int. 2023;103(2):261–75.
12. Sriyuktasuth A, Vongsirimas N, Praha N, Prapaiwong P. Quality of life and related factors in women receiving hemodialysis and continuous ambulatory peritoneal dialysis: a comparative study. J Nurs Sci. 2017;35(1):72–84.
13. Phuka W, Vongsirimas N, Thanoi W. Factors correlated with psychological well-being in patients receiving hemodialysis. Nurs Sci J Thailand. 2020;38(1):73–85.
14. Ryff CD. Happiness is everything, or is it? Explorations on the meaning of psychological well-being. J Pers Soc Psychol. 1989;57(6):1069–81.
15. Ryan RM, Deci EL. On happiness and human potentials: a review of research on hedonic and eudaimonic well-being. Annu Rev Psychol. 2001;52:141–66.
16. Marin A-E, Redolat R, Gil-Gómez J-A, Mesa-Gresa P. Addressing cognitive function and psychological well-being in chronic kidney disease: a systematic review on the use of technology-based interventions. Int J Environ Res Public Health. 2023;20(4):3342.

17. Musa AS. Spiritual well-being, quality of life and depression among patients with end-stage renal disease undergoing hemodialysis. Scand J Caring Sci. 2017;31(4):745–53.
18. Sin NL, Lyubomirsky S. Enhancing well-being and alleviating depressive symptoms with positive psychology interventions: a practice-friendly meta-analysis. J Clin Psychol. 2009;65(5):467–87.
19. Seligman MEP, Steen TA, Park N, Peterson C. Positive psychology progress: empirical validation of interventions. Am Psychol. 2005;60(5):410–21.
20. Carr A, Cullen K, Keeney C, Canning C, Mooney O, Chinseallaigh E, *et al.* Effectiveness of positive psychology interventions: a systematic review and meta-analysis. J Posit Psychol. 2021;16(6):749–69.
21. Huffman JC, DuBois CM, Healy BC, Boehm JK, Kashdan TB, Celano CM, *et al.* Feasibility and utility of positive psychology exercises for suicidal inpatients. Gen Hosp Psychiatry. 2015;37(1):88–93.
22. Moskowitz JT, Carrico AW, Duncan LG, *et al.* Randomized controlled trial of a positive affect intervention for people newly diagnosed with HIV. J Consult Clin Psychol. 2017;85(5):409–23.
23. Bolier L, Haverman M, Westerhof GJ, Riper H, Smit F, Bohlmeijer E. Positive psychology interventions: a meta-analysis of randomized controlled studies. BMC Public Health. 2014;13:119.
24. Schueller SM, Parks AC, Pekka K. Disseminating self-help: positive psychology exercises in an online trial. J Med Internet Res. 2013;15(2):e36.
25. Gander F, Proyer RT, Ruch W, Wyss T. Strength-based positive interventions: further evidence for their potential in enhancing well-being and alleviating depression. J Happiness Stud. 2013;14:1241–59.
26. Chakhssi F, Kraiss JT, Sommers-Spijkerman M, Bohlmeijer ET. The effect of positive psychology interventions on well-being and distress in clinical samples with psychiatric or somatic disorders: a systematic review and meta-analysis. BMC Psychiatry. 2018;18(1):211.
27. Moskowitz JT, Carrico AW, Duncan LG, Cohn MA, Cheung EO, Batchelder A, *et al.* Randomized controlled trial of a positive affect intervention for people newly diagnosed with HIV. J Consult Clin Psychol. 2017;85(5):409–23.
28. Punyabati O, Chanu LB, Devi NS. Effect of a positive psychology intervention on psychological distress and quality of life in patients undergoing hemodialysis. Soc Work Health Care. 2020;59(9):635–49.
29. Mehta S, Peynenburg VA, Hadjistavropoulos HD. Internet-delivered cognitive behaviour therapy for chronic health conditions: a systematic review and meta-analysis. J Behav Med. 2019;42(2):169–87.

30. Adhikary D, Barman S, Ranjan R. Internet-based cognitive behavioural therapy for individuals with depression and chronic health conditions: a systematic review. Cureus. 2023;15(4):e37014.
31. Hernandez R, Burrows B, Wilund K, Cohn M, Xu S, Moskowitz JT. Feasibility of an internet-based positive psychological intervention for hemodialysis patients with symptoms of depression. Soc Work Health Care. 2018;57(10):864–79.

https://doi.org/10.1142/9789819817320_0012

Chapter 12

The Effectiveness of Psychosocial Interventions for Depression in Caregivers of Stroke Survivors: A Systematic Review

Jasmine Keh[1], Liberty Neo[2], and Jeanette Ignacio[3,*]

[1]*Ng Teng Fong General Hospital, 1 Jurong East Street 21, Singapore 609606*

[2]*Khoo Teck Puat Hospital, Singapore, 90 Yishun Central, Singapore 768828*

[3]*Alice Lee Centre for Nursing Studies, Yong Loo Lin School of Medicine, National University of Singapore, 10 Medical Drive, Singapore 117597*

**Corresponding author: nurimjj@nus.edu.sg*

12.1 Background

Stroke is known as a disturbance to the neurological function caused by an injury to the brain and resulting in impairment of function and mortality around the world [1]. According to the World Health Organisation [2], stroke is ranked the second top reason in causing mortality and third for causing disability worldwide. Additionally, the risk of having a stroke is one in four people [2]. According to the National Registry of Disease Office [3], there was a rising trend of stroke incidence from 2010 to 2019 which was also strongly impacted by the growing ageing population, with older adults showing a larger stroke occurrence in Singapore. This shows an evident disease burden caused by stroke and the growing number of stroke survivors present.

Also, many individuals who survived stroke suffer long-term impairments of the condition. The long-lasting complications include impairments affecting the individual's health condition such as seizures, affecting the function of the muscles and limbs, and causing changes in the emotions of the individual [4]. These complications can appear shortly after the acute episode or even many years later [4]. As a result, the stroke becomes a long-term condition with long-lasting implications affecting the loved ones around them, especially their caregiver.

Individuals with stroke are often supported and taken care of by their caregivers. The caregiver is an individual taking on the role of taking care of one who is sick, disabled or with a mental disorder, where the person is not able to perform self-care [5]. There are two types of caregivers: informal carers who help individuals with long-term conditions by providing them continuous, free assistance with their daily routines, and formal carers who provide care for the individuals in exchange for monetary benefits [6]. In this review, we focused solely on informal carers who are unpaid in their care. These caregiver roles can be taken up by the spouse, family members and relatives of stroke survivors providing long-term and unpaid care.

The caring process can be a demanding one with the unexpected effects of the condition. After the acute episode of the stroke, care for the stroke condition by healthcare professionals is often targeted towards the diseased individual with the priority of the acute management of stroke and its side effects. After the acute episode, the individual goes for rehabilitation and eventually back to the community, where the responsibility lies on the caregiver to care for their loved ones. However, given the unexpectedness of the complications of stroke and the demanding and extended period of the caring process, this adds to the burden of the caregivers.

Carers play an important part in the journey of stroke survivors, but their presence is often overlooked. The sudden and shocking characteristics of knowing the stroke condition drive the loved ones of the stroke survivor to take on the responsibility of the caregiver when they are unprepared [7]. The new roles force the carers to adapt and learn quickly before they return home from the hospital. Mostly, the majority of the individuals who suffer from stroke will be taken care of by their family members with insufficient training back in their homes [8]. Additionally, the caring role consists of not only the caregiver's responsibilities but also other implications to their own such as the carers' physical and mental well-being, affecting their social skills and connections, switches in their responsibilities, giving up on their freedom and monetary aspect gained from their careers, etc. [9]. This causes great disruption and changes to the carers' life in a short amount of time and might cause them to feel overly stressed in caregiving. Furthermore, even for carers who had prior knowledge and encounters, the requirements and attentiveness needed to provide sufficient caregiving at home are overly demanding and taxing [10]. Given the overwhelming caregiver burden, it is important to recognise the carers' roles and crucial to have interventions to assist them. The taxing conditions of the carers can affect them mentally and physically and turn into a vicious cycle.

Depression is a mental condition of having traits of lasting sadness and having no interest or feelings of happiness when involved in fun and fulfilling events [11]. In caregiving, the family carers may undergo depression, stress and other issues affecting mental stability [12]. In the study done by Loh *et al.* [13], it was reported that carers of people with stroke had a high percentage of 40.2% of depressive symptoms and 21.4% of anxiety symptoms. Additionally, in a study by Byun *et al.* [14], it was noted that depressive symptoms were already present in the early-stage caregiving of an individual post-stroke. Additionally, the impact of depression can influence an individual's capability to function and enjoy life which subsequently can affect their caregiver journey [11]. Hence, the incidence of depression is a potential issue that affects caregivers and should be prioritised, i.e., support should be provided for them.

One way of assisting the carers will be through psychosocial interventions (PIs) to help to manage the depressive symptoms. PIs including behavioural, psychological, and social aspects were reviewed [7, 15]. PIs would include many different interventions that can target various aspects. A search of the existing literature revealed one systematic review by Eldred and Sykes [16] where they reviewed the PIs for carers of stroke survivors. However, their study was focused on the burden of caring and helping to relieve the care burden; depression was not covered. Additionally, this previous review included only those interventions consisting of a theoretical framework, which resulted in only seven included studies. On the other hand, most recent reviews regarding PIs on stroke are mainly focused on its effects on both stroke survivors and their carers, and on the overall different effects that the various interventions can bring. The two systematic reviews by Mou and Wong [17] and Pucciarelli *et al.* [18] show the trend of PIs moving towards dyadic interventions due to the connected relationship between the carers and stroke survivors. However, the results are often generalised toward multiple outcomes and are difficult to conclude on a single outcome or population. Similarly, the systematic review by Cheng *et al.* [19] focuses on both impacts on dyads with a larger number of studies on interventions involving the family caregiver. However, with a combination of interventions only targeting one or both parties and the different types of PIs, the effectiveness of one of the interventions, known as psychoeducation, on depression was small and not significant [19]. As a result, it is difficult to conclude the effectiveness of the PIs acting on depression of the carer themselves.

Furthermore, most research involving depression as an outcome is mostly catered for caregivers of people with dementia as there is much evidence to support the effectiveness of PIs and known for their vital role in carers of individuals with dementia [20, 21]. Like dementia, stroke is also a chronic illness that results in long-term impact on both the individual suffering from the disease and the family. However, as the symptoms of dementia are more visible and stroke is perceived to be an acute condition rather than a long-term disease, the caregivers assisting stroke patients are often neglected.

With the rising trend of an ageing population and people living a longer lifespan, society will face the problem of more people living with disabilities caused by stroke [19]. This would mean that there will be a larger caregiver burden and stress to carers of stroke patients causing them to be more vulnerable towards having depressive symptoms. As a result, there is a gap in research evaluating PIs that focus solely on the carer and specifically target depression as an outcome. Moreover, more studies are now available compared to the previous systematic review on the same topic, allowing for a more comprehensive and up-to-date evaluation of PIs. Hence, a systematic review would be crucial to find out all the relevant PIs available targeting depression specific to carers of people with stroke.

12.1.1 *Review Question*

What is the effectiveness of PIs for depression in caregivers of stroke survivors?

12.1.2 *Review Aim*

The aim of the review is to synthesise the finest and latest accessible evidence to find out the effectiveness of PIs for caregivers of stroke survivors on the outcome of depression.

12.2 Methods

This systematic review was done in accordance with the Preferred Reporting Items for Systematic reviews and Meta-Analyses (PRISMA) checklist [22].

12.2.1 *Selection Criteria*

Studies fulfilling all the inclusion requirements stated below were included:

- Population: Carers, especially referring to informal carers, of stroke survivors who are aged 18 years and above, regardless of their gender. Caregivers may include their family members or their assigned primary caregiver.

- Intervention: PIs include any interventions covering the psychological and social aspects. PIs can include interventions such as counselling, peer support group, skill training, psychoeducation, cognitive and behavioural interventions [7, 19]. There is no limit on the frequency, location, timeframe and personnel carrying out the intervention.
- Comparator: No intervention, placebo or usual care.
- Outcomes: The primary outcome of depression will have to be one of the presented outcomes of the included studies. Secondary outcomes may include anxiety and caregiver burden. All measures of depression, anxiety and caregiver burden were accepted as long as they were validated tools.
- Study type: Randomised controlled trials (RCTs) only

Studies included are available in English and have no date restriction. Studies were excluded if:

i. study population involved paid carers;
ii. they combined the results of the PIs for stroke survivors and carers, where the outcomes of the carers cannot be isolated;
iii. they did not report carers' depression as an outcome of their PIs;
iv. they were duplicated studies;
v. there was no randomisation;
vi. they were quasi-experimental design, case-control studies, prospective and retrospective cohort studies;
vii. they were not published in English; and
viii. they were studies written in books.

12.2.2 *Search Strategy*

In this review, a systematic JBI three-step search strategy was used to identify all eligible studies [23]. An initial search was done in Nov 2022 in PubMed and Embase to identify all relevant keywords from the title, abstract and index terms which were then collated and analysed from all the relevant studies. The search terms identified were based on the population, intervention, comparator and outcome (PICO) framework where P: caregivers of stroke survivors, I: psychosocial intervention, C: no intervention, and O: depression. It was then followed by a search consisting of all the collated keywords and index terms identified across all six databases which were PubMed, Embase, CINAHL, Cochrane, PsycInfo and Scopus. Lastly, reference lists of all the included articles were reviewed. The search for eligible studies was restricted to those available in English unless there was a translated review. Additionally, grey literature was searched to locate any other relevant articles using Google Scholar.

12.2.3 *Study Selection*

After collating all eligible articles, all citations were uploaded into EndNote and duplicates removed via the software. Two reviewers independently screened the titles and abstracts of the studies to determine their eligibility, without influence from the other. Subsequently, the full texts of the included articles were retrieved and independently screened by the same two reviewers using the inclusion criteria. Any discrepancy on whether to include an article was resolved through a discussion between the two reviewers.

12.2.4 *Data Extraction*

Data were independently extracted by two reviewers using a modified Cochrane data collection form, with no mutual influence during the process. The form was modified to include the different details for this systematic review. The data collected was separated into two forms consisting of the study characteristics and the details of the intervention. Study characteristics included items such as study ID, setting and country, participants, intervention, significant outcome measures and findings while the details of interventions included items such as study

ID, intervention details, a framework for intervention, control details, mode of delivery, timepoint measuring outcomes and their providers. Pilot testing of the forms was carried out by the same two reviewers independently to refine any missing items before carrying out for all the included studies. Any discrepancy on whether to include an article was resolved through discussion between the two reviewers.

12.2.5 *Assessment of Methodological Quality*

The two reviewers who carried out the study selection continued to independently evaluate the quality of the articles included in this study. Any discrepancies among the two reviewers were settled through a discussion session. The methodological quality of the included articles was rated via JBI critical appraisal tool catered for RCTs as all the included studies were RCTs [24]. According to Tufanaru *et al.* [24], the methodological quality was assessed using 13 questions and elaborations provided on the criteria of each question. Each question could be responded with "Yes", "No" or "Unclear". To ensure comprehensive inclusion of all available PIs, the results of the critical appraisal did not influence study inclusion. Instead, appraisal outcomes were used to highlight limitations when interpreting the study findings.

12.2.6 *Data Synthesis*

Quantitative data were statistically analysed by meta-analysis using Review Manager software (RevMan). The summarised data were presented with the standardised mean difference (SMD) showing the effect size with a 95% confidence interval (CI) and were shown for the secondary outcomes of anxiety and caregiver burden. Outcomes measures of anxiety and caregiver burden were treated as continuous data. As a result of the different types of interventions included in the study, the random-effects model was selected to analyse data. The amount of heterogeneity of the data was evaluated using the I^2 statistics. Due to the heterogeneity of the intervention data, narrative synthesis was used for the primary outcome of depression. According to Sterne *et al.* [25], funnel plots are not recommended for assessing publication bias in meta-analyses with fewer than 10 studies. As such, there were insufficient studies in this review to generate a funnel plot.

12.2.7 *GRADE Assessment of Findings*

The Grading of Recommendations, Assessment, Development and Evaluation (GRADE) tool was used to assess the quality of evidence for the reported outcomes, particularly those included in the meta-analysis [26]. According to Meader *et al.* [26], reviews consisting of RCTs initially begin with a high-quality evidence rating, which may then be downgraded based on five domains: study design, risk of bias, inconsistency, indirectness, and imprecision. The quality of outcomes is ultimately rated as 'high,' 'moderate,' 'low,' or 'very low.' The evidence rating can be improved by the large magnitude of effect, dose response and through a reduction of the effect of other potential confounding factors [27]. Depression, anxiety and caregiver burden were the outcomes assessed by GRADE. The quality of evidence was independently assessed by two reviewers, with any disagreements resolved through discussion and consensus.

12.3 Results

12.3.1 *Search Results*

The entire search process and findings are presented in Figure 12.1. There were in total 1,917 eligible studies identified. Of these, 545 duplicate records were removed via EndNote before screening. The remaining 1,372 records were screened for their title and abstract by two independent reviewers, of which 1,310 records were excluded. After screening, 62 articles were left eligible and were identified to retrieve the full text of the articles; however, three records were excluded as we were unable

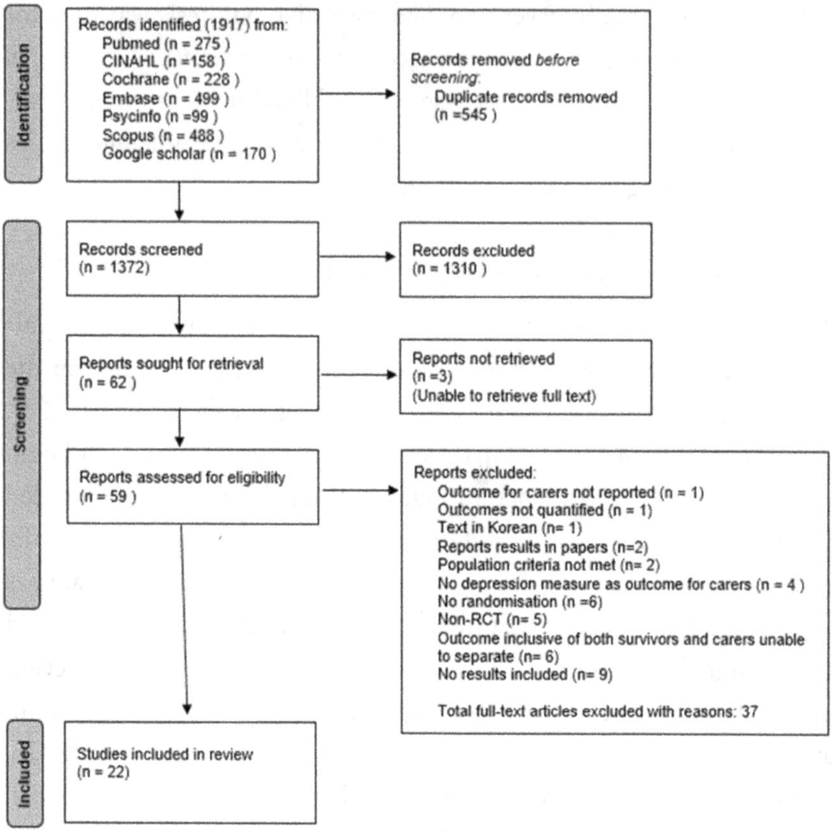

Figure 12.1 PRISMA flowchart consisting of the full search process and results.

to retrieve the full text for screening. Then the full text of the remaining 59 reports were screened for eligibility by the same two reviewers. Out of the 59 reports, only 22 studies fulfilled the inclusion criteria. Specific reasons for exclusion and the corresponding number of reports are presented in Figure 12.1.

12.3.2 *Methodological Quality*

Methodological quality was assessed for all the 22 RCT studies and Table 12.1 presents the results of the appraisal, with the legend listing the

Table 12.1 Critical appraisal of all the included studies.

Study	Q1	Q2	Q3	Q4	Q5	Q6	Q7	Q8	Q9	Q10	Q11	Q12	Q13
Wang, J., *et al.* (2021)	Y	Y	Y	N	N	N	Y	Y	Y	Y	Y	Y	Y
Pfeiffer, K., *et al.* (2014)	Y	Y	Y	N	N	Y	Y	Y	Y	Y	Y	Y	Y
Grant, J. S., *et al.* (2002)	U	N	Y	N	Y	Y	Y	Y	N	Y	Y	Y	Y
Bakas, T., et al (2015)	Y	Y	Y	Y	Y	Y	Y	Y	Y	Y	Y	Y	Y
Yilmaz, C. K., *et al.* (2019)	N	Y	Y	N	N	N	Y	Y	U	Y	Y	Y	Y
Kootker, J. A., *et al.* (2019)	Y	Y	Y	Y	N	Y	Y	Y	Y	Y	Y	Y	Y
Smith, G. C., et al (2012)	Y	Y	Y	Y	N	Y	Y	Y	Y	Y	Y	Y	Y
Beauchamp, J. E. S., *et al.* (2023)	Y	Y	Y	N	Y	N	Y	Y	Y	Y	Y	Y	Y
Mou, H., *et al.* (2022)	Y	Y	Y	N	N	Y	Y	Y	Y	Y	Y	Y	Y
Minshall, C., *et al.* (2020)	Y	Y	Y	N	N	N	Y	Y	N	Y	Y	Y	Y
Cheng, H. Y., *et al.* (2018)	Y	Y	Y	N	N	Y	Y	Y	Y	Y	Y	Y	Y
Ostwald, S. K., *et al.* (2014)	Y	U	Y	N	N	Y	Y	Y	Y	Y	Y	Y	Y
Perrin, P. B., *et al.* (2010)	U	U	Y	N	N	Y	Y	Y	N	Y	Y	Y	Y
Pierce, L. L., *et al.* (2009)	Y	N	Y	N	N	N	Y	Y	N	Y	Y	Y	Y
Kalra, L., *et al.* (2004)	Y	Y	Y	N	N	Y	Y	Y	Y	Y	Y	Y	Y
Hartke, R. J. and R. B. King (2003)	U	N	Y	N	N	N	Y	Y	N	Y	Y	Y	Y
Grant, J. S. (1999)	U	N	Y	N	N	N	Y	N	N	Y	Y	Y	Y

(*Continued*)

Table 12.1 (*Continued*)

Study	Q1	Q2	Q3	Q4	Q5	Q6	Q7	Q8	Q9	Q10	Q11	Q12	Q13
Patchwood, E., *et al.* (2021)	Y	Y	Y	Y	N	N	Y	Y	Y	Y	Y	Y	Y
Woodward, A. T., *et al.* (2021)	Y	N	Y	N	N	N	Y	Y	N	Y	Y	Y	Y
McCarthy, M. J., *et al.* (2021)	Y	N	Y	N	N	Y	Y	Y	N	Y	Y	Y	Y
Goudarzian, M., *et al.* (2018)	Y	N	Y	N	N	N	Y	Y	N	Y	Y	Y	Y
Bakas, T., *et al.* (2009)	Y	N	Y	U	N	Y	Y	Y	N	Y	Y	Y	Y

Legend:
Y = Yes, N = No, U = Unclear
Q1: Was true randomisation used for assignment of participants to treatment groups?
Q2: Was allocation to treatment groups concealed?
Q3: Were treatment groups similar at the baseline?
Q4: Were participants blind to treatment assignment?
Q5: Were those delivering treatment blind to treatment assignment?
Q6: Were outcomes assessors blind to treatment assignment?
Q7: Were treatment groups treated identically other than the intervention of interest?
Q8: Was follow-up complete and if not, were differences between groups in terms of their follow-up adequately described and analysed?
Q9: Were participants analysed in the groups to which they were randomised?
Q10: Were outcomes measured in the same way for treatment groups?
Q11: Were outcomes measured in a reliable way?
Q12: Was appropriate statistical analysis used?
Q13: Was the trial design appropriate, and any deviations from the standard RCT design (individual randomisation, parallel groups) accounted for in the conduct and analysis of the trial?

13 questions (Q1 to Q13) and the rating of each question. The process of true randomisation was not clearly reported in one study [28] despite being a randomised trial and was unclear in four studies for Q1 [29–32]. Concealment of the respective intervention and control group was not reported in eight studies [29–31, 33–37] and unclear description in two studies [32, 38] for Q2. For Q4, 17 studies [28–32, 34–45] did not have

participants blinded to the intervention and one [33] was unclear in its blinding of participants; for Q5, 19 studies consisted of the party giving the intervention not being blinded to the assignment [28, 29, 31–44, 46–48]. For Q4 and Q5, it was difficult for the included studies to blind the participants and the one guiding the intervention as most of the participants in the intervention group had to attend additional interventions while those guiding the intervention only met up with those in the intervention group. Ten studies [28, 29, 31, 34, 35, 37, 42, 43, 45, 48] had researchers collecting the outcomes not blinded to the intervention groups (Q6). One study [29] did not include explanations on whether follow-up was done and the reasons for any dropouts (Q8). Ten studies [29–37, 42] lacked analysis of the participants and one study [28] was unclear in its explanation (Q9). Regardless of the quality, all studies were included in the review for a comprehensive review.

12.3.3 *GRADE Assessment*

The summary of findings table was created via GRADEpro, including only the studies with the relevant data of mean and standard deviation reported. GRADE was used to assess the outcomes from the findings of the studies. The following outcomes of depression, anxiety and caregiver burden were reported as very low, low and low quality of evidence respectively as shown in Table 12.2. This translates to the three outcomes having low or very low quality of evidence, showing that PIs were effective in reducing the three outcomes as compared to usual care, placebo or no treatment.

12.3.4 *Characteristics of Studies Included*

There were a total of 22 studies ranging from the year 1999 to 2023, where they were all RCTs and published in English. Most of the included studies were from the United States, with ten included [31–34, 36–39, 45, 49]. There were three from China [41, 43, 44], three from the United

Table 12.2 Summary of findings via GRADE assessment.

Certainty assessment							No of patients		Effect			
No of studies	Study design	Risk of bias	Inconsistency	Indirectness	Imprecision	Other considerations	Psychosocial interventions	Usual care or placebo or no interventions	Relative (95% CI)	Absolute (95% CI)	Certainty	Importance
Depression												
13	randomised trials	not serious	serious[a]	not serious	serious[b]	publication bias strongly suspected[c]	705	703	—	see comment	⊕○○○ Very low	IMPORTANT
Anxiety												
6	randomised trials	serious[c]	not serious	not serious	not serious	publication bias strongly suspected[c]	414	413	—	SMD 0.22 SD lower (0.42 lower to 0.02 lower)	⊕⊕○○ Low	IMPORTANT
Caregiver burden												
5	randomised trials	serious[c]	not serious	not serious	not serious	publication bias strongly suspected[c]	242	239	—	SMD 0.015 SD lower (0.33 lower to 0.03 higher)	⊕⊕○○ Low	IMPORTANT

CI: confidence interval; SMD: standardised mean difference

a. This is due to the result of the heterogeneity of interventions.

b. No effect size generated due to no meta-analysis done.

c. Due to some studies not having allocation concealment of the treatment group and blinding of participants and researchers.

Kingdom [29, 30, 48], one from Australia [42], one from Germany [40], one from Iran [35], one from Turkey [28], one from the Netherlands [47] and one study did not specify which country it was conducted in [46]. Interventions were mostly carried out either in the stroke rehabilitation unit or after the patients were discharged back to their homes.

12.3.5 *Participants*

There were a total of 2,449 caregivers included in the 22 studies. The average age of the caregiver was highlighted in all trials except the article by Kalra *et al.* [39] which only highlighted the mean age of stroke survivors. The mean age range for all studies ranged from 26 to 89 years old. In general, apart from the study by Smith *et al.* [46] involving only female carers, most of the studies reported more female carers in comparison to male carers.

12.3.6 *Details About the Interventions*

A summary of the interventions is presented in Table 12.3. Out of the 22 studies, 12 interventions were provided for carers, eight for dyads, one for only stroke patients and one for female carers only. Of the 22 studies, only nine employed a guiding framework for their intervention. Unlike the previous review by Eldred and Sykes [16], this review did not restrict inclusion to studies with a framework, allowing for a broader range of studies to be included. Due to the variations in interventions, all the interventions were classified under their psychosocial components for clarity.

12.3.7 *Outcomes*

All studies included the primary outcome of depression and for secondary outcomes, eight studies reported the outcome of anxiety and nine studies reported about caregiver burden.

Table 12.3 Summary of the interventions delivered.

Study	**Intervention Catered to**	**Outcomes Included**	**Psychosocial Components of Intervention**
Wang, J., *et al.* (2021)	Carers	Depression, anxiety, caregiver burden	Relaxation program and education
Pfeiffer, K., *et al.* (2014).	Carers	Depressive symptoms	Problem-solving skills
Grant, J. S., *et al.* (2002).	Carers	Depression, caregiver burden	Problem-solving skills
Bakas, T., *et al.* (2015)	Carers	Depression	Education
Yilmaz, C. K., *et al.* (2019)	Carers	Depression, caregiver burden	Relaxation
Kootker, J. A., *et al.* (2019)	Stroke patients	Depression, anxiety	Cognitive behavioural therapy
Smith, G. C., *et al.* (2012)	Female carers	Depression	Education and problem-solving skills
Beauchamp, J. E. S., *et al.* (2023)	Dyads	Depression, anxiety	Mediation
Mou, H., *et al.* (2022)	Dyads	Depression, anxiety, caregiver burden	Education and problem-solving skills
Minshall, C., *et al.* (2020)	Dyads	Depression, anxiety	Psychosocial support
Cheng, H. Y., *et al.* (2018)	Carers	Depressive symptoms, caregiving burden	Education and problem-solving skills
Ostwald, S. K., *et al.* (2014)	Dyads	Depression, caregiver burden	Education, support and problem-solving skills
Perrin, P. B., *et al.* (2010)	Dyads	Depression	Education and problem-solving skills
Pierce, L. L., *et al.* (2009)	Cares	Depression	Education and support
Kalra, L., *et al.* (2004)	Dyads	Depression, anxiety, caregiver burden	Support and training

Table 12.3 (*Continued*)

Study	**Intervention Catered to**	**Outcomes Included**	**Psychosocial Components of Intervention**
Hartke, R. J. and King, R. B. (2003)	Carers	Depression, caregiver burden	Education and skill
Grant, J. S. (1999)	Carers	Depression, caregiver burden	Problem-solving skills
Patchwood, E., *et al.* (2021)	Carers	Depression, anxiety	Support
Woodward, A. T., *et al.* (2021)	Dyads	Depressive symptoms	Education
McCarthy, M. J., *et al.* (2021)	Dyads	Depression	Education and support
Goudarzian, M., *et al.* (2018)	Carers	Depression, anxiety	Support
Bakas, T., *et al.* (2009)	Carers	Depressive symptoms	Support and skills

12.3.7.1 *Depression (Primary Outcome)*

All studies in the review investigated the outcome of depression. However, due to the heterogeneity of the PIs, a meta-analysis was not conducted for the effects of depression. For effects ranging from immediately after the intervention to about one month after intervention, nine studies showed a decrease in depression or depressive symptoms [29, 30, 32, 33, 35–37, 39, 46]. For long-term effects of the intervention beyond one month, three studies found that depression was significantly reduced [40, 43, 49]. On the other hand, ten studies reported no statistically significant difference in the outcome of depression between treatment and control before treatment and after [28, 31, 34, 38, 41, 42, 44, 45, 47, 48].

Study or Subgroup	psychosocial intervention Mean	SD	Total	Control Mean	SD	Total	Weight	Std. Mean Difference IV, Random, 95% CI
Goudarzian, M., et al. 2018	30.18	5.52	76	33.59	6.4	76	20.7%	-0.57 [-0.89, -0.24]
Kootker, J. A., et al. 2019	6.6	4.5	20	6.9	4.7	27	9.4%	-0.06 [-0.64, 0.51]
Minshall, C., et al. 2020	6.1	3.39	35	6.9	4.05	29	12.0%	-0.21 [-0.71, 0.28]
Mou, H., et al. 2022	3.45	3.39	20	4.65	4.07	20	8.4%	-0.31 [-0.94, 0.31]
Patchwood, E., et al. 2021	8.2	4.73	208	8.34	4.51	206	32.0%	-0.03 [-0.22, 0.16]
Wang, J., et al. 2021	5.8	2.7	55	6.4	3	55	17.5%	-0.21 [-0.58, 0.17]
Total (95% CI)			**414**			**413**	**100.0%**	**-0.22 [-0.42, -0.02]**

Heterogeneity: $Tau^2 = 0.02$; $Chi^2 = 8.18$, $df = 5$ ($P = 0.15$); $I^2 = 39\%$
Test for overall effect: $Z = 2.17$ ($P = 0.03$)

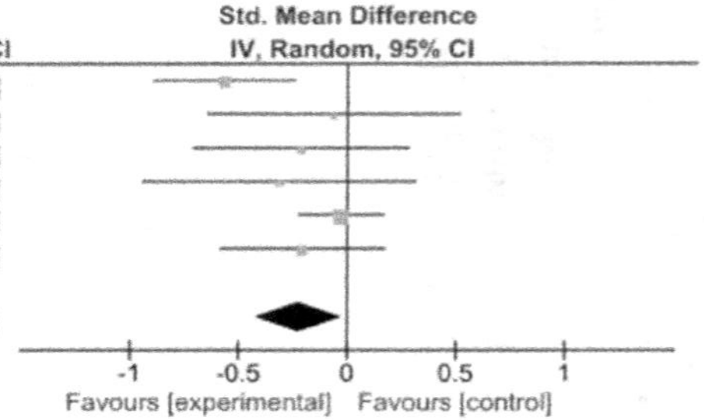

Figure 12.2 Forest plot of six studies reporting on the effects of PIs on anxiety post-intervention.

Study or Subgroup	psychosocial intervention Mean	SD	Total	Control Mean	SD	Total	Weight	Std. Mean Difference IV, Random, 95% CI
Cheng, H. Y., et al. 2018	6.19	3.26	64	6.79	3.58	64	26.6%	-0.17 [-0.52, 0.17]
Mou, H., et al. 2022	32.45	15.86	20	44.4	16.5	20	8.0%	-0.72 [-1.37, -0.08]
Ostwald, S. K., et al. 2014	25.36	14.47	80	26.43	15.26	79	32.9%	-0.07 [-0.38, 0.24]
Wang, J., et al. 2021	42.6	13.9	55	44.6	12.7	55	23.0%	-0.15 [-0.52, 0.23]
Yilmaz, C. K., et al. 2019	42.89	10.86	23	41.33	15.24	21	9.4%	0.12 [-0.48, 0.71]
Total (95% CI)			**242**			**239**	**100.0%**	**-0.15 [-0.33, 0.03]**

Heterogeneity: $Tau^2 = 0.00$; $Chi^2 = 4.11$, $df = 4$ ($P = 0.39$); $I^2 = 3\%$
Test for overall effect: $Z = 1.62$ ($P = 0.10$)

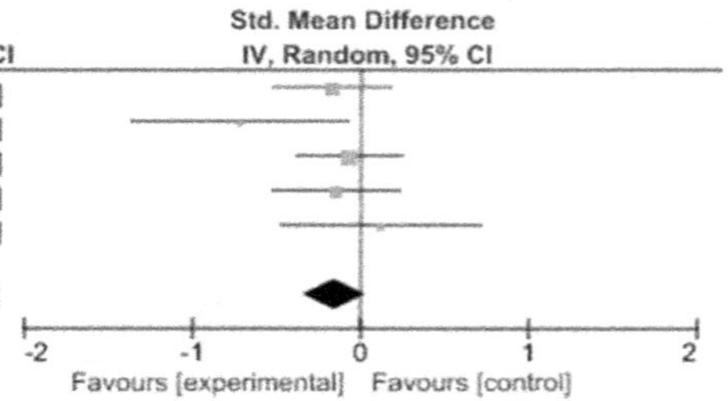

Figure 12.3 Forest plot of five studies reporting on the effects of PIs on caregiver burden post-intervention.

12.3.7.2 *Anxiety (Secondary Outcome)*

Out of the eight studies, six reported the outcome of anxiety with sufficient data of mean and standard deviation after intervention and were pooled for meta-analysis shown in Figure 12.2 [35, 42–44, 47, 48]. The results indicated that PIs had statistically significant small effects on the anxiety of stroke survivors (SMD = −0.22, 95% CI: −0.42, −0.02, p = 0.03) with a low heterogeneity ($Chi^2 = 8.18$, df = 5 (p = 0.15); $I^2 = 39\%$). For the remaining two studies not included in the meta-analysis, Kalra *et al.* [39] showed significant effects of reduction of anxiety (anxiety score 3 v4; P = 0.0001) while Beauchamp *et al.* [45] showed a reduction of anxiety but was not significant (mean difference = −11.7500, 95% CI: −24.419, 0.919, p = 0.0644).

12.3.7.3 *Caregiver Burden (Secondary Outcome)*

Out of the nine studies, five reported the outcomes of caregiver burden with sufficient data for meta-analysis shown in Figure 12.3 [28, 38, 41, 43, 44]. The results revealed a small but not significant effect on PIs acting on caregiver burden (SMD = −0.15, 95% CI: −0.33, 0.03, p = 0.10) with a low heterogeneity ($Chi^2 = 4.41$, df = 4 (p = 0.39); $I^2 = 3\%$).

For the four remaining studies, two studies reported no significant difference between control versus treatment parties on caregiver burden [29, 30]. However, the other two studies by Kalra *et al.* [39] and Hartke and King [31] showed a significant effect on decreasing caregiver burden.

12.4 Discussion

This systematic review evaluated the effectiveness of PIs for carers of stroke survivors, focusing on depression as the primary outcome, along with secondary outcomes of anxiety and caregiver burden, using evidence from the past 24 years. The primary outcome of depression had varied results with nine studies showing reduction of depression and ten studies showing no effect at all. Long-term effects of PIs were found to be effective in reducing depression in carers in three studies. For the secondary outcome of anxiety, meta-analysis of five out of nine studies showed that PIs were effective in reducing anxiety among carers. However, analysis of five out of nine studies reporting caregiver burden indicated that PIs had no significant effect on this outcome.

Although there were 22 studies included, the differences in the types of psychosocial components of interventions and in the mode of delivery among the studies made it difficult to directly compare their results and conclude their effectiveness. Similar to the findings of Eldred and Sykes [16], comparing results across studies was challenging due to variations in the interventions. Likewise, Qureshi *et al.* [7], in their review of PIs, concluded that no specific treatment could be recommended because of the diversity in interventions. Consequently, mixed outcomes across the included PIs were expected. Additionally, the included studies varied in their intervention durations and follow-up periods, making direct comparisons difficult. In contrast, Pucciarelli *et al.* [18] limited outcomes to those measured between three and six months, resulting in more homogeneous data that allowed for more effective comparison.

12.4.1 *Strengths*

This review synthesises the latest evidence on PIs specifically targeting carers of stroke survivors — a focus not addressed in recent studies that emphasised dyads or in the previous review conducted over a decade ago. By concentrating solely on depression as the primary outcome, this review highlights interventions that may effectively support stroke caregivers.

12.4.2 *Limitations*

A key limitation across the literature and in this review is the lack of a clear definition or criteria for what constitutes a PI, making article inclusion somewhat subjective. This may have led to the inadvertent exclusion of relevant studies, potentially impacting the evaluation of intervention effectiveness. Additionally, this review included all studies regardless of methodological quality. Several studies lacked critical information, particularly regarding allocation concealment and blinding of participants and intervention personnel, which may affect the overall quality and reliability of the findings.

12.4.3 *Implications*

From a clinical perspective, one implication is the need for healthcare professionals to recognise the risk of depression among carers and offer targeted support, such as ward-based education or problem-solving interventions, to help them better adapt to their caregiving role. Additionally, this review provides an updated synthesis of the latest clinical evidence on PIs specifically for carers, offering a valuable foundation for researchers to develop new interventions or refine existing ones to more effectively address depression in caregivers of stroke survivors.

12.4.4 *Conclusion*

This review evaluated PIs designed for caregivers of stroke survivors, with a primary focus on reducing depression and additional attention to secondary outcomes. However, the wide variation in the psychological and social components of the interventions led to inconclusive findings regarding their overall effectiveness.

References

1. Sacco RL, Kasner SE, Broderick JP, Caplan LR, Connors JJ, Culebras A, *et al.* An updated definition of stroke for the 21st century: a statement for healthcare professionals from the American Heart Association/American Stroke Association. Stroke. 2013;44(7):2064–89.
2. World Health Organization. World Stroke Day [Internet]. Geneva: World Health Organization; 2021 Oct 28 [cited 2022 Dec 8]. Available from: https://www.who.int/southeastasia/news/detail/28-10-2021-world-stroke-day

3. National Registry of Diseases Office. Singapore Stroke Registry Annual Report 2019 [Internet]. Singapore: National Registry of Diseases Office; 2021 Nov 3 [cited 2022 Dec 9]. Available from: https://www.nrdo.gov.sg/
4. Chohan SA, Venkatesh PK, How CH. Long-term complications of stroke and secondary prevention: an overview for primary care physicians. Singapore Med J. 2019;60(12):616.
5. Agency for Integrated Care. Roles of a caregiver [Internet]. Singapore: Agency for Integrated Care; 2022 [cited 2022 Dec 9]. Available from: https://www.aic.sg/caregiving/caregiver-role
6. Roth DL, Fredman L, Haley WE. Informal caregiving and its impact on health: a reappraisal from population-based studies. Gerontologist. 2015;55(2):309–19.
7. Qureshi A, Hargest C, Swain N, Aldabe D, Hale L. Psychosocial interventions for building resilience of informal carers of people living with stroke: a systematic review. Disabil Rehabil. 2022;1–14.
8. Creasy KR, Lutz BJ, Young ME, Stacciarini JMR. Clinical implications of family-centered care in stroke rehabilitation. Rehabil Nurs. 2015;40(6):349–59.
9. Hall JF, Crocker TF, Clarke DJ, Forster A. Supporting carers of stroke survivors to reduce carer burden: development of the Preparing is Caring intervention using Intervention Mapping. BMC Public Health. 2019;19(1):1–16.
10. Lutz BJ, Young ME, Cox KJ, Martz C, Creasy KR. The crisis of stroke: experiences of patients and their family caregivers. Top Stroke Rehabil. 2011;18(6):786–97.
11. World Health Organization. Depression [Internet]. Geneva: World Health Organization; [cited 2022 Dec 9]. Available from: https://www.who.int/health-topics/depression#tab=tab_1
12. Omar O, Aziz AFA, Ali MF, Ja SEHA, Izzudin MPE. Caregiver depression among home-bound stroke patients in an urban community. Cureus. 2021;13(9):e17948.
13. Loh AZ, Tan JS, Zhang MW, Ho RC. The global prevalence of anxiety and depressive symptoms among caregivers of stroke survivors. J Am Med Dir Assoc. 2017;18(2):111–6.
14. Byun E, Evans L, Sommers M, Tkacs N, Riegel B. Depressive symptoms in caregivers immediately after stroke. Top Stroke Rehabil. 2019;26(3):187–94.
15. Minshall C, Pascoe MC, Thompson DR, Castle DJ, McCabe M, Chau JP, *et al.* Psychosocial interventions for stroke survivors, carers and survivor-carer dyads: a systematic review and meta-analysis. Top Stroke Rehabil. 2019;26(7):554–64.
16. Eldred C, Sykes C. Psychosocial interventions for carers of survivors of stroke: a systematic review of interventions based on psychological principles and theoretical frameworks. Br J Health Psychol. 2010;13(3):563–81.

17. Mou H, Wong MS. Effectiveness of dyadic psychoeducational intervention for stroke survivors and family caregivers on functional and psychosocial health: a systematic review and meta-analysis. Int J Nurs Stud. 2021;120:103969.
18. Pucciarelli G, Lommi M, Magwood GS, Simeone S, Colaceci S, Vellone E, *et al.* Effectiveness of dyadic interventions to improve stroke patient–caregiver dyads' outcomes after discharge: a systematic review and meta-analysis study. Eur J Cardiovasc Nurs. 2021;20(1):14–33.
19. Cheng HY, Chair SY, Chau JPC. The effectiveness of psychosocial interventions for stroke family caregivers and stroke survivors: a systematic review and meta-analysis. Patient Educ Couns. 2014;95(1):30–44.
20. McDermott O, Charlesworth G, Hogervorst E, Stoner C, Moniz-Cook E, Spector A, *et al.* Psychosocial interventions for people with dementia: a synthesis of systematic reviews. Aging Ment Health. 2019;23(4):393–403.
21. Dickinson C, Dow J, Gibson G, Hayes L, Robalino S, Robinson L. Psychosocial intervention for carers of people with dementia: what components are most effective and when? A systematic review of systematic reviews. Int Psychogeriatr. 2017;29(1):31–43.
22. Page MJ, McKenzie JE, Bossuyt PM, Boutron I, Hoffmann TC, Mulrow CD, *et al.* The PRISMA 2020 statement: an updated guideline for reporting systematic reviews. Syst Rev. 2021;10(1):1–11.
23. Peters MDJ, Godfrey C, McInerney P, Munn Z, Tricco AC, Khalil H. Chapter 11: Scoping reviews (2020 version). In: Aromataris E, Munn Z, editors. JBI Manual for Evidence Synthesis. Adelaide: JBI; 2020. Available from: https://synthesismanual.jbi.global
24. Tufanaru C, Munn Z, Aromataris E, Campbell J, Hopp L. Chapter 3: Systematic reviews of effectiveness. In: Aromataris E, Munn Z, editors. JBI Manual for Evidence Synthesis. Adelaide: JBI; 2020. Available from: https://synthesismanual.jbi.global
25. Sterne JA, Sutton AJ, Ioannidis JP, Terrin N, Jones DR, Lau J, *et al.* Recommendations for examining and interpreting funnel plot asymmetry in meta-analyses of randomised controlled trials. BMJ. 2011;343:d4002.
26. Meader N, King K, Llewellyn A, Norman G, Brown J, Rodgers M, *et al.* A checklist designed to aid consistency and reproducibility of GRADE assessments: development and pilot validation. Syst Rev. 2014;3:82.
27. Ryan R, Hill S. How to GRADE the quality of the evidence. Cochrane Consumers and Communication Group; 2016 [cited 2025 May 19]. Version 3.0. Available from: http://cccrg.cochrane.org/author-resources
28. Yilmaz CK, Aşiret GD, Çetinkaya F, Oludağ G, Kapucu S. Effect of progressive muscle relaxation on the caregiver burden and level of depression among

caregivers of older patients with a stroke: a randomized controlled trial. Jpn J Nurs Sci. 2019;16(2):202–11.

29. Grant JS. Social problem-solving partnerships with family caregivers. Rehabil Nurs. 1999;24(6):254–60.
30. Grant JS, Elliott TR, Weaver M, Bartolucci AA, Giger JN. Telephone intervention with family caregivers of stroke survivors after rehabilitation. Stroke. 2002;33(8):2060–5.
31. Hartke RJ, King RB. Telephone group intervention for older stroke caregivers. Top Stroke Rehabil. 2003;9(4):65–81.
32. Perrin PB, Johnston A, Vogel B, Heesacker M, Vega-Trujillo M, Anderson J, *et al.* A culturally sensitive transition assistance program for stroke caregivers: examining caregiver mental health and stroke rehabilitation. J Rehabil Res Dev. 2010;47(7):605–15.
33. Bakas T, Farran CJ, Austin JK, Given BA, Johnson EA, Williams LS. Stroke caregiver outcomes from the Telephone Assessment and Skill-Building Kit (TASK). Top Stroke Rehabil. 2009;16(2):105–21.
34. Pierce LL, Steiner VL, Khuder SA, Govoni AL, Horn LJ. The effect of a web-based stroke intervention on carers' well-being and survivors' use of healthcare services. Disabil Rehabil. 2009;31(20):1676–84.
35. Goudarzian M, Fallahi-Khoshknab M, Dalvandi A, Delbari A, Biglarian A. Effect of telenursing on levels of depression and anxiety in caregivers of patients with stroke: a randomized clinical trial. Iran J Nurs Midwifery Res. 2018;23(4):248–52.
36. McCarthy MJ, Sanchez A, Garcia YE, Lyons KS, Bakas T. Feasibility of the Hand in Hand Relationship Intervention for Stroke Survivor–Caregiver Dyads: A randomized trial. Res Soc Work Pract. 2021;31(1):75–89.
37. Woodward AT, Fritz MC, Hughes AK, Coursaris CK, Swierenga SJ, Freddolino PP, *et al.* Effect of transitional care stroke case management interventions on caregiver outcomes: the MISTT randomized trial. Soc Work Health Care. 2021;60(10):642–55.
38. Ostwald SK, Godwin KM, Cron SG, Kelley CP, Hersch G, Davis S. Home-based psychoeducational and mailed information programs for stroke-caregiving dyads post-discharge: a randomized trial. Disabil Rehabil. 2014;36(1):55–62.
39. Kalra L, Evans A, Perez I, Melbourn A, Patel A, Knapp M, *et al.* Training caregivers of stroke patients: randomised controlled trial. BMJ. 2004;328(7448):1099–101.
40. Pfeiffer K, Beische D, Hautzinger M, Berry JW, Wengert J, Hoffrichter R, *et al.* Telephone-based problem-solving intervention for family caregivers of stroke survivors: a randomized controlled trial. J Consult Clin Psychol. 2014;82(4): 628–43.

41. Cheng HY, Chair SY, Chau JPC. Effectiveness of a strength-oriented psychoeducation on caregiving competence, problem-solving abilities, psychosocial outcomes and physical health among family caregiver of stroke survivors: a randomised controlled trial. Int J Nurs Stud. 2018;87:84–93.
42. Minshall C, Castle DJ, Thompson DR, Pascoe M, Cameron J, McCabe M, *et al.* A psychosocial intervention for stroke survivors and carers: 12-month outcomes of a randomized controlled trial. Top Stroke Rehabil. 2020;27(8):563–76.
43. Wang J, Liu J, Li L, Man J, Yue S, Liu Z. Effect of education and muscle relaxation program on anxiety, depression and care burden in caregivers of acute stroke survivors: a randomized, controlled study. Medicine (Baltimore). 2021;100(4):e24154.
44. Mou H, Lam SKK, Chien WT. Effects of family-focused dyadic psychoeducational intervention for stroke survivor-caregiver dyads: A randomised controlled trial [conference abstract]. Int J Stroke. 2022;17(3):72.
45. Beauchamp JES, Sharrief A, Chaoul A, Casameni Montiel T, Love MF, Cron S, *et al.* Feasibility of a meditation intervention for stroke survivors and informal caregivers: a randomized controlled trial. BMC Psychol. 2023;11(1):9.
46. Smith GC, Egbert N, Dellman-Jenkins M, Nanna K, Palmieri PA. Reducing depression in stroke survivors and their informal caregivers: a randomized clinical trial of a web-based intervention. Rehabil Psychol. 2012;57(3):196–206.
47. Kootker JA, van Heugten CM, Kral B, Rasquin SM, Geurts AC, Fasotti L. Caregivers' effects of augmented cognitive-behavioural therapy for post-stroke depressive symptoms in patients: secondary analyses to a randomized controlled trial. Clin Rehabil. 2019;33(6):1056–65.
48. Patchwood E, Woodward-Nutt K, Rhodes SA, Batistatou E, Camacho E, Knowles S, *et al.* Organising Support for Carers of Stroke Survivors (OSCARSS): a cluster randomised controlled trial with economic evaluation. BMJ Open. 2021;11(1):e038777.
49. Bakas T, Austin JK, Habermann B, Jessup NM, McLennon SM, Mitchell PH, *et al.* Telephone Assessment and Skill-Building Kit for Stroke Caregivers: A randomized controlled clinical trial. Stroke. 2015;46(12):3478–87.

https://doi.org/10.1142/9789819817320_0013

Chapter 13*

Effects of Virtual Reality Intervention on Cognitive, Physical, and Psychological Outcomes Among Individuals with Mild Cognitive Impairment or Dementia: A Systematic Review and Meta-Analysis

Ser Ning Lua[1], Han Peng Benedict[2], Vivien Xi Wu[3], and Piyanee Klainin-Yobas[3,*]

[1]*Khoo Teck Puat Hospital, Singapore, 90 Yishun Central, Singapore 768828*

[2]*Tan Tock Seng Hospital, 11 Jln Tan Tock Seng, Singapore 308433*

[3]*Alice Lee Centre for Nursing Studies, Yong Loo Lin School of Medicine, National University of Singapore, Level 5, Centre of Translational Medicine, Block MD6, 14 Medical Drive, Singapore 117599*

**Corresponding author: nurpk@nus.edu.sg*

13.1 Introduction

Dementia, also known as major neurocognitive disorder, is an umbrella term for conditions with pronounced deficits in cognitive domains, which interfere significantly with an individual's independence and functional abilities [1]. Individuals with dementia often experience behavioural and psychological symptoms of dementia [2]. Globally, in 2020, over 50 million people live with dementia. This number is projected to double every two decades [3].

---

*Appendices to this chapter are available for download at https://www.worldscientific.com/worldscibooks/10.1142/14420#t=suppl.

Mild cognitive impairment (MCI), or minor neurocognitive disorder, is a stage of cognitive deterioration between normal cognition and dementia, which requires compensatory strategies to preserve independence [4]. Individuals with MCI encounter neuropsychiatric symptoms, such as depression and anxiety, and they are slower in executing complex activities [5]. Nearly 15% of older adults are affected by MCI [6] and many of them experience cognitive deterioration and later develop dementia [7].

There is no known cure for MCI or dementia. Pharmacological methods are commonly used for symptomatic treatments. Nonetheless, their limited efficacy warrants the use of non-pharmacological interventions to ameliorate the symptoms of MCI and dementia [8]. Such interventions include cognitive stimulation, cognitive remediation therapy, and exercise, which help prevent functional decline, and improve cognition, mood, and quality of life (QoL) [9]. Recently, virtual reality (VR) technology shows the potential in enhancing non-pharmacological treatments [10].

VR technology utilises computer technology to create artificial environments that provide interaction and real-time feedback through multiple sensory channels [11]. The fundamentals of VR technology — immersion and interactivity — allow users to feel present in and connected to the virtual world [12]. VR encompasses mixed and augmented realities, and is classified as non-immersive and immersive [13]. Immersive VR utilises sophisticated technologies such as Cave Automatic Virtual Environment systems and head-mounted devices. VR achieves interactivity by tracking head and hand positions in real time. In contrast, non-immersive VR has a smaller field of regard and displays virtual environments on screens. Gamepads, computer mouse or keyboards are used to control interactions [14, 15].

VR has gained popularity for exergaming and cognitive rehabilitation of phobia, anxiety and amnesia [16, 17]. Sensory stimulation and real-time feedback allow motor learning and improvements in emotional states and interpersonal interactions [18, 19]. Moreover, VR eliminates physical dangers and provides safe environments to train situations that are typically perceived as dangerous (e.g., wayfinding, fire safety) [20]. Hence, VR may be a judicious alternative to traditional rehabilitation for people with MCI.

Six systematic reviews (Appendix A) examined the effects of VR interventions on people with MCI or dementia. However, the intervention effects of VR remain inconclusive in three systematic reviews [17, 21, 22] as meta-analysis was not undertaken. Through statistical integration of findings from multiple primary studies, meta-analysis generated a quantitative estimate of VR interventions, thereby boosting the review's power and precision [23]. While [24] performed meta-analysis, the methodological diversity was high due to the inclusion of non-randomised controlled trials (non-RCTs). Furthermore, [24] did not include specific cognitive and physical outcomes. References [25] and [26] performed meta-analysis of RCTs. However, they did not include grey literature, which may contribute to publication bias [27]. Moreover, [25] included only interventions with drill-and-practice of standardised tasks, while [26] omitted the possible benefits of VR interventions on mood and well-being. These literature gaps can be plugged with a more thorough systematic review to guide the use of VR among patients with MCI or dementia.

To minimise the aforementioned knowledge gaps, this systematic review aimed to synthesise the best available evidence regarding the effectiveness of VR interventions on cognitive, physical, and psychological outcomes of individuals with dementia or MCI. The review questions are:

1. What is the magnitude of the effect of VR interventions, in comparison to controls, on cognitive outcomes (attention, executive function, language, memory, sensation/perception, and processing speed) among individuals with MCI or dementia?
2. What is the magnitude of the effect of VR interventions, in comparison to controls, on physical outcomes (physical functions, mobility and balance) and psychological outcomes (depression and QoL) among individuals with MCI or dementia?

3. To what extent does the level of immersivity (non-immersive, immersive) affect the cognitive, physical and psychological outcomes among individuals with MCI or dementia?

13.2 Method

This review was developed in accordance with the PRISMA (Preferred Reporting Items for Systematic Reviews and Meta-Analysis) Checklist [28] and Cochrane Handbook for Systematic Reviews of Interventions [29].

13.2.1 *Eligibility Criteria*

Inclusion criteria included studies utilising: (a) participants with any type of MCI or dementia using validated diagnostic tools, (b) immersive or non-immersive VR interventions as a single intervention or as co-interventions alongside conventional interventions, (c) comparison group in terms of placebo, waitlist, no intervention, usual care or other non-VR interventions, (d) outcomes concerning cognitive, physical and psychological domains, and (e) published and unpublished randomised RCTs from inception to 2022. Only studies reported in English were considered due to logistic issues and no associated systematic bias from such language restrictions [30].

13.2.2 *Search Strategy*

A preliminary search was initially conducted on PubMed, CINAHL and EMBASE to identify possible key terms. We used terms such as "virtual reality", "augmented reality", "mixed reality", "dementia", "major neurocognitive disorder", "mild cognitive impairment" and "mild neurocognitive disorder". Using appropriate Boolean operators and truncations, keywords and index terms derived from eligible articles of the preliminary search were compiled into a search strategy (Appendix D) [31]. Using the Peer Review of Electronic Search Strategies (PRESS) checklist (Appendix E), two reviewers independently reviewed the search strategy, which was subsequently vetted by an experienced librarian. Afterward, eight electronic databases were searched for published studies: PubMed, CINAHL, PsychInfo, EMBASE, Web of Science, Scopus, CENTRAL and IEEE. Then, two Trial protocols were searched from ClinicalTrials.gov and WHO International Clinical Trials Registry Platform. Next, grey literature was searched using ProQuest Dissertations and Theses and Google Scholar. Finally, handsearching on topic-related journals and manual examination of reference lists were also performed.

13.2.3 *Selection Process*

Search results were collated and uploaded into EndNote X9.3.3 [32], where duplicated records were removed using EndNote feature and manually. After excluding irrelevant titles and abstracts, two reviewers independently screened the full texts of the remaining references to ensure compliance with the eligibility criteria. Inter-rater agreement between the two reviewers was high ($k = 0.860$) [33]. Authors of unpublished trials and articles without full texts or missing data were contacted, but none provided useful data (Appendix F).

13.2.4 *Methodological Quality and Data Extraction*

Two reviewers independently evaluated the included RCTs using the Cochrane Collaboration Risk-of-Bias tool Version 1.0 (Appendix G) by assessing random sequence generation; allocation concealment; participant and personnel blinding; outcome assessment blinding; incomplete outcome data; and selective reporting [34]. Inter-rater agreement was substantial ($k = 0.713$) [33].

A data extraction form adapted from the Cochrane Handbook for Systematic Reviews of Interventions was piloted independently by two reviewers [35]. Subsequently, using the modified form (Appendix H), the two reviewers independently completed data extraction. For studies with multiple publications, the reviewers inspected all papers and extracted the most complete dataset [35].

13.2.5 *Data Analysis*

Meta-analysis was performed using RevMan 5.4 software [36] to consolidate the intervention effects of VR among included studies. A random-effect model was used to permit variations of effect sizes across studies [37]. The effects of VR interventions were calculated by applying inverse-variance weighting to standardised mean differences (SMD) or mean differences (MD) for continuous variables. The effect sizes were interpreted the same as Hedge's g (Appendix I) [38]. Particularly, the value of 0.2, 0.5, 0.8 and 1.2 would be interpreted as small, medium, large, and very large effect size respectively.

Heterogeneity was determined by statistically significant Chi^2 and high percentage of I^2 statistics (Appendix J) [23]. Reasons underlying high heterogeneity ($I^2 > 60\%$) were explored using sensitivity analysis and subgroup analysis. If applicable, sensitivity analysis was performed by removing outliers to determine the impact on overall heterogeneity [39]. Where possible, subgroup analyses were conducted based on types of participants (MCI or dementia), immersivity of VR interventions, and measurements. Additionally, publication bias was examined through generating and visually assessing funnel plots when minimally ten studies were pooled in the meta-analysis [7]. The overall certainty of evidence was evaluated using the Grading of Recommendations, Assessments, Development and Evaluation (GRADE) approach (GRADEpro Guideline Developmental Tool) [40].

13.3 Results

A summary of search results was portrayed using the PRISMA flowchart (Appendix K). From the 16,816 articles initially retrieved,

7,689 duplicates were removed. Six additional studies were identified from handsearching. Based on the relevancy of title and abstracts, 154 full-text articles were assessed for compliance to the eligibility criteria, and 123 articles were excluded. Ultimately, the review included 28 studies.

Across the 28 studies published from 2012 to 2021, there were 1,367 participants from 16 countries. Sample sizes ranged from ten to 115, with the mean age of participants ranging between 68 and 87.65 years old. Studies recruited participants with MCI ($n = 15$), dementia ($n = 11$), or both diagnoses ($n = 2$). Three studies implemented immersive VR, while 25 studies utilised non-immersive VR. Study characteristics are summarised in Appendix M, with a substantial inter-rater agreement ($k = 0.762$).

13.3.1 *Quality Assessment*

Methodological quality is illustrated in a risk of bias graph and summary (Appendix N). All studies performed appropriate randomisation. Adequate allocation concealment and blinding of outcome assessment were, respectively, found in seven and eight studies. 15 open-label trials were subjected to high performance bias. Attrition bias was established in ten studies that did not account for missing data. 12 studies had low attrition bias as studies either performed intention-to-treat or had no missing data. Where protocols and trial registries were accessible, no reporting bias was identified.

According to GRADE criteria (Appendix P), all outcomes were downgraded due to lack of participants, personnel and outcome assessments blinding, heterogeneity, differences in interventions and wide confidence intervals, resulting in "low" and "very low" outcomes. The only outcome scoring "moderate" was the mean difference in global cognition. As all outcomes could influence recommendations for intervention use, they were given "important" ratings [41].

13.3.2 *Effects of Virtual Reality Interventions*

13.3.2.1 *Global Cognition*

Twenty studies measured global cognition and 18 studies (24 comparisons) involving 773 participants were submitted in meta-analysis. As results indicated substantial heterogeneity across effect sizes ($Chi^2 = 159.35, p < 0.00001, I^2 = 86\%$) (Appendix Q1), a pooled effect size was not used. The funnel plot of the studies (Appendix O) showed a symmetric distribution, indicating no publication bias.

A subgroup analysis was performed based on medical diagnosis (Figure 13.1) and heterogeneity is still observed in both subgroups. The MCI subgroup had variation in effect sizes (SMDs ranged from

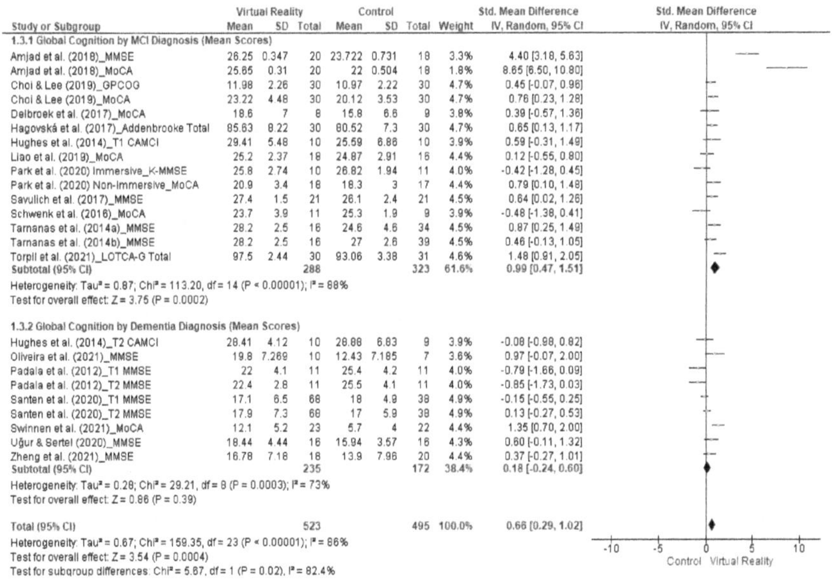

Figure 13.1 Effects of virtual reality on global cognition (based on medical diagnosis). Note: CAMCI: Computer Assessment of Mild Cognitive Impairment; GPCOG: General Practitioner Assessment of Cognition; K-MMSE: Mini-Mental State Exam (Korean Version); LOTCA-G: Loewenstein Occupational Therapy Cognitive Assessment Geriatric Version; MMSE: Mini-Mental State Exam; MoCA: Montreal Cognitive Assessment.

−0.48 to 8.65) with [42] showing the strongest effect size (SMD = 8.65, SMD = 4.40), followed by [43] (SMD = 1.48). The dementia subgroup showed SMD in the range of −0.08 to 1.35. Afterward, subgroup analysis was conducted according to VR immersivity and assessment points (Appendix Q2). The subgroup of non-immersive VR at post-intervention assessment demonstrated positive findings with [42] showing the largest effect size (SMD = 8.65, SMD = 4.40), followed by [43] (SMD = 1.48).

The two remaining studies (five comparisons) reported mean differences, and they were submitted to a separate meta-analysis (Appendix Q2). A small, pooled effect ($SMD = 0.36$, 95% $CI = 0.01, 0.71$) was found with homogeneity of effect sizes ($Chi^2 = 1.19$, $p = 0.88$, $I^2 = 0\%$). In sum, 16 out of 20 studies indicated small to large effect sizes of VR interventions on global cognition.

13.3.2.2 *Attention*

Four studies measured attention. Two studies, comprising of 121 participants, were pooled for meta-analysis, which suggested substantial heterogeneity across effect size ($Chi^2 = 16.35$, $p < 0.0001$, $I^2 = 94\%$) (Appendix R1). Subsequently, subgroup analysis was conducted according to measurements (Appendix R2). A study using observation-based assessment subgroup ($SMD = 1.79$, 95% $CI = 1.19, 2.39$) had a larger effect size than that using the task-based assessment ($SMD = 0.17$, 95% $CI = -0.34, 0.68$). Another two studies, involving 28 participants, reported mean difference. A separate meta-analysis revealed small size ($SMD = 0.45$, 95% $CI = -0.31, 1.20$) with effect size homogeneity ($Chi^2 = 0.16$, $p = 0.69$, $I^2 = 0\%$) (Appendix R2). Again, small to large effect sizes of VR interventions were observed on attention.

13.3.2.3 *Executive Function*

Ten studies evaluated executive function, where nine studies (12 comparisons) involving 465 participants were pooled into the meta-analysis

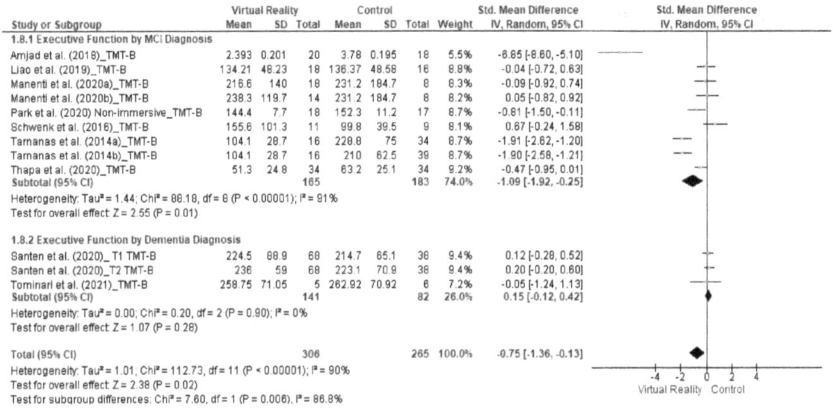

Figure 13.2 Effects of virtual reality on executive function (based on medical diagnosis).

(Appendix S1). Trail Making Test Part B (TMT-B) was used as a measurement, where shorter time indicates better executive function [44]. Considerable heterogeneity was observed across the studies (*Chi*^{2} = 112.73, $p < 0.00001$, $I^2 = 90\%$). Therefore, a subgroup analysis was performed based on medical diagnosis (Figure 13.2). The MCI subgroup had SMDs ranging from −6.85 to 0.67, which appear larger than those of the dementia subgroup (SMD range from −0.15 to 0.20). Reference [42] had the largest effect size (*SMD* = −6.85, 95% *CI* = −8.60, −5.10), followed by [45] (*SMD* = −1.91, 95% *CI* = −2.62, −1.20), and [45] (*SMD* = −1.90, 95% *CI* = −2.58, −1.21).

Subgroup analysis was conducted based on VR immersivity (Appendix S1–S3). While results indicated no significant difference between the two subgroups (*Chi*^{2} = 1.60, $p = 0.021$), the non-immersive VR subgroup (*SMD* = −0.89, 95% *CI* = −1.66, −0.11) had a larger pooled effect size than the immersive VR subgroup (*SMD* = −0.32, 95% *CI* = −0.72, 0.07). Note that the non-immersive VR subgroup had substantial heterogeneity (*Chi*^{2} = 112.73, $p < 0.00001$, $I^2 = 92\%$). Additionally, the study excluded from meta-analysis [43] measured executive function using the

LOTCA-G thinking operation domain and reported a very large effect size of 2.34, highlighting the effectiveness of VR in improving executive functions. In sum, 6 out of 10 studies showed positive effects of VR on executive function.

13.3.2.4 *Language*

Eight studies (22 comparisons) comprising 369 participants assessed language abilities, and were included in the meta-analysis. Three subgroups were created according to language domains: comprehension, naming and fluency (Figure 13.3). Significant difference in effect size was noticed among the three subgroups ($Chi^2 = 18.54$, $p < 0.0001$). The naming subgroup had the largest pooled effect size ($SMD = 1.94$, 95%

	Virtual Reality			Control				Std. Mean Difference
Study or Subgroup	Mean	SD	Total	Mean	SD	Total	Weight	IV, Random, 95% CI
1.9.1 Comprehension								
Hagovská et al. (2017)_Language	22.73	3.49	30	20.37	3.44	30	5.6%	0.67 [0.15, 1.19]
Subtotal (95% CI)			30			30	5.6%	0.67 [0.15, 1.19]
Heterogeneity: Not applicable								
Test for overall effect: Z = 2.53 (P = 0.01)								
1.9.2 Naming								
Tarnanas et al. (2014a)_BNT	15.4	2.4	16	10	2.2	34	4.0%	2.35 [1.58, 3.11]
Tarnanas et al. (2014b)_BNT	15.4	2.4	16	12	2	39	4.7%	1.58 [0.92, 2.24]
Subtotal (95% CI)			32			73	8.7%	1.94 [1.19, 2.69]
Heterogeneity: Tau² = 0.16; Chi² = 2.23, df = 1 (P = 0.14); I² = 55%								
Test for overall effect: Z = 5.07 (P < 0.00001)								
1.9.3 Fluency								
Hagovská et al. (2017)_VF	13.87	2.72	30	12.33	2.17	30	5.7%	0.62 [0.10, 1.14]
Manenti et al. (2020a)_FPC	30.8	6.8	18	29.4	6	9	3.8%	0.21 [-0.60, 1.01]
Manenti et al. (2020a)_FPL	31.5	9.1	18	31.7	8.8	9	3.8%	-0.02 [-0.82, 0.78]
Manenti et al. (2020b)_FPC	29.2	6.8	14	29.4	6	8	3.5%	-0.03 [-0.90, 0.84]
Manenti et al. (2020b)_FPL	33.4	8.4	14	31.7	8.8	8	3.5%	0.19 [-0.68, 1.06]
Park et al. (2020) Immersive_WF Animal	11.6	3.53	10	11	3.79	11	3.5%	0.16 [-0.70, 1.01]
Park et al. (2020) Immersive_WF-G	8	3.27	10	6	3.35	11	3.5%	0.58 [-0.30, 1.46]
Park et al. (2020) Immersive_WF-O	6.2	4.71	10	5.09	2.43	11	3.5%	0.29 [-0.57, 1.15]
Park et al. (2020) Immersive_WF-S	7.7	4.81	10	5.82	2.48	11	3.5%	0.48 [-0.39, 1.35]
Tarnanas et al. (2014a)_CF	13.4	5.7	16	11.6	4.8	34	5.1%	0.35 [-0.25, 0.95]
Tarnanas et al. (2014a)_LF	8.6	4.8	16	6	5	34	5.0%	0.52 [-0.09, 1.12]
Tarnanas et al. (2014b)_CF	13.4	5.7	16	13.2	4.4	39	5.2%	0.04 [-0.54, 0.62]
Tarnanas et al. (2014b)_LF	8.6	4.8	16	7.6	2.9	39	5.2%	0.28 [-0.31, 0.86]
Tominari et al. (2021)_WF Animals	7.14	3.04	21	5.58	2.15	24	5.1%	0.59 [-0.01, 1.19]
Tominari et al. (2021)_WF Fruits	5	2.1	21	4.29	1.97	24	5.1%	0.34 [-0.25, 0.93]
Tominari et al. (2021)_WF-I	3.71	2.61	21	2.96	2.24	24	5.1%	0.30 [-0.28, 0.89]
Tominari et al. (2021)_WF-re	2.33	1.91	21	2.38	1.84	24	5.2%	-0.03 [-0.61, 0.56]
Tominari et al. (2021)_WF-shi	3	3.24	21	2.38	2.14	24	5.2%	0.22 [-0.36, 0.81]
Tominari et al. (2021)_WF Vehicles	4.62	2.56	21	3.58	1.93	24	5.1%	0.46 [-0.14, 1.05]
Subtotal (95% CI)			324			398	85.6%	0.31 [0.16, 0.46]
Heterogeneity: Tau² = 0.00; Chi² = 7.09, df = 18 (P = 0.99); I² = 0%								
Test for overall effect: Z = 4.01 (P < 0.0001)								
Total (95% CI)			386			501	100.0%	0.46 [0.25, 0.67]
Heterogeneity: Tau² = 0.13; Chi² = 46.07, df = 21 (P = 0.001); I² = 54%								
Test for overall effect: Z = 4.31 (P < 0.0001)								
Test for subgroup differences: Chi² = 18.54, df = 2 (P < 0.0001), I² = 89.2%								

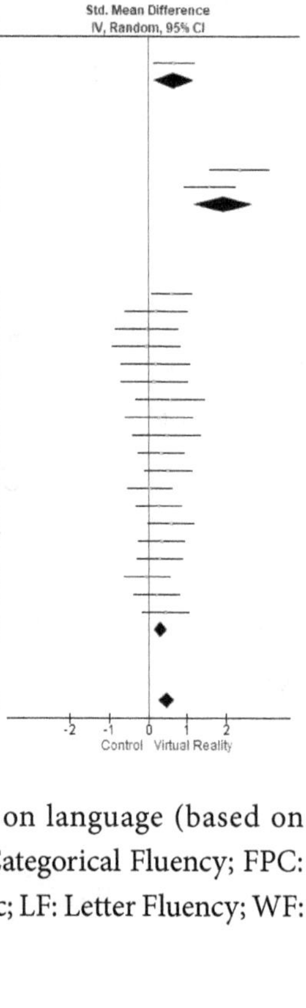

Figure 13.3 Effects of virtual reality intervention on language (based on measurements). Note: BNT: Boston Naming Test; CF: Categorical Fluency; FPC: Verbal Fluency, Semantic; FPL: Verbal Fluency, Phonemic; LF: Letter Fluency; WF: Word Fluency.

CI = 1.19, 2.69), followed by the comprehension subgroup (*SMD* = 0.67, 95% *CI* = 0.15, 1.19) and the fluency subgroup (*SMD* = 0.31, 95% *CI* = 0.16, 0.46). The naming subgroup was moderately heterogeneous ($Chi^2 = 2.23$, $p < 0.00001$, $I^2 = 55\%$), possibly due to the difference in controls.

Subgroup analysis was performed to assess the effects of VR immersivity on language fluency (Appendix T2). Results showed no significant difference between the two subgroups ($Chi^2 = 0.09$, $p = 0.76$). Both non-immersive (*SMD* = 0.30, 95% *CI* = 0.14, 0.46) and immersive VR (*SMD* = 0.37, 95% *CI* = –0.06, 0.81) subgroups had small pooled effect sizes. Additionally, two studies (three comparisons) reported mean difference in language fluency. The separate meta-analysis did not favour VR interventions (*SMD* = –0.12, 95% *CI* = –0.69, 0.45). Homogeneity of effect sizes was observed ($Chi^2 = 0.77$, $p = 0.68$, $I^2 = 0\%$) (Appendix T3).

13.3.2.5 *Memory*

Twelve studies examined memory. Ten studies (34 comparisons) involving 498 participants were pooled into the meta-analysis. Three subgroups were created: immediate memory, delayed memory, and combined immediate and delayed memory (Appendix U1). Significant difference in effect size was not observed among the three subgroups ($Chi^2 = 6.07$, $p = 0.05$). The combined memory subgroup had variation in effect sizes (SMD ranged from –0.70 to 1.22) with high heterogeneity ($Chi^2 = 30.76$, $p < 0.0001$, $I^2 = 87\%$). The immediate memory subgroup had a small pooled effect size favouring VR interventions (*SMD* = 0.35, 95% *CI* = 0.13, 0.58).

Subgroup analysis conducted to examine the effects of immersivity VR on immediate memory showed no significant difference between the two subgroups ($Chi^2 = 0.11$, $p = 0.74$) (Appendix U2). Both non-immersive (*SMD* = 0.36, 95% *CI* = 0.10, 0.62) and immersive VR (*SMD* = 0.27, 95% *CI* = –0.18, 0.73) subgroups had small pooled effect sizes. Moreover, two studies (five comparisons) reported mean difference. The separate meta-analysis found a small pooled effect size (*SMD* = 0.44,

95% *CI* = –0.02, 0.90) with homogeneity across effect sizes ($Chi^2 = 1.73$, $p = 0.79$, $I^2 = 0\%$) (Appendix U3).

13.3.2.6 *Sensation and Perception*

Three studies (four comparisons) comprising 117 participants measured sensation and perception (Appendix V1). Meta-analysis highlighted the effectiveness of VR interventions in improving sensation and perception with a moderate effect size ($SMD = 0.71$, 95% $CI = 0.38, 1.04$) with low heterogeneity ($Chi^2 = 4.71$, $p = 0.19$, $I^2 = 36\%$).

13.3.2.7 *Processing Speed*

Processing speed was evaluated in ten studies. Nine studies (15 comparisons) involving 444 participants were submitted into the meta-analysis. As processing speed is a measure of time, shorter time indicates faster processing speed. Meta-analysis revealed substantial heterogeneity across effect size ($Chi^2 = 105.51$, $p < 0.00001$, $I^2 = 81\%$) (Appendix V2). Sensitivity analysis identified one study [42] as the outlier. This study made "slight modifications" to the assessment tool, which could affect the test validity. Subsequently, heterogeneity across effect size dropped ($Chi^2 = 13.16$, $p = 0.44$, $I^2 = 1\%$) (Appendix V3). However, results suggested that VR interventions had very weak pooled effects ($SMD = -0.08$, 95% $CI = -0.23, 0.07$) on processing speed. Additionally, a study [46] excluded from the meta-analysis reported mean difference in processing speed. This study suggested that the VR training group did not show significant improvements in processing speed ($d = -0.03 \pm 0.57$, $p = 1.00$).

13.3.2.8 *Physical Function*

Physical function was assessed by six studies (12 comparisons), where 343 participants were pooled in a meta-analysis. Pooled effect size was not used due to substantial heterogeneity across the studies ($Chi^2 = 28.52$, $p = 0.001$, $I^2 = 65\%$) (Appendix W1). Following subgroup analysis based on medical diagnosis, homogeneity was observed ($Chi^2 = 4.29$, $p = 0.83$, $I^2 = 0\%$) (Appendix W2). Thus, medical diagnosis could be an appropriate explanation for the previous heterogeneity. Furthermore, there was significant difference between the three subgroups ($Chi^2 = 24.23$, $p < 0.0001$). The institutionalised dementia subgroup ($SMD = 1.85$, 95% $CI = 1.14, 2.55$) had the largest effect size, followed by the institutionalised MCI subgroup ($SMD = 0.54$, 95% $CI = -0.44, 1.51$) and the community dementia subgroup ($SMD = 0.04$, 95% $CI = -0.14, 0.22$).

13.3.2.9 *Mobility*

Eight studies (24 comparisons) comprising 360 participants measured mobility. Results showed that that VR interventions had a very weak pooled effect size ($SMD = -0.08$, 95% $CI = -0.21, 0.04$), with homogeneity across studies ($Chi^2 = 22.79$, $p = 0.49$, $I^2 = 0\%$) (Appendix W3).

13.3.2.10 *Balance*

Four studies including 284 participants examined balance. Meta-analysis of two studies (three comparisons) using mean/SD yielded a very large pooled effect size ($SMD = 3.32$, 95% $CI = 2.24, 4.39$) with homogeneity across studies ($Chi^2 = 1.16$, $p < 0.00001$, $I^2 = 0\%$) (Appendix X1). Another study used mean difference at two timepoints [47] (Figure 13.4). While meta-analysis showed no significant difference between the two subgroups ($Chi^2 = 1.34$, $p = 0.25$), the post-intervention subgroup ($SMD = 2.14$, 95% $CI = 0.13, 4.15$) had a larger effect size than the follow-up subgroup ($SMD = 0.91$, 95% $CI = 0.37, 1.44$). The remaining study [48] found a small but significant reduction in Center of Mass sway area ($r^2 = 0.224$, $p = 0.041$), suggesting balance improvement.

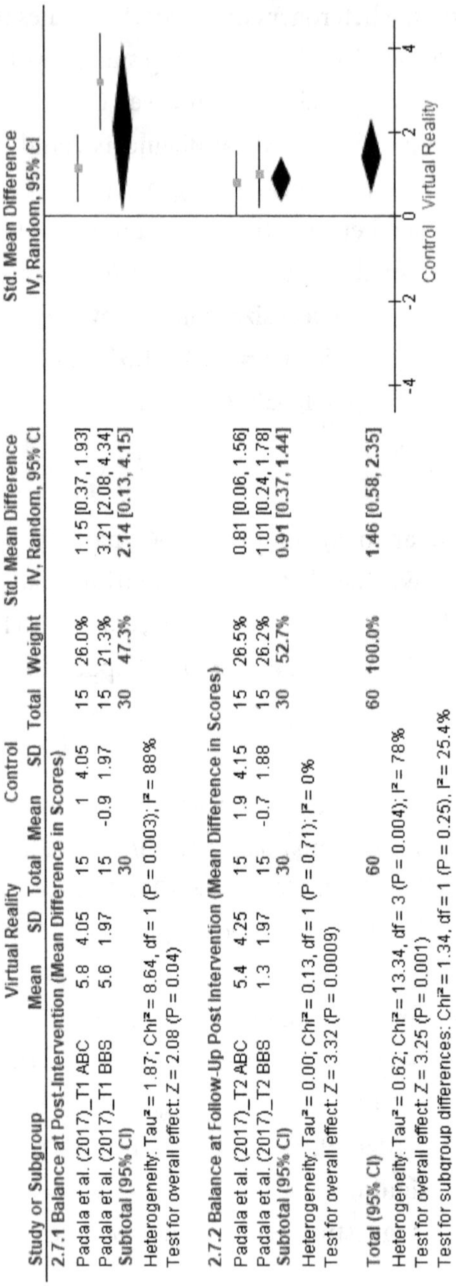

Figure 13.4 Forest plot for balance (mean difference). Note: ABC: Activities-Specific Balance Confidence Scale; BBS: Berg Balance Test.

13.3.2.11 *Depression*

Six studies measured depression. Meta-analysis of four studies using Mean/SD, involving 141 participants, suggested substantial heterogeneity across the studies ($Chi^2 = 12.94$, $p = 0.005$, $I^2 = 77\%$) (Appendix W3). Subsequently, subgroup analysis was performed according to measurements (Figure 13.5) and I^2 of both groups became 0%. Henceforth, it is reasonable to conclude that measurement types explained the previous heterogeneity. Furthermore, there was significant difference between the two subgroups ($Chi^2 = 12.91$, $p = 0.0003$). The dementia-specific tool subgroup ($SMD = -1.14$, 95% $CI = 1.60, -0.67$) had a larger effect size than the general tool subgroup ($SMD = 0.18$, 95% $CI = -0.36, 0.73$). Additionally, two studies are reported in narrative analysis. Reference [68] reported a larger effect of the computerised cognitive stimulation intervention on depression ($Eta^2 = 0.35$) as compared to controls ($Eta^2 = 0.01$). However, [49] did not find significant improvement ($F(1, 40) = 3.59, p = 0.074$) after delivering iPad-based cognitive training.

13.3.2.12 *Quality of Life*

Seven studies assessed QoL. Meta-analysis of six studies (nine comparisons) involving 326 participants revealed substantial heterogeneity ($Chi^2 = 51.92, p = 0.34, I^2 = 85\%$) (Appendix Z1). Thereafter, a subgroup analysis conducted based on measurements (Appendix Z1) found significant difference among the three subgroups ($Chi^2 = 30.94, p < 0.00001$). The cancer-specific tool subgroup had the largest pooled effect size ($SMD = 1.92$, 95% $CI = 1.30, 2.54$), followed by the dementia-specific tool subgroup ($SMD = 0.19$, 95% $CI = -0.23, 0.61$). Additionally, the study excluded from the meta-analysis [47] used mean difference in QoL at two time-points. Compared to the walking control group, the Wii-Fit group did not show significant change in QoL at post-intervention and follow-up.

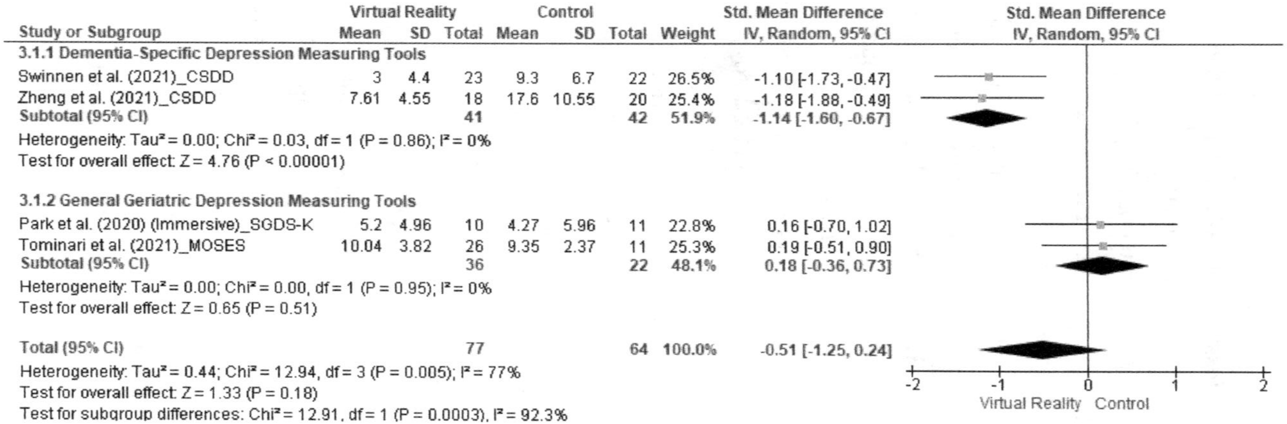

Figure 13.5 Effects of virtual reality on depression (based on measurements). Note: CSDD: Cornell Scale for Depression in Dementia; MOSES: Multidimensional Observation *Scale* for Elderly Subjects; SGDS-K: Short Form Geriatric Depression Scale Korean Version.

13.4 Discussion

The results of this review showed that VR interventions had small to very large effects on global cognition, cognitive domains (attention, executive function, language, immediate memory, sensation and perception), physical function, balance and depression. However, very weak effects were observed on delayed memory, processing speed, mobility and QoL.

This review found that VR interventions improved global cognition among people with MCI and dementia, which is consistent with a previous meta-analysis [26]. This is not surprising as VR interventions provide stimulating effects on the mind [50], where increased engagements in mental stimulation are associated with reduced cognitive decline [51]. This is possibly due to a mechanism of enriched environments (Appendix AA), which postulated that additional environmental exposure to various stimuli helps in enhancing neuroplasticity [52, 53]. Nevertheless, VR interventions had stronger effects on MCI than dementia. This finding concurs with a meta-analysis assessing the efficacy of computerised cognitive training [25] and suggested that the intervention was more beneficial for those with less severe cognitive failure, and thus early intervention is crucial.

Our review supports the beneficial effects of VR technology on cognitive domains (attention, executive function, language, sensation and perception, and immediate memory). This is not surprising as enriched environments activate the hippocampus and cerebral cortex, which contain crucial areas responsible for the functioning of such cognitive domains [54, 55]. On the contrary, [25] did not find significant improvements in executive function, language, and visuospatial skills (subdomain of sensation and perception) in both MCI and dementia groups. This could be attributable to [25]'s inclusion of traditional computerised cognitive training approaches, which were reported to be less clinically meaningful as compared to more stimulating and engaging VR interventions.

Interestingly, [42] and [45], which had the largest effects for executive function, incorporated training content for specific cognitive domains in their intervention designs, with executive function being one of the chosen domains. This suggested that VR interventions, designed with content intended to train specific cognitive domains, may be more beneficial. In terms of memory, our review found that immediate memory improved with a small effect. However, another systematic review [26] revealed significant and moderate improvements in memory. The larger effects in [26] could be due to the study's inclusion of language abilities tests (e.g., Boston Naming Test) in the memory domain. Although working memory is involved in language processing [56], this review classified language as an independent outcome as patients with dementia commonly experience aphasia [57].

Unexpectedly, VR interventions did not show significant effects on processing speed or delayed memory. Another meta-analysis [25] also suggested that VR interventions did not improve processing speed and attributed the finding to insufficient training content on processing speed. However, [25] reported that VR interventions significantly improved working memory with moderate effects. The lack of beneficial effects in our review could be attributed to the limited studies assessing delayed memory (n = 3). Hence, more RCTs are needed to draw conclusions on delayed memory. The significant difference between immediate and delayed memory could be explained by [58]'s Decay Theory, which states that memories may decay over the short term. Therefore, it could be helpful for future studies to explore the effects of both immediate and delayed memory.

This review demonstrated small to moderate effects of VR interventions on physical functions, which concur with two previous meta-analyses [24, 26]. Furthermore, VR interventions demonstrated the largest effect on institutionalised participants with dementia. As motor deficits typically affect patients with later stages of dementia, neurogenesis and motor cortex stimulation by enriched environments would offer more prominent effects in physical function for those who are more cognitively and physically incapacitated [59]. Therefore, VR interventions were more beneficial in the later stages of disease progression. Moreover, the findings on balance and mobility agree with another meta-analysis [26]. VR interventions had very large effects on balance, but a non-significant and weak effect on mobility. Reference [26] explained that single walking tasks was unable to show motor function deficits and dual tasking would be required to effectuate compensatory efforts.

Depression is associated with further cognitive deterioration [60]. Our findings suggested that dementia-specific measurement (Cornell Scale for Depression in Dementia) might be more sensitive in detecting depression amongst people with MCI or dementia. Unlike other depression tools, dementia-specific tools use observational and interview data from both client and caregiver and make minimal use of subjective responses. Furthermore, VR interventions utilise enriched environments to stimulate neural mechanisms of recovery connected to stress management. They produce structural and neurochemical changes (e.g., decrease catecholamines) in the nervous system, thereby facilitating greater social, emotional and psychological well-being [50, 61].

QoL is a person's outlook of their life relating to their standards, goals, concerns and expectations based on their culture and value systems [62]. Surprisingly, this review showed a weak effect of VR interventions on QoL; nevertheless, studies using the cancer-specific QoL tool generated the largest effect. A possible explanation is that the tool captured the aspect of 'activity', which was likely to receive higher ratings due to participation in the VR intervention [63]. Furthermore, dementia-specific tools might be biased as they involve proxy-reported assessments, where outcomes could be influenced by the proxy's personal burdens. Interpretation of self-reported QoL may also be affected by severe cognitive impairments [64].

Subgroup analyses examined the effects of different levels of VR immersion on global cognition, executive function, language and memory. Global cognition observed significant subgroup differences in post-intervention effects, favouring non-immersive VR. The remaining outcomes suggested that both immersive and non-immersive VR produced similar effects. Although higher levels of immersivity may enhance the virtual experience, our findings aligned with [24], which concluded that non-immersive VR is more effective, as it is more user-friendly.

13.4.1 *Limitations*

This review objectively assessed the targeted outcomes with minimal publication bias by considering only RCTs from various published and non-published databases. Nonetheless, this review has some limitations. Firstly, the included studies utilised different VR mediums and software for varying durations and frequencies. Optimal intervention design should be explored to maximise intervention effects [65]. Secondly, it was difficult to ascertain the long-term effects of VR interventions as the timepoints of follow-up assessments were inconsistent across studies. Finally, the applicability and accuracy of results may be compromised due to the relatively small sample sizes for most trials [66].

More rigorous studies are required to explore the effects of VR interventions on specific cognitive and physical functioning domains. Future studies may also evaluate the effects on specific memory types, such as episodic and working memory, which are most frequently compromised amongst people with MCI [67]. To examine long-term effects, longitudinal studies with larger sample sizes should be studied. Future trials could also present neuroimaging and biomarkers as outcome measures to investigate physiological changes.

13.4.2 *Relevance to Clinical Practice*

The aggregated findings highlight the potential of VR interventions on people with MCI and dementia. Non-immersive VR, which is more cost-effective than immersive VR, may be disseminated to various healthcare institutions and community-based senior activity centres. Healthcare and gaming companies may collaborate to develop domain-specific training content, where physicians and therapists may prescribe VR-based rehabilitation according to patients' conditions. Taking real-world constraints (such as limitations of manpower and VR hardware) into consideration, this review recommends 30 minutes of supervised VR-based rehabilitation sessions held twice weekly for 12 weeks. To preserve their cognitive functions, people with MCI may focus on cognitive training. In addition to cognitive training, people with dementia may be prescribed balance and mobility training to minimise functional decline. With the ubiquity of mobile devices (such as tablets, smartphones), it is conceivable to develop a mobile application to facilitate remote VR-based cognitive rehabilitation, which could reduce the workload of healthcare professionals and caregivers [20].

13.4.3 *Recommendations for Future Research*

Future research may examine the effect of VR interventions on attention, delayed memory, processing speed, mobility, and QoL given the small number of existing studies and unclear effects using RCTs with large sample size and multiple research settings. Non-immersive VR can be further tested in comparison with immersive VR on their effects on cognitive, physical and psychological outcomes. The use of mobile applications can be examined as an alternative mode to deliver VR-based interventions. The mixed method can be used and qualitative data can be added to explore perceptions of people receiving VR technology. Further evidence is needed to ascertain the long-term effects of VR interventions.

13.5 Conclusion

This review provided evidence to support the effects of VR interventions in improving cognitive (global cognition, attention, executive function, language, immediate memory, sensation and perception), physical (physical function and balance) and psychological outcomes (depression). Non-immersive VR interventions, which are less costly, had similar effects to immersive VR interventions. Nonetheless, findings should be interpreted with caution due to heterogeneity in intervention designs. Rigorous RCTs with specific cognitive and physical domains, memory types, neuroimaging and biomarkers are required in future studies to gain insights into the effects and mechanisms of VR interventions among individuals with MCI or dementia.

References

1. Hugo J, Ganguli M. Dementia and cognitive impairment: Epidemiology, diagnosis, and treatment. Clin Geriatr Med. 2014;30(3):421–42. https://doi.org/10.1016/j.cger.2014.04.001
2. Nakamura K, Kumai K, Takada J, Chida K, Kato Y, Takahashi Y, *et al.* Behavioural and psychological symptoms of dementia (BPSD) in Alzheimer disease is "cognitive" symptoms? The Osaki-Tajiri Project. Alzheimer Dement. 2017;13(7 Suppl):375–76. https://doi.org/10.1016/j.jalz.2017.06.332
3. Alzheimer's Disease International. Dementia statistics [Internet]. [cited 2025 Jul 28]. Available from: https://www.alzint.org/about/dementia-facts-figures/dementia-statistics/
4. American Psychiatric Association. Mild neurocognitive disorder [Internet]. 2013. Available from: https://www.psychiatry.org/File%20Library/Psychiatrists/Practice/DSM/APA_DSM-5-Mild-Neurocognitive-Disorder.pdf
5. Langa KM, Levine DA. The diagnosis and management of mild cognitive impairment: A clinical review. JAMA. 2014;312(23):2551–61. https://doi.org/10.1001/jama.2014.13806
6. Lu Y, Liu C, Yu D, Fawkes S, Ma J, Zhang M, Li C. Prevalence of mild cognitive impairment in community-dwelling Chinese populations aged over 55 years: A meta-analysis and systematic review. BMC Geriatr. 2021;21(1):10. https://doi.org/10.1186/s12877-020-01948-3
7. Boutron I, Page MJ, Higgins JPT, Altman DG, Lundh A, Hróbjartsson A. Chapter 7: Considering bias and conflicts of interest among the included studies. In: Higgins JPT, Thomas J, Chandler J, *et al.*, editors. Cochrane Handbook for Systematic Reviews of Interventions version 6.2 (updated Feb 2021). Available from: www.training.cochrane.org/handbook

8. Shigihara Y, Hoshi H, Poza J, Rodríguez-González V, Gómez C, Kanzawa T. Predicting the outcome of non-pharmacological treatment for patients with dementia-related mild cognitive impairment. Aging (Albany NY). 2020;12(23):24101-16. https://doi.org/10.18632/aging.202270
9. Zucchella C, Sinforiani E, Tamburin S, Federico A, Mantovani E, Bernini S, *et al.* The multidisciplinary approach to Alzheimer's disease and dementia: A narrative review of non-pharmacological treatment. Front Neurol. 2018;9:1058. https://doi.org/10.3389/fneur.2018.01058
10. Tieri G, Morone G, Paolucci S, Iosa M. Virtual reality in cognitive and motor rehabilitation: Facts, fiction and fallacies. Expert Rev Med Devices. 2018;15(2):107-17. https://doi.org/10.1080/17434440.2018.1425613
11. Tominari M, Uozumi R, Becker C, Kinoshita A. Reminiscence therapy using virtual reality technology affects cognitive function and subjective well-being in older adults with dementia. Cogent Psychol. 2021;8(1):1968991. https://doi.org/10.1080/23311908.2021.1968991
12. Kardong-Edgren S, Farra SL, Alinier G, Young HM. A call to unify definitions of virtual reality. Clin Simul Nurs. 2019;31:28–34. https://doi.org/10.1016/j.ecns.2019.02.006
13. Ryan ML. Narrative as virtual reality 2: Revisiting immersion and interactivity in literature and electronic media. 2nd ed. Baltimore (MD): Johns Hopkins University Press; 2015.
14. Skarbez R, Smith M, Whitton MC. Revisiting Milgram and Kishino's reality-virtuality continuum. Front Virtual Realit. 2021;2(27). https://doi.org/10.3389/frvir.2021.647997
15. Swinnen N, Vandenbulcke M, de Bruin ED, Akkerman R, Stubbs B, Firth J, *et al.* The efficacy of exergaming in people with major neurocognitive disorder residing in long-term care facilities: A pilot randomized controlled trial. Alzheimer Res Ther. 2021;13(1):70. https://doi.org/10.1186/s13195-021-00806-7
16. Peukert C, Pfeiffer J, Meißner M, Pfeiffer T, Weinhardt C. Shopping in virtual reality stores: The influence of immersion on system adoption. J Manag Inf Syst. 2021;36(3):755–88. https://doi.org/10.1080/07421222.2019.1628889
17. Robert P, Albrengues C, Fabre R, Derreumaux A, Pancrazi MP, Luporsi I, *et al.* Efficacy of serious exergames in improving neuropsychiatric symptoms in neurocognitive disorders: Results of the X-TORP cluster randomized trial. Alzheimer Dement (NY). 2021;7(1):e12149. https://doi.org/10.1002/trc2.12149
18. Ventura S, Brivio E, Riva G, Baños RM. Immersive versus non-immersive experience: Exploring the feasibility of memory assessment through 360° technology. Front Psychol. 2019;10:2509. https://doi.org/10.3389/fpsyg.2019.02509

19. García-Betances RI, Jiménez-Mixco V, Arredondo MT, Cabrera-Umpiérrez MF. Using virtual reality for cognitive training of the elderly. Am J Alzheimer Dis Other Dement. 2015;30(1):49–54. https://doi.org/10.1177/1533317514545866
20. Zhao Y, Feng H, Wu X, Du Y, Yang X, Hu M, *et al.* Effectiveness of exergaming in improving cognitive and physical function in people with mild cognitive impairment or dementia: Systematic review. JMIR Serious Games. 2020;8(2):e16841. https://doi.org/10.2196/16841
21. Zheng JY, Yu P, Chen XP. An evaluation of the effects of active gameplay on cognition, quality of life and depression for older people with dementia. Clin Gerontol. 2021;1–10. https://doi.org/10.1080/07317115.2021.1980170
22. Kim JH, Park S, Lim H. Developing a virtual reality for people with dementia in nursing homes based on their psychological needs: A feasibility study. BMC Geriatr. 2021;21(1):167. https://doi.org/10.1186/s12877-021-02125-w
23. Sánchez A, Millán-Calenti JC, Lorenzo-López L, Maseda A. Multisensory stimulation for people with dementia: A review of the literature. Am J Alzheimer Dis Other Dement. 2013;28(1):7–14.
24. Santen J, Dröes RM, Twisk JWR, Blanson Henkemans OA, van Straten A, Meil FJM. Effects of exergaming on cognitive and social functioning of people with dementia: A randomized controlled trial. J Am Med Dir Assoc. 2020;21(12):1958. https://doi.org/10.1097/TGR.0000000000000285
25. Santen J, Meil FJM, Dröes RM, Straten A, Bosmans JE. Cost-effectiveness of exergaming compared to regular day-care activities in dementia: Results of a randomised controlled trial in the Netherlands. Health Soc Care Community. 2021. https://doi.org/10.1111/hsc.13608
26. Bauer ACM, Andringa G. The potential of immersive virtual reality for cognitive training in elderly. Gerontology. 2020;66(6):614–23. https://doi.org/10.1159/000509830
27. Clay F, Howett D, FitzGerald J, Fletcher P, Chan D, Price A. Use of immersive virtual reality in the assessment and treatment of Alzheimer's disease: A systematic review. J Alzheimer Dis. 2020;75(1):23–43. https://doi.org/10.3233/JAD-191218
28. Sayma M, Tuijt R, Cooper C, Walters K. Are we there yet? Immersive virtual reality to improve cognitive function in dementia and mild cognitive impairment. Gerontologist. 2020;60(7):e502–12. https://doi.org/10.1093/geront/gnz132
29. Deeks JJT, Higgins JPT, Altman DG. Chapter 10: Analysing data and undertaking meta-analyses. In: Higgins JPT, Thomas J, Chandler J, et al, editors. Cochrane Handbook for Systematic Reviews of Interventions version 6.2 (updated Feb 2021). Available from: www.training.cochrane.org/handbook

30. Delbroek T, Vermeylen W, Spildooren J. The effect of cognitive-motor dual task training with the biorescue force platform on cognition, balance and dual task performance in institutionalized older adults: A randomized controlled trial. J Phys Ther Sci. 2017;29(7):1137–44.
31. Kim O, Pang Y, Kim JH. The effectiveness of virtual reality for people with mild cognitive impairment or dementia: A meta-analysis. BMC Psychiatry. 2019;19(1):1–10. https://doi.org/10.1186/s12888-019-2180-x
32. Hill NT, Mowszowski L, Naismith SL, Chadwick VL, Valenzuela M, Lampit A. Computerized cognitive training in older adults with mild cognitive impairment or dementia: A systematic review and meta-analysis. Am J Psychiatry. 2017;174(4):329–40. https://doi.org/10.1176/appi.ajp.2016.16030360
33. Hughes TF, Flatt JD, Fu B, Butters MA, Chang CCH, Ganguli M. Interactive video gaming compared with health education in older adults with mild cognitive impairment: A feasibility study. Int J Geriatr Psychiatry. 2014;29(9):890–98. http://dx.doi.org/10.1002/gps.4075
34. Zhu S, Sui Y, Shen Y, Zhu Y, Ali N, Guo C, Wang T. Effects of virtual reality intervention on cognition and motor function in older adults with mild cognitive impairment or dementia: A systematic review and meta-analysis. Front Aging Neurosci. 2021;13:217.
35. Lefebvre C, Glanville J, Briscoe S, Littlewood A, Marshall C, Metzendorf MI, *et al.* Chapter 4: Searching for and selecting studies. In: Higgins JPT, Thomas J, Chandler J, et al, editors. Cochrane Handbook for Systematic Reviews of Interventions version 6.2 (updated Feb 2021). Available from: www.training.cochrane.org/handbook
36. Page MJ, McKenzie JE, Bossuyt PM, Boutron I, Hoffmann TC, Mulrow CD, *et al.* The PRISMA 2020 statement: An updated guideline for reporting systematic reviews. BMJ. 2021;372:n71. https://doi.org/10.1136/bmj.n71
37. Park JH. Effects of virtual reality-based spatial cognitive training on hippocampal function of older adults with mild cognitive impairment. Int Psychogeriatr. 2020;1–7. https://doi.org/10.1017/S1041610220001131
38. Park JS, Jung YJ, Lee G. Virtual reality-based cognitive-motor rehabilitation in older adults with mild cognitive impairment: A randomized controlled study on motivation and cognitive function. Healthcare (Basel). 2020;8(3):335. https://doi.org/10.3390/healthcare8030335
39. Park JH, Liao Y, Kim DR, Song S, Lim JH, Park H, *et al.* Feasibility and tolerability of a culture-based virtual reality (VR) training program in patients with mild cognitive impairment: A randomized controlled pilot study. Int J Environ Res Public Health. 2020;17(9):3030. https://doi.org/10.3390/ijerph17093030

40. Higgins JPT, Thomas J, Chandler J, Cumpston M, Li T, Page MJ, Welch VA, editors. Cochrane Handbook for Systematic Reviews of Interventions version 6.2 (updated Feb 2021). Available from: www.training.cochrane.org/handbook
41. Morrison A, Polisena J, Husereau D, Moulton K, Clark M, Fiander M, Mierzwinski-Urban M, Clifford T, Hutton B, Rabb D. The effect of English-language restriction on systematic review-based meta-analyses: A systematic review of empirical studies. Int J Technol Assess Health Care. 2012;28(2):138–44. https://doi.org/10.1017/S0266462312000086
42. McGowan J, Sampson M, Salzwedel DM, Cogo E, Foerster V, Lefebvre C. PRESS Peer Review of Electronic Search Strategies: 2015 guideline statement. J Clin Epidemiol. 2016;75:40–46. https://doi.org/10.1016/j.jclinepi.2016.01.021
43. The EndNote Team. EndNote. Version X9 [software]. Clarivate Analytics; 2013. Available from: https://endnote.com/
44. McHugh ML. Interrater reliability: The kappa statistic. Biochem Med (Zagreb). 2012;22(3):276–82.
45. McMaster University. GRADEpro GDT: GRADEpro Guideline Development Tool [Software]. 2021. Available from: https://gradepro.org
46. Higgins JPT, Savović J, Page MJ, Elbers RG, Sterne JAC. Chapter 8: Assessing risk of bias in a randomized trial. In: Higgins JPT, Thomas J, Chandler J, et al, editors. Cochrane Handbook for Systematic Reviews of Interventions version 6.2 (updated Feb 2021). Available from: www.training.cochrane.org/handbook
47. Li T, Higgins JPT, Deeks JJ. Chapter 5: Collecting data. In: Higgins JPT, Thomas J, Chandler J, et al, editors. Cochrane Handbook for Systematic Reviews of Interventions version 6.2 (updated Feb 2021). Available from: www.training.cochrane.org/handbook
48. Liao YY, Chen IH, Lin YJ, Chen Y, Hsu WC. Effects of virtual reality-based physical and cognitive training on executive function and dual-task gait performance in older adults with mild cognitive impairment: A randomized controlled trial. Front Aging Neurosci. 2019;10:162. http://dx.doi.org/10.3389/fnagi.2019.00162
49. Liao YY, Tseng HY, Lin YJ, Wang CJ, Hsu WC. Using virtual reality-based training to improve cognitive function, instrumental activities of daily living and neural efficiency in older adults with mild cognitive impairment. Eur J Phys Rehabil Med. 2020;56(1):47–57.
50. The Cochrane Collaboration. Review Manager (RevMan) Version 5.4 [Software]. 2020. Available from: https://community.cochrane.org/help/tools-and-software/revman-5
51. Langan D, Higgins JPT, Jackson D, Bowden J, Veroniki AA, Kontopantelis E, Viechtbauer W, Simmonds M. A comparison of heterogeneity variance

estimators in simulated random-effects meta-analyses. Res Synth Methods. 2019;10(1):83–98. https://doi.org/10.1002/jrsm.1316
52. Hedges LV, Olkin I. Statistical methods for meta-analysis. San Diego (CA): Academic Press; 2014.
53. Bown MJ, Sutton AJ. Quality control in systematic reviews and meta-analyses. Eur J Vasc Endovasc Surg. 2010;40(5):669–77. https://doi.org/10.1016/j.ejvs.2010.07.011
54. Breton A, Casey D, Arnaoutoglou NA. Cognitive tests for the detection of mild cognitive impairment (MCI), the prodromal stage of dementia: meta-analysis of diagnostic accuracy studies. Int J Geriatr Psychiatry. 2019;34(2):233–42. https://doi.org/10.1002/gps.5016
55. Atkins D, Best D, Briss PA, Eccles M, Falck-Ytter Y, Flottorp S, *et al.* Grading quality of evidence and strength of recommendations. BMJ. 2004;328(7454):1490. https://doi.org/10.1136/bmj.328.7454.1490
56. Schünemann H, Brożek J, Guyatt G, Oxman A. GRADE handbook for grading quality of evidence and strength of recommendations [Internet]. 2013. Available from: https://gdt.gradepro.org/app/handbook/handbook.html
57. Amjad I, Toor H, Niazi IK, Pervaiz S, Jochumsen M, Shafique M, Haavik H, Ahmed T. Xbox 360 Kinect cognitive games improve slowness complexity of EEG, and cognitive functions in subjects with mild cognitive impairment: A randomized control trial. Games Health J. 2018. Available from: https://www.cochranelibrary.com/central/doi/10.1002/central/CN-01649110/full
58. Torpil B, Azahin S, Pekçetin S, Uyanlık M. The effectiveness of a virtual reality-based intervention on cognitive functions in older adults with mild cognitive impairment: A single-blind, randomized controlled trial. Games Health J. 2021;10(2):109–14. https://doi.org/10.1089/g4h.2020.0086
59. Uğur F, Sertel M. The effect of virtual reality applications on balance and gait speed in individuals with Alzheimer dementia. Top Geriatr Rehabil. 2020;36(4):221–29.
60. Arbuthnott K, Frank J. Trail making test part B as a measure of executive control: Validation using a set-switching paradigm. J Clin Exp Neuropsychol. 2000;22(4):518–28. https://doi.org/10.1076/1380-3395(200008)22:4;1-0;ft518
61. Tarnanas I, Tsolakis A, Tsolaki M. Assessing virtual reality environments as cognitive stimulation method for patients with MCI. In: Brooks A, Brahnam S, Jain L, editors. Technologies of Inclusive Well-Being. Stud Comput Intell. Vol 536. Berlin, Heidelberg: Springer; 2014. p 1092–1103. https://doi.org/10.1007/978-3-642-45432-5_4
62. Thapa N, Park HJ, Yang JG, Son H, Jang M, Lee J, Kang SW, Park KW, Park H. The effect of a virtual reality-based intervention program on cognition in older

adults with mild cognitive impairment: A randomized control trial. J Clin Med. 2020;9(5):1283. https://doi.org/10.3390/jcm9051283

63. Mrakic-Sposta S, Di Santo SG, Franchini F, Arlati S, Zangiacomi A, Greci L, *et al.* Effects of combined physical and cognitive virtual reality-based training on cognitive impairment and oxidative stress in MCI patients: A pilot study. Front Aging Neurosci. 2018;10:282.
64. Muhanna MA. Virtual reality and the CAVE: Taxonomy, interaction challenges and research directions. J King Saud Univ Comput Inf Sci. 2015;27(3):344–61. https://doi.org/10.1016/j.jksuci.2014.03.023
65. Padala KP, Padala P, Lensing SY, Dennis RA, Bopp MM, Parkes CM, *et al.* Home-based exercise program improves balance and fear of falling in community dwelling older adults with mild Alzheimer's disease. J Am Geriatr Soc. 2017;65 Suppl S9–S10. Available from: https://www.cochranelibrary.com/central/doi/10.1002/central/CN-01376948/full
66. Schwenk M, Sabbagh M, Lin I, Morgan P, Grewal GS, Mohler J, Coon DW, Najafi B. Sensor-based balance training with motion feedback in people with mild cognitive impairment. J Rehabil Res Dev. 2016;53(6):945–58. https://doi.org/10.1682/jrrd.2015.05.0089
67. Serino S, Pedroli E, Tuena C, De Leo G, Stramba-Badiale M, Goulene K, Mariotti NG, Riva G. A novel virtual reality-based training protocol for the enhancement of the "mental frame syncing" in individuals with Alzheimer's disease: A development-of-concept trial. Front Aging Neurosci. 2017;9:240.
68. Savulich G, Piercy T, Fox C, Suckling J, Rowe JB, O'Brien JT, Sahakian BJ. Cognitive training using a novel memory game on an iPad in patients with amnestic mild cognitive impairment: aMCI. Int J Neuropsychopharmacol. 2017;20(8):624–33. https://doi.org/10.1093/ijnp/pyx040
69. Georgiev DD, Georgieva I, Gong Z, Nanjappan V, Georgiev GV. Virtual reality for neurorehabilitation and cognitive enhancement. Brain Sci. 2021;11(2):221. Available from: https://www.mdpi.com/2076-3425/11/2/221

https://doi.org/10.1142/9789819817320_0014

Chapter 14*

Effectiveness of Telemedicine on Health-Related Outcomes Among Patients Undergoing Major Elective Surgery: A Systematic Review and Meta-Analysis

Claudia Loh Hwee Tze[1], Ong Qian Ying[2], and Piyanee Klainin-Yobas[3,*]

[1]*Tan Tock Seng Hospital, 11 Jln Tan Tock Seng, Singapore 308433*

[2]*Ng Teng Fong General Hospital, 1 Jurong East Street 21, Singapore 609606*

[3]*Alice Lee Centre for Nursing Studies, Yong Loo Lin School of Medicine, National University of Singapore, Level 5, Centre of Translational Medicine, Block MD6, 14 Medical Drive, Singapore 117599*

**Corresponding author: nurpk@nus.edu.sg*

14.1 Introduction

More than 312 million major surgeries are performed yearly worldwide [1]. Major surgery refers to procedures in hospital operating rooms involving manipulation of tissue and usually require regional or general anaesthesia [2]. Elective surgery can be scheduled in advance due to the lack of a medical emergency [3, 4]. Major elective surgeries include any pre-scheduled cardiac, abdominal, orthopaedic, gastrointestinal, cancer, neurological, spinal, transplant and urological surgeries.

The initial wave of the COVID-19 pandemic in 2020 overwhelmed healthcare systems globally and temporarily halted non-emergency

---

*Appendices to this chapter are available for download at https://www.worldscientific.com/worldscibooks/10.1142/14420#t=suppl.

surgeries [5, 6]. Consequently, a staggering estimated 72% of elective operations were cancelled, leading to a massive backlog requiring years to clear [7]. Delayed surgical treatment for conditions such as cancer and organ failure worsened patients' health and quality of life (QOL) [8]. It is therefore imperative to explore avenues to support major elective surgery in this current context [9].

Telemedicine reflects the utilisation of modern information and communication technologies to overcome geographical barriers and deliver healthcare services to people [10]. With the ubiquity of telecommunication and its ability to minimise physical contact between persons, telemedicine use has skyrocketed since the pandemic to substitute many face-to-face healthcare services [11, 12]. Telemedicine can be subdivided into three categories: synchronous, asynchronous and remote monitoring [13]. Synchronous telemedicine involves real-time communication (e.g., teleconsultation). Asynchronous telemedicine refers to store-and-forward communication (e.g., text messaging). Remote monitoring is the continuous tracking of patients' real-time condition (e.g., remote tracking of vital signs).

The perioperative period refers to pre- and postoperative care [14]. Prior to surgery, patients usually undergo pre-anaesthetic evaluation [15]. Some require additional preoperative interventions such as weight-loss programmes [16]. Telemedicine can deliver preoperative education, exercise programs and pre-anaesthetic evaluation to improve patient preparation for surgery [17–19]. Postoperatively, discharge care transitions patients from hospital to home [20]. However, patients often lack understanding towards their discharge care plan, feel uncertain and commit errors, increasing their likelihood of visiting the emergency department (ED) [21–23]. Telemedicine can improve post-discharge communication with healthcare providers, increase therapy adherence and satisfaction while reducing healthcare resource utilisation [24, 25]. After discharge, patients often return to the hospital for follow-up assessments. This can be disruptive and difficult if they need to travel long distances or face mobility issues, affecting their QOL [26, 27]. Teleconsultations allow patients to attend their appointments with greater ease without compromising on quality of care [28].

About 4–25% of postoperatively discharged patients require rehospitalisation due to complications such as pain, infection and gastrointestinal problems [29, 30]. Additional follow-ups and remote monitoring technologies can enable healthcare providers to assess patients closely and intervene timely, preventing further escalation and usage of healthcare resources [31]. Some surgeries such as knee arthroplasty also require long rehabilitation periods for successful outcomes [32]. Rapid ageing has increased the number of orthopaedic surgeries performed, placing a heavy burden on healthcare systems [33]. Consequently, telerehabilitation has been highlighted as a viable alternative to traditional in-person rehabilitation [34].

Therapy adherence, hospital readmissions and ED visits are common clinical indicators of postoperative recovery [25, 35, 36]. Therapy adherence refers to the extent to which patients follow recommendations by healthcare providers [37]. Health-related quality of life (HRQOL) refers to one's perceived physical and mental well-being [38]. HRQOL is a significant measure of population health and strongly correlates to morbidity and mortality [39]. Patient satisfaction refers to patients' thoughts and feelings towards their care experience [40]. Higher patient satisfaction links to greater success in care implementation and may improve clinical outcomes [41, 42]. Collectively, we term all the outcomes as health-related outcomes.

14.1.1 *Existing Systematic Reviews*

Currently, no known systematic review was reported on the effectiveness of telemedicine on health-related outcomes among patients following major elective surgery. Among nine systematic reviews identified regarding telemedicine use in perioperative care, most focused on either major or elective surgeries, not concurrently on both. Intervention-wise, four of them included all types of telemedicine [43–46], while others focused on specific forms such as messaging, mobile apps, telephone and video consultations, telemonitoring and telerehabilitation [19, 25, 26, 47, 48].

Seven of the nine systematic reviews did not conduct meta-analysis due to heterogeneity [19, 25, 43, 45, 47, 48]. One systematic review [46] performed a meta-analysis examining the effectiveness of telerehabilitation; nevertheless some outcomes (physical functioning, pain level and mental well-being) were not synthesised due to heterogeneity. Another systematic review [26] conducted a meta-analysis but included only seven randomised controlled trials (RCTs). Additionally, two systematic reviews [43, 45] searched only four databases each and did not cover grey literature, and two systematic reviews [19, 47] covered only three databases, which may lead to publication bias.

14.1.2 *Review Objective*

This review minimised the knowledge gaps in the literature by covering all relevant databases. It aimed to synthesise the best available evidence concerning the effectiveness of telemedicine on health-related outcomes among patients following major elective surgery. The review question is: In comparison with controls, what is the effectiveness of telemedicine on therapy adherence, hospital readmissions, ED visits, HRQOL and patient satisfaction among patients following major elective surgery?

14.2 Methods

This review followed the Cochrane Handbook for Systematic Reviews of Interventions and the PRISMA 2020 statement [49, 50]. It has been registered with PROSPERO (Registration number CRD42022299360).

14.2.1 *Eligibility Criteria*

This review considered studies that: (a) used RCTs, which represent the best available literature on this topic [51], (b) recruited participants aged

18 years and above who underwent major elective surgery, (c) examined any telemedicine intervention in perioperative care (both pre- and post-operative periods), such as teleconsultation, mobile apps and remote monitoring devices, and (d) compared outcomes with no-intervention control, standard care and/or active control group. Furthermore, primary outcomes would be therapy adherence, hospital readmissions, ED visits and HRQOL; and secondary outcome included patient satisfaction. Only studies in English conducted from 2011 to 2021 were considered to reflect up-to-date information on telemedicine [11].

14.2.2 *Information Sources*

A comprehensive search was conducted on 10 electronic databases. PubMed/MEDLINE, EMBASE, CINAHL, Scopus, Web of Science, CENTRAL, and IEEE Xplore were searched for published studies. Google Scholar, OpenGrey and ProQuest Dissertations & Theses Global were unpublished reports and ongoing trials [52]. Handsearching on reference lists of existing systematic reviews, including articles and targeted journals (*Journal of Telemedicine and Telecare* and *Telemedicine and e-Health*), were performed [53, 54]. Study authors would be contacted for missing information.

14.2.3 *Search Strategy*

A search strategy was developed using the concepts "telemedicine" and "major elective surgery". Free-text terms and subject headings were combined using relevant Boolean operators [52]. Word variations with syntaxes and truncation were used [55]. Wherever possible, searches were limited to the title and abstract fields. A medical librarian was consulted and the search strategy was peer-reviewed using the PRESS 2015 Evidence-Based Checklist [55].

The selection process was guided by the Cochrane Handbook [52]. Records were downloaded into EndNoteX20, where duplicates were removed [56]. These citations were exported to Rayyan for title/abstract screening [57]. One reviewer performed the initial title/abstract screening and removed clearly irrelevant articles. Thereafter, two reviewers pilot-tested the eligibility criteria on six articles and independently screened full texts for inclusion [52]. Disagreements were resolved by discussions with the third reviewer wherever consensus was not reached.

14.2.4 *Quality Appraisal and Data Extraction*

The Cochrane Collaboration's tool for assessing risk of bias (ROB 1) was used to assess individual study quality [58]. Domains assessed included: random sequence generation, allocation concealment, blinding of participants and personnel, blinding of outcome assessment, incomplete outcome data and selective outcome reporting. Domains were rated low, unclear or high risk of bias and the overall risk was determined by the worst rating across all domains [59]. Additionally, the Grading of Recommendations Assessment, Development, and Evaluation (GRADE) criteria [61, 62] was used to assess the certainty of evidence for all outcomes using the GRADEpro tool [63]. Certainty of evidence was graded high, moderate, low, or very low.

The modified Cochrane data extraction form for RCT [64] was used. The data extraction form was piloted on six articles [65] and modified through discussion between CL and QY, with disagreements resolved by PY. CL carried out the rest of the data extraction and attempted to contact study authors for missing information [60].

14.2.5 *Data Synthesis*

Meta-analysis was performed using Review Manager software [66]. The Mantel-Haenszel method was used to analyse dichotomous data while the inverse-variance method was used for continuous data [67]. Continuous data were summarised using standardised mean difference (SMD) [67]. Effect size (Cohen's d) was defined as small = 0.20,

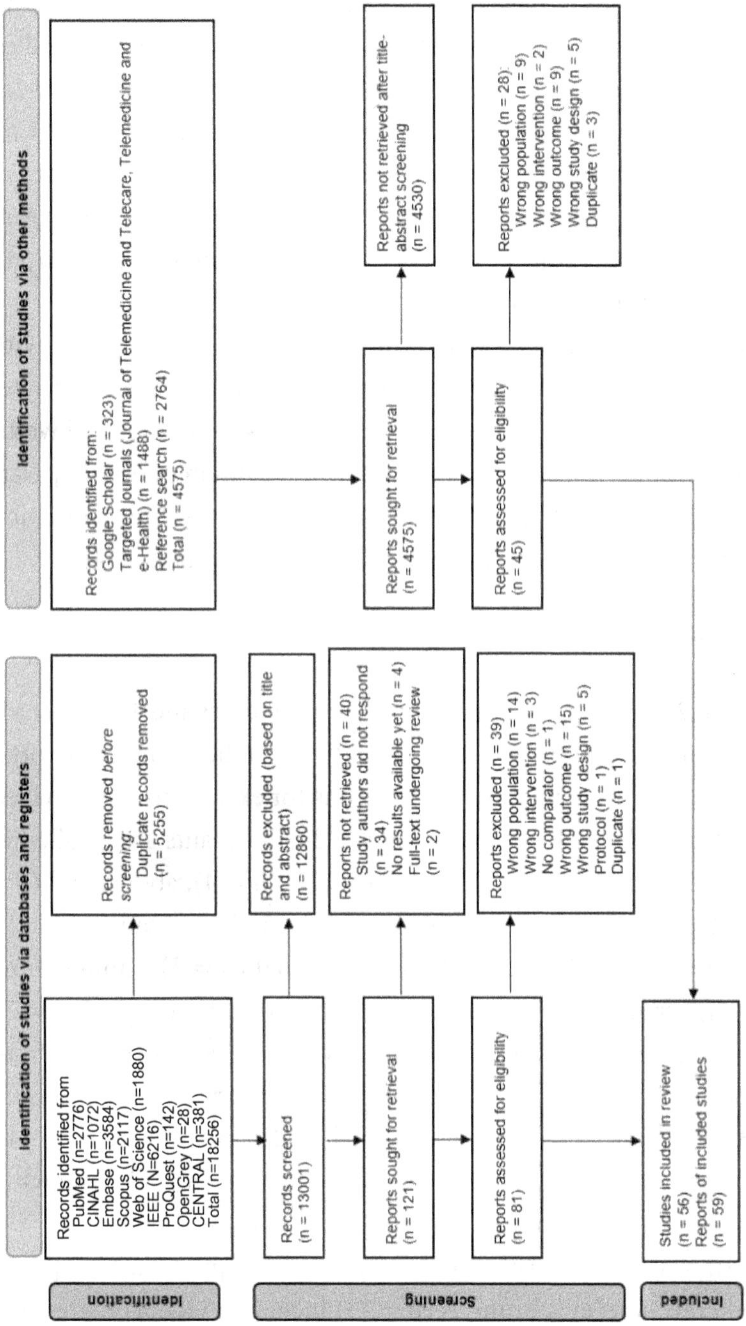

Figure 14.1 PRISMA flow diagram presenting the search process.

medium = 0.50, large = 0.80 and very large = 1.30 [68, 69]. Dichotomous data were summarised using risk ratio (RR) [67]. For multi-arm studies, groups were combined to create pairwise comparison using the RevMan calculator [66, 70]. Heterogeneity was assessed using I^2 statistics and Chi^2 test with $I^2 > 60\%$ and Chi^2 test of $p < 0.10$ suggesting the presence of substantial heterogeneity [67]. Publication bias was assessed via Egger's test and visual inspection of funnel plots created in Jamovi [71] when ≥10 studies were included in a forest plot [72, 73].

Sensitivity analysis was conducted by excluding studies with lower quality to determine the robustness of results [67]. Subgroup analyses were performed based on surgery types and assessment points to investigate sources of heterogeneity and compare between subgroups [67]. Narrative summary was undertaken by describing study characteristics, assessing quality and investigating sources of heterogeneity [74].

14.3 Results

In total, 18,256 records were identified from databases and 4,575 records were identified from other sources. Finally, 56 studies (with 59 reports) [28, 36, 75, 129] were included and reasons for exclusions are provided (Figure 14.1). The 56 RCTs involving 9,093 participants are detailed in Appendix A. Surgery types included cardiac (n = 4), abdominal (n = 11), head and neck (n = 3), orthopaedic (n = 15), breast cancer (n = 2), brain tumour resection (n = 1), lumbar spinal (n = 3), thoracotomy (n = 1), transplant (n = 6), hysterectomy (n = 3) and urological (n = 7). Participants' ages ranged from 42 to 76 years old. Education ranged from 4.4 to 16 years and proportion of those below tertiary education ranged from 3.75% to 89.15%. Comparators included standard care (n = 44), active control (n = 8) and no-intervention control (n = 4). Follow-up assessments ranged from one day to 24 months postoperatively.

A summary of interventions is provided in Appendix B. Types of telemedicine were: synchronous (n = 23) including videoconferencing and phone calls; asynchronous (n = 17) consisting mostly of app-based interventions; remote monitoring (n = 1); and a combination of types (n = 14). The contents of telemedicine interventions were: educational (n = 7), self-monitoring/management (n = 10), follow-up (n = 15), rehabilitation (n = 9), preoperative assessment (n = 1) and mixed interventions (n = 12). Telemedicine was used as a complement (n = 19) or replacement (n = 37) to usual care. Most interventions occurred in the community (n = 51, 91%), followed by inpatient (n = 4, 7%) and outpatient settings (n = 1, 2%). Five interventions were provided preoperatively, six perioperatively and the rest postoperatively (n = 45, 80%).

14.3.1 *Methodological Quality Assessment*

The ROB graph and summary are illustrated in Appendix C. All studies had low risk for randomisation except one which was unclear and 61% (34/56) had low risk for allocation concealment. 80% (45/56) had high risk for failing to blind participants, personnel and outcome assessors. 88% (49/56) had low risk for attrition bias [130, 131]. Reporting bias was high risk in 20% (11/56) of studies for reporting primary outcomes in non-prespecified ways.

The overall certainty of all outcomes was very low, except ED visits which was low (Appendix D). Therapy adherence, hospital readmissions and ED visits were rated critical because they directly impacted patients' clinical condition [132]. HRQOL and patient satisfaction were gradsed important due to their patient-centred nature [133].

14.3.2 *Effectiveness of telemedicine interventions on outcomes*

14.3.2.1 *Therapy Adherence*

Fourteen studies assessed therapy adherence, 11 of which used dichotomous outcomes. A meta-analysis involving 2,095 participants showed considerable heterogeneity ($I^2 = 92\%$, $Chi^2 = 118.91$, $p < 0.00001$)

Study or Subgroup	Telemedicine Events	Telemedicine Total	Comparator Events	Comparator Total	Weight	Risk Ratio M-H, Random, 95% CI
1.3.1 Transplant						
DeVito Dabbs et al., 2016	31	74	20	83	7.4%	1.74 [1.09, 2.77]
Reese et al., 2017	65	79	21	38	9.3%	1.49 [1.10, 2.02]
Schmid et al., 2017	19	23	10	23	7.1%	1.90 [1.15, 3.14]
Subtotal (95% CI)		**176**		**144**	**23.8%**	**1.62 [1.29, 2.04]**
Total events	115		51			
Heterogeneity: Tau² = 0.00; Chi² = 0.78, df = 2 (P = 0.68); I² = 0%						
Test for overall effect: Z = 4.18 (P < 0.0001)						
1.3.2 Abdominal						
Downey et al., 2020	43	60	65	65	10.7%	0.72 [0.61, 0.84]
Mata et al., 2020	30	50	31	50	9.2%	0.97 [0.71, 1.32]
Subtotal (95% CI)		**110**		**115**	**19.9%**	**0.81 [0.60, 1.10]**
Total events	73		96			
Heterogeneity: Tau² = 0.03; Chi² = 3.15, df = 1 (P = 0.08); I² = 68%						
Test for overall effect: Z = 1.34 (P = 0.18)						
1.3.3 Cardiac						
Lindman et al., 2021	23	25	21	25	10.3%	1.10 [0.89, 1.35]
Yu et al., 2020	58	493	58	494	8.9%	1.00 [0.71, 1.41]
Subtotal (95% CI)		**518**		**519**	**19.2%**	**1.07 [0.90, 1.28]**
Total events	81		79			
Heterogeneity: Tau² = 0.00; Chi² = 0.39, df = 1 (P = 0.53); I² = 0%						
Test for overall effect: Z = 0.75 (P = 0.46)						
1.3.4 Orthopedic						
Prvu Bettger et al., 2019	126	143	94	144	10.9%	1.35 [1.18, 1.54]
Subtotal (95% CI)		**143**		**144**	**10.9%**	**1.35 [1.18, 1.54]**
Total events	126		94			
Heterogeneity: Not applicable						
Test for overall effect: Z = 4.40 (P < 0.0001)						
1.3.5 Spinal						
He et al., 2020	42	48	29	48	9.9%	1.45 [1.12, 1.86]
Subtotal (95% CI)		**48**		**48**	**9.9%**	**1.45 [1.12, 1.86]**
Total events	42		29			
Heterogeneity: Not applicable						
Test for overall effect: Z = 2.87 (P = 0.004)						
1.3.6 Neurosurgery						
van de Linden et al., 2021	31	31	31	31	11.3%	1.00 [0.94, 1.06]
Subtotal (95% CI)		**31**		**31**	**11.3%**	**1.00 [0.94, 1.06]**
Total events	31		31			
Heterogeneity: Not applicable						
Test for overall effect: Z = 0.00 (P = 1.00)						
1.3.7 Oral						
Wang et al., 2019	32	34	6	34	5.0%	5.33 [2.57, 11.08]
Subtotal (95% CI)		**34**		**34**	**5.0%**	**5.33 [2.57, 11.08]**
Total events	32		6			
Heterogeneity: Not applicable						
Test for overall effect: Z = 4.49 (P < 0.00001)						
Total (95% CI)		**1060**		**1035**	**100.0%**	**1.28 [1.03, 1.59]**
Total events	500		386			
Heterogeneity: Tau² = 0.11; Chi² = 118.91, df = 10 (P < 0.00001); I² = 92%						
Test for overall effect: Z = 2.24 (P = 0.03)						
Test for subgroup differences: Chi² = 55.74, df = 6 (P < 0.00001), I² = 89.2%						

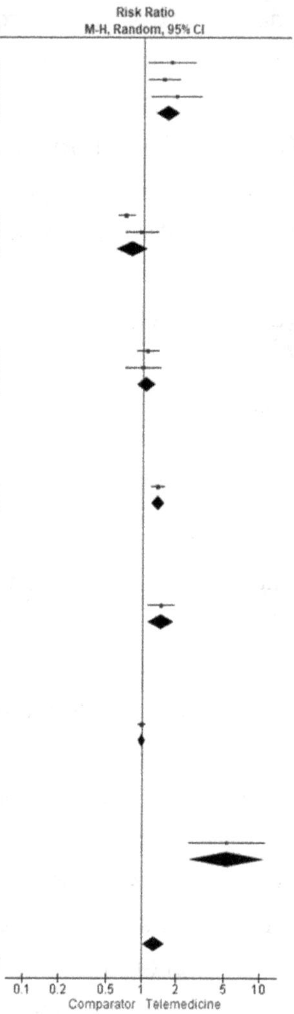

Figure 14.2 Effects of telemedicine on therapy adherence (categorical outcomes).

(Appendix B8) and thus the pool effect size will not be used. Therefore, subgroup analysis by type of surgery was performed (Figure 14.2).

Results suggested that the differences among subgroups achieved statistical significance ($Chi^2 = 55.74$, $p < 0.00001$). The oral surgery subgroup had the largest effect size (RR = 5.33, 95% CI = 2.57 to 11.08) and the study [125] used a weekly follow-up and rehabilitation intervention on oral cancer surgery patients. Furthermore, the transplant (RR = 1.62, 95% CI = 1.29 to 2.04), spinal (RR = 1.45, 95% CI = 1.12 to 1.86) and orthopaedic (RR = 1.35, 95% CI = 1.18 to 1.54) surgery subgroups had large effect size. Nevertheless, one study by subgroup analysis by assessment time-points showed no notable differences (Appendix B10).

Three studies reported continuous outcomes. A meta-analysis on 154 participants (Figure 14.3) showed considerable heterogeneity ($I^2 = 83\%$, $Chi^2 = 11.60$, $p = 0.003$) and therefore, a pooled effect size was not used. Examination of individual study suggested that one RCT [105] (using a daily self-monitoring/management intervention for renal transplant patients) showed a very large effect size (SMD = 3.15, 95% CI = 1.71 to 4.59). Moderate effects (SMD = 0.51–0.73) were found in two RCTs that used telerehabilitation on orthopaedic surgery.

14.3.2.2 *Hospital Readmissions*

Twenty studies assessed hospital readmission and 18 reported dichotomous outcomes. Telemedicine including education (n = 2), self-monitoring/management (n = 4), follow-up (n = 7), rehabilitation (n = 1) and mixed interventions (n = 4) were delivered. A meta-analysis on 4,029 participants (Figure 14.4) showed non-substantial heterogeneity ($I^2 = 24\%$, $Chi^2 = 22.49$, $p = 0.17$). A pooled effect size suggested 12% reduction in hospital readmissions (RR = 0.88, 95% CI = 0.74 to 1.06).

Two RCTs (using telerehabilitation and follow-up interventions) reported continuous outcomes. A meta-analysis on 389 participants showed homogeneity ($I^2 = 0\%$, $Chi^2 = 0.76$, $p = 0.38$) and a small pooled effect (SMD = –0.29, 95% CI = –0.49 to –0.09). One RCT [114] was excluded from meta-analysis due to the use of median and interquartile range [70]. It showed that telemedicine reduced readmissions compared to standard care ($F(1,\infty) = 6.59$, $p = 0.01$).

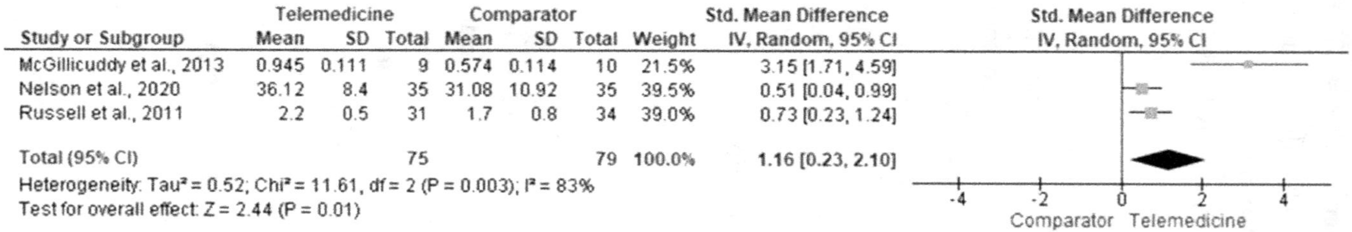

Figure 14.3 Effect of telemedicine on therapy adherence (continuous outcomes).

Study or Subgroup	Telemedicine Events	Telemedicine Total	Comparator Events	Comparator Total	Weight	Risk Ratio M-H, Random, 95% CI
Bednarski et al., 2019	2	14	0	16	0.4%	5.67 [0.29, 108.91]
Clari et al., 2015	1	136	2	139	0.6%	0.51 [0.05, 5.57]
Crawford et al., 2021a	5	208	13	244	2.9%	0.45 [0.16, 1.24]
Crawford et al., 2021b	7	116	3	137	1.7%	2.76 [0.73, 10.42]
DeVito Dabbs et al., 2016	80	99	87	102	28.8%	0.95 [0.84, 1.07]
Downey et al., 2020	6	60	5	65	2.3%	1.30 [0.42, 4.04]
Harrison et al., 2011	14	37	17	36	8.4%	0.80 [0.47, 1.37]
Inman et al., 2011	1	30	0	30	0.3%	3.00 [0.13, 70.83]
Kane et al., 2020	1	21	0	20	0.3%	2.86 [0.12, 66.44]
Keeping-Burke et al., 2013	14	84	8	84	4.3%	1.75 [0.78, 3.95]
Kleinpell et al., 2015	18	134	13	72	6.2%	0.74 [0.39, 1.43]
Lee et al., 2019	14	50	29	50	9.3%	0.48 [0.29, 0.80]
Lee et al., 2021	1	26	3	26	0.7%	0.33 [0.04, 3.00]
Mata et al., 2020	4	50	0	47	0.4%	8.47 [0.47, 153.18]
Moffet et al., 2015	7	104	5	101	2.4%	1.36 [0.45, 4.14]
Vesterby et al., 2017	1	36	0	36	0.3%	3.00 [0.13, 71.28]
Young et al., 2013	96	375	99	355	21.0%	0.92 [0.72, 1.17]
Yu et al., 2020	26	496	37	496	9.7%	0.70 [0.43, 1.14]
Total (95% CI)		**2076**		**2056**	**100.0%**	**0.88 [0.74, 1.06]**
Total events	298		321			

Heterogeneity: Tau² = 0.03; Chi² = 22.49, df = 17 (P = 0.17); I² = 24%
Test for overall effect: Z = 1.37 (P = 0.17)

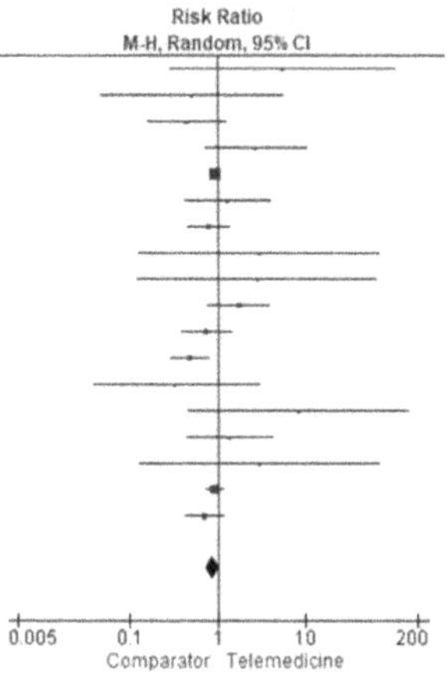

Figure 14.4 Effect of telemedicine on hospital admission.

14.3.2.3 *Emergency Department Visits*

Twelve RCTs assessed the number of ED visits. They used educational (n = 1), self-monitoring/management (n = 1), follow-up (n = 5), rehabilitation (n = 1) and mixed interventions (n = 4). A meta-analysis involving 2,449 participants (Figure 14.5) showed 6% reduction on ED visits (RR = 0.94, 95% CI = 0.79 to 1.12) and homogeneity ($I^2 = 0\%$).

14.3.2.4 *Health-Related Quality Of Life*

Thirty studies reported HRQOL outcomes, presented in three categories: Overall HRQOL, HRQOL-related physical health and HRQOL-related mental health.

Overall HRQOL. 12 studies assessed overall HRQOL. A meta-analysis on 2,683 participants showed considerable heterogeneity ($I^2 = 89\%$, $Chi^2 = 104.65$, $p < 0.00001$). A subgroup analysis by surgery types (Figure 14.6) showed unimportant heterogeneity across subgroups with significant test for differences ($Chi^2 = 92.96$, $p < 0.00001$, $I^2 = 97.2\%$). Hence, it is reasonable to conclude that type of surgery was an underlying reason for the heterogeneity. One RCT [93] (using a daily rehabilitation

Study or Subgroup	Telemedicine Events	Telemedicine Total	Comparator Events	Comparator Total	Weight	Risk Ratio M-H, Random, 95% CI
Bednarski et al., 2019	2	14	1	16	0.6%	2.29 [0.23, 22.59]
Crawford et al., 2021a	5	208	16	244	3.1%	0.37 [0.14, 0.98]
Crawford et al., 2021b	11	116	10	137	4.5%	1.30 [0.57, 2.95]
Harrison et al., 2011	8	37	12	36	5.2%	0.65 [0.30, 1.40]
Inman et al., 2011	2	30	3	30	1.0%	0.67 [0.12, 3.71]
Keeping-Burke et al., 2013	29	84	23	84	14.7%	1.26 [0.80, 1.99]
Kleinpell et al., 2015	19	134	17	72	8.8%	0.60 [0.33, 1.08]
Lee et al., 2021	4	26	5	26	2.1%	0.80 [0.24, 2.65]
Mata et al., 2020	10	50	9	47	4.7%	1.04 [0.47, 2.34]
Prvu Bettger et al., 2019	10	143	14	144	5.0%	0.72 [0.33, 1.57]
Radtke et al. 2021	0	16	1	25	0.3%	0.51 [0.02, 11.80]
Young et al., 2013	97	375	90	355	49.9%	1.02 [0.80, 1.31]
Total (95% CI)		**1233**		**1216**	**100.0%**	**0.94 [0.79, 1.12]**
Total events	197		201			

Heterogeneity: $Tau^2 = 0.00$; $Chi^2 = 10.75$, $df = 11$ ($P = 0.46$); $I^2 = 0\%$
Test for overall effect: $Z = 0.71$ ($P = 0.47$)

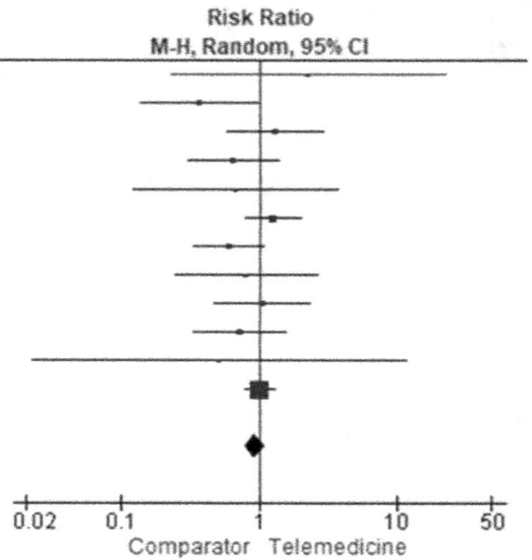

Figure 14.5 Effect of telemedicine on emergency department visit.

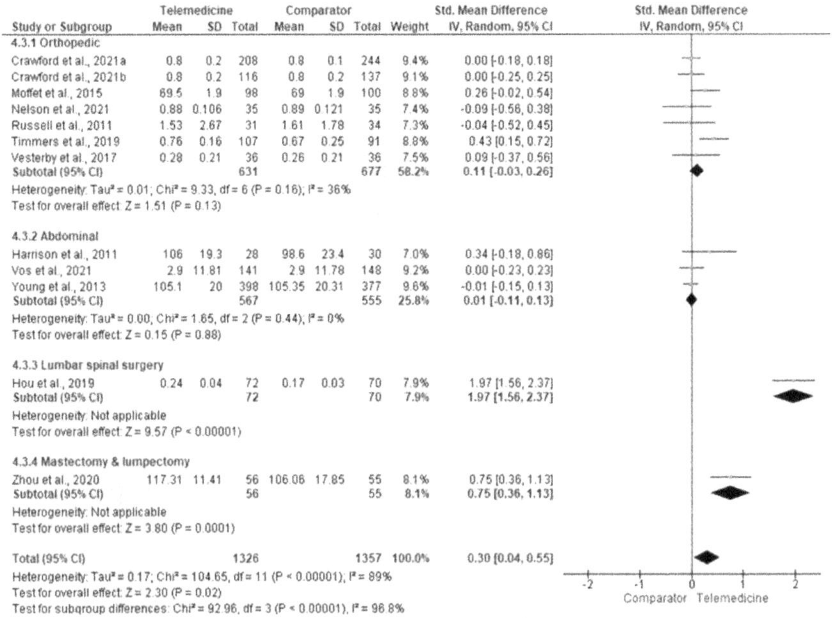

Figure 14.6 Effect of telemedicine on health-related quality of life.

and follow-up intervention) on spinal surgery patients showed a very large effect (SMD = 1.97, 95% CI = 1.56 to 2.37). Another RCT [129] (using daily educational, self-monitoring/management and follow-up interventions for breast cancer) on surgery patients also generated a moderate effect (SMD = 0.75, 95% CI = 0.36 to 1.13). Nevertheless, other subgroups had small effects.

HRQOL-related Physical Health. A meta-analysis on nine studies containing 1,358 participants showed moderate heterogeneity ($I^2 = 47\%$, $Chi^2 = 15.15$, p = 0.06) and a small pooled effect size (SMD = 0.18, 95% CI = 0.01 to 0.35). One RCT [36] was excluded from meta-analysis as it was the sole study using dichotomous outcomes. It reported non-significant differences between intervention and control (p = 0.820; p = 0.615) (F-test was not reported).

Study or Subgroup	Telemedicine Mean	Telemedicine SD	Telemedicine Total	Comparator Mean	Comparator SD	Comparator Total	Weight	Std. Mean Difference IV, Random, 95% CI
Dallimore et al., 2017	25.1	4.3	16	16.6	7.4	26	18.3%	1.30 [0.61, 1.99]
Halder et al., 2021	4.8	0.5	63	4.8	0.4	69	20.8%	0.00 [-0.34, 0.34]
Lee et al., 2021	80.7	2.6	26	81.2	2.8	26	19.4%	-0.18 [-0.73, 0.36]
van der Meij et al., 2018	7.2	1.7	163	6.3	2.4	167	21.4%	0.43 [0.21, 0.65]
Zhang et al., 2013	3.55	0.0858	59	2.96	0.38	60	20.1%	2.12 [1.67, 2.57]
Total (95% CI)			327			348	100.0%	0.72 [-0.02, 1.46]

Heterogeneity: $Tau^2 = 0.65$; $Chi^2 = 68.97$, $df = 4$ ($P < 0.00001$); $I^2 = 94\%$

Test for overall effect: $Z = 1.92$ ($P = 0.06$)

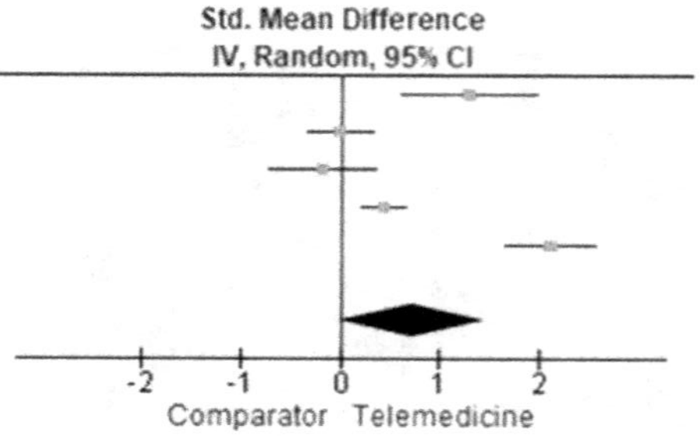

Figure 14.7 Effect of telemedicine on patient satisfaction.

HRQOL-related Mental Health. A meta-analysis on eight studies with 1,237 participants showed moderate heterogeneity ($I^2 = 39\%$, $Chi^2 = 11.50$, $p = 0.12$). A small pooled effect size was small (SMD = 0.10, 95% CI = −0.07 to 0.27).

14.3.2.5 *Patient Satisfaction*

22 studies reported patient satisfaction. A meta-analysis on five studies comprising 675 participants (Figure 14.7) showed considerable heterogeneity ($I^2 = 94\%$, $Chi^2 = 68.97$, $p < 0.00001$). Therefore, the pooled effect size was not used. Examination of individual effect size suggested two RCTs had a large effect size. One RCT [128] utilised a follow-up intervention on abdominal surgery patients (SMD = 2.12, 95% CI = 1.67 to 2.57) and another RCT [85] used an inpatient educational intervention on orthopaedic surgery patients (SMD = 1.30, 95% CI = 0.61 to 1.99). Furthermore, one RCT [120] (using daily self-monitoring/management on abdominal surgery patients) showed a small effect (SMD = 0.43, 95% CI = 0.21 to 0.65).

Additionally, 17 RCTs were excluded from meta-analysis due to heterogeneity in outcome reporting [74], six of which reported higher levels of satisfaction following telemedicine interventions using self-monitoring/management ($n = 1$), follow-up ($n = 4$) and rehabilitation ($n = 1$). 11 RCTs reported non-significant findings.

14.3.3 *Publication Bias*

Four outcomes had ≥10 studies each. Visual inspection of funnel plots for hospital readmissions and ED visits revealed slight asymmetry (Appendix E1 and E2) with $p = 0.411$ and $p = 0.259$ for Egger's test respectively, indicating no publication bias. Visual inspection of funnel plots for therapy adherence and overall HRQOL revealed asymmetry with both $p < 0.001$ for Egger's test, suggesting the presence of publication bias (Appendices E3 and E4).

14.4 Discussion

This review suggested that telemedicine generated small-to-very large effects on improving therapy adherence, HRQOL and patient satisfaction among people undergoing major elective surgery. Telemedicine also produced small-to-moderate effects in reducing hospital readmissions and ED visits.

Regarding therapy adherence, patients who underwent transplant, oral cancer and orthopaedic surgeries had the highest effectiveness. Specifically, telemedicine with regular self-monitoring/management and follow-up produced the greatest benefits. Previous systematic reviews also suggested the benefits of eHealth among patients undergoing transplant and oral cancer surgery [134, 135]. Such patients tend to lack knowledge of their treatments and forget the regime [136–138], which may explain why telemedicine was especially useful in increasing adherence. Furthermore, another review revealed that orthopaedic surgery patients demonstrated better adherence with close follow-up [139].

For HRQOL, telemedicine demonstrated the greatest effects on spinal and breast cancer surgery patients. Daily rehabilitation, self-monitoring/management interventions with frequent follow-up were beneficial. An explanation is that spinal surgery patients might fulfil their needs for social support and physical activity via telemedicine, and might overcome factors predisposing poorer HRQOL such as fear of movement [140]. Furthermore, among patients undergoing breast cancer surgery, telemedicine facilitating comprehensive self-management is known to improve their HRQOL [141]. Additionally, a previous meta-analysis on lung cancer patients showed that HRQOL continued to increase even three months after telemedicine [142]. This evidence suggested that HRQOL, being a subjective experience, requires time to change [38, 143].

Telemedicine improved patient satisfaction with small to large effect size, which agrees with previous systematic reviews [19, 26, 135]. Specifically, abdominal and orthopaedic surgery patients who used self-monitoring/management, educational and follow-up telemedicine interventions experienced higher satisfaction. This may be because such telemedicine interventions raised self-efficacy and social participation, particularly in abdominal surgery patients, which was linked to satisfaction [120, 128, 144, 145]. Certain orthopaedic surgeries require months for full recovery and patients continued their lives through the use of telemedicine [32]. While one previous systematic review supports our findings for abdominal surgery [146], other systematic reviews disagree [147, 148]. This could be explained by the presence of ceiling effects, which are especially prevalent in patient satisfaction measurement tools [149]. Beyond a certain threshold, patient satisfaction tools are unable to detect differences in two groups of relatively satisfied patients even if differences actually exist [149]. In one systematic review [148], patients expressed preference to use telemedicine over standard care in the future.

In hospital readmissions and ED visits, telemedicine generated small-to-moderate effects across surgery types, coinciding with previous systematic reviews that revealed slight reductions in those outcomes [25, 45, 150, 151]. Telemedicine interventions that helped reduce hospital readmissions and ED visits encompassed self-monitoring/management, education and follow-up. These components have shown to improve management of post-discharge complications and prevent further escalation in previous systematic reviews [25, 29, 43].

14.4.1 *Strengths and Limitations*

A comprehensive search yielded many studies, enabling us to analyse large samples across various demographics and countries for a globally representative perspective [152, 153]. The use of RCTs may reduce bias and enhance rigor in determining the effectiveness of telemedicine [51]. Nevertheless, this review has limitations. First, many studies had high or unclear risk of bias due to the lack of blinding. Secondly, publication bias was also detected, but likely minimised due to a comprehensive search over published and unpublished sources [52]. Thirdly, only articles in English were included which may have induced language bias [70]. However, evidence suggests that exclusion of non-English articles did not significantly impact overall conclusions [154, 155]. Finally, all outcomes had low and very low certainty of evidence. Therefore, our results should be interpreted with caution [61].

14.4.2 *Implications on Clinical Practice*

With the COVID-19 pandemic and rapid progression of technology having ushered in a paradigm shift in how society operates, telemedicine use in surgical care will continue being highly relevant [156]. To enhance therapy adherence, telemedicine with self-monitoring/management, personalised daily medication alert systems, and weekly follow-up via phone/videoconferences may be offered to patients following transplant, oral cancer and orthopaedic surgery. To improve HRQOL among patients undergoing breast cancer and spinal surgery, mobile application-based or website-based telerehabilitation programs may be delivered. In the programs, patients can carry out personalised plans and goals set by healthcare providers, communicate with healthcare providers regarding their recovery and access educational resources concerning self-management. Additionally, to reduce hospital readmissions and ED visits and raise patient satisfaction, telemedicine with self-monitoring/management, daily or weekly assessment by healthcare providers, education by healthcare providers via calls/messages and regular follow-up can be offered to patients with ongoing abdominal and orthopaedic surgery. Such telemedicine can be provided until the patient fully recovers or becomes competent in caring for themselves.

14.4.3 *Recommendations for Future Research*

Future RCTs may consider ways to identify strategies to ensure blinding of personnel, participants and outcome assessors (such as using active controls like apps with only basic functions, to reduce bias and improve reliability of conclusions) [70]. Future studies and systematic reviews may analyse a variety of aspects of patient satisfaction to avoid ceiling effects and obtain a more meaningful analysis [149]. Publication bias may also be better averted by searching in more trial registries for future systematic reviews [160].

14.5 Conclusion

Against the painful experience of the COVID-19 pandemic, backlog of elective surgeries and limited healthcare resources, telemedicine has never been more relevant in the surgical care setting. This systematic review and meta-analysis of a large number of RCTs has shown that telemedicine improves therapy adherence, hospital readmissions, ED visits, HRQOL and patient satisfaction in patients who undergo major elective surgery. Telemedicine intervention components such as self-monitoring/management, education and follow-up show greatest benefit when conducted regularly and are thus recommended for future clinical practice. While findings are promising, they should be interpreted with caution and future studies should look to improve the comprehensiveness in analysing patient satisfaction and methodological quality.

References

1. Weiser TG, Haynes AB, Molina G, Lipsitz SR, Esquivel MM, Uribe-Leitz T, *et al.* Estimate of the global volume of surgery in 2012: an assessment supporting improved health outcomes. Lancet. 2015;385 Suppl 2:S11.
2. Weiser TG, Regenbogen SE, Thompson KD, Haynes AB, Lipsitz SR, Berry WR, *et al.* An estimation of the global volume of surgery: a modelling strategy based on available data. Lancet. 2008;372(9633):139–44.
3. Diaz A, Sarac BA, Schoenbrunner AR, Janis JE, Pawlik TM. Elective surgery in the time of COVID-19. Am J Surg. 2020;219(6):900–2.
4. Stahel PF. How to risk-stratify elective surgery during the COVID-19 pandemic? Patient Saf Surg. 2020;14(1):8.

5. American College of Surgeons. COVID-19: Elective case triage guidelines for surgical care [Internet]. [cited 2022 Jul 4]. Available from: https://www.facs.org/covid-19/clinical-guidance/elective-case
6. COVIDSurg Collaborative. Global guidance for surgical care during the COVID-19 pandemic: Surgical care during the COVID-19 pandemic. Br J Surg. 2020;107(9):1097–103.
7. COVIDSurg Collaborative. Elective surgery cancellations due to the COVID-19 pandemic: global predictive modelling to inform surgical recovery plans. Br J Surg. 2020;107(11):1440–9.
8. Fu SJ, George EL, Maggio PM, Hawn M, Nazerali R. The consequences of delaying elective surgery: Surgical perspective. Ann Surg. 2020;272(2):e79–80.
9. Meredith JW, High KP, Freischlag JA. Preserving elective surgeries in the COVID-19 pandemic and the future. JAMA. 2020;324(17):1725–6.
10. World Health Organization. Telemedicine: Opportunities and developments in member states. Genève, Switzerland: World Health Organization; 2010.
11. Anderson M. Mobile Technology and Home Broadband 2019 [Internet]. Pew Research Center. 2019 [cited 2022 Jul 4]. Available from: https://www.pewresearch.org/internet/2019/06/13/mobile-technology-and-home-broadband-2019/
12. Gajarawala SN, Pelkowski JN. Telehealth benefits and barriers. J Nurse Pract. 2021;17(2):218–21.
13. Mechanic OJ, Persaud Y, Kimball AB. Telehealth Systems [Internet]. Treasure Island (FL): StatPearls Publishing; 2022 Jan-. [cited 2022 Jul 4]. Available from: https://www.ncbi.nlm.nih.gov/books/NBK459384/
14. Goodman T, Spry C. Essentials of perioperative nursing. 6th ed. Sudbury, MA: Jones and Bartlett; 2016.
15. American Society of Anesthesiologists. Distinguishing between a pre-anesthesia evaluation and a separately reportable evaluation and management service [Internet]. [cited 2022 Jul 4]. Available from: https://www.asahq.org/quality-and-practice-management/managing-your-practice/timely-topics-in-payment-and-practice-management/distinguishing-between-a-pre-anesthesia-evaluation-and-a-separately-reportable-evaluation-and-management-service
16. Keeney BJ, Austin DC, Jevsevar DS. Preoperative weight loss for morbidly obese patients undergoing total knee arthroplasty: Determining the necessary amount. J Bone Joint Surg Am. 2019;101(16):1440–50.
17. De La Cruz Monroy MFI, Mosahebi A. The use of smartphone applications (apps) for enhancing communication with surgical patients: A systematic review of the literature. Surg Innov. 2019;26(2):244–59.

18. Morsli H, Mathew D. CRT-708 development and evaluation of a smartphone application for the perioperative care of patients undergoing routine cardiology procedures. JACC Cardiovasc Interv. 2015;8(2):S46.
19. Schoen DC, Prater K. Role of telehealth in pre-anesthetic evaluations. AANA J. 2019;87(1):43–9.
20. Berian JR, Rosenthal RA, Baker TL, Coleman J, Finlayson E, Katlic MR, *et al.* Hospital standards to promote optimal surgical care of the older adult: A report from the coalition for quality in geriatric surgery. Ann Surg. 2018;267(2):280–90.
21. Newnham H, Barker A, Ritchie E, Hitchcock K, Gibbs H, Holton S. Discharge communication practices and healthcare provider and patient preferences, satisfaction and comprehension: A systematic review. Int J Qual Health Care. 2017;29(6):752–68.
22. Vonk Noordegraaf A, Anema JR, Louwerse MD, Heymans MW, van Mechelen W, Brölmann HAM, *et al.* Prediction of time to return to work after gynaecological surgery: a prospective cohort study in the Netherlands. BJOG. 2014;121(4):487–97.
23. Sandberg EH, Sharma R, Sandberg WS. Deficits in retention for verbally presented medical information. Anesthesiology. 2012;117(4):772–9.
24. Felbaum DR, Stewart JJ, Anaizi AN, Sandhu FA, Nair MN, Voyadzis J-M. Implementation and evaluation of a smartphone application for the perioperative care of neurosurgery patients at an academic medical center: Implications for patient satisfaction, surgery cancelations, and readmissions. Oper Neurosurg (Hagerstown). 2018;14(3):303–11.
25. Lu K, Marino NE, Russell D, Singareddy A, Zhang D, Hardi A, *et al.* Use of short message service and smartphone applications in the management of surgical patients: A systematic review. Telemed J E Health. 2018;24(6):406–14.
26. Oates EV, Lim GHC, Nevins EJ, Kanakala V. Are surgical patients satisfied with remote consultations? A comparison of remote versus conventional outpatient clinic follow-up for surgical patients: A systematic review and meta-analysis of randomized controlled trials. J Patient Exp. 2021;8.
27. Thatcher MD, Thatcher MW, Smith MC, McCarron M, Reed J. Opportunity costs of attending surgical clinic appointments and experiences with telemedicine for follow-up care. SAGE Open Med. 2021;9.
28. Augestad KM, Sneve AM, Lindsetmo R-O. Telemedicine in postoperative follow-up of STOMa PAtients: a randomized clinical trial (the STOMPA trial): Assessment of the feasibility of telemedicine in postsurgical care. Br J Surg. 2020;107(5):509–18.

29. Morris MS, Graham LA, Richman JS, Hollis RH, Jones CE, Wahl T, *et al.* Postoperative 30-day readmission: Time to focus on what happens outside the hospital. Ann Surg. 2016;264(4):621–31.
30. Tevis SE, Kohlnhofer BM, Weber SM, Kennedy GD. Postdischarge complications are an important predictor of postoperative readmissions. Am J Surg. 2014;208(4):505–10.
31. McElroy I, Sareh S, Zhu A, Miranda G, Wu H, Nguyen M, *et al.* Use of digital health kits to reduce readmission after cardiac surgery. J Surg Res. 2016;204(1):1–7.
32. Dávila Castrodad IM, Recai TM, Abraham MM, Etcheson JI, Mohamed NS, Edalatpour A, *et al.* Rehabilitation protocols following total knee arthroplasty: a review of study designs and outcome measures. Ann Transl Med. 2019;7 Suppl 7:S255.
33. Jiang S, Xiang J, Gao X, Guo K, Liu B. The comparison of telerehabilitation and face-to-face rehabilitation after total knee arthroplasty: A systematic review and meta-analysis. J Telemed Telecare. 2018;24(4):257–62.
34. Shukla H, Nair SR, Thakker D. Role of telerehabilitation in patients following total knee arthroplasty: Evidence from a systematic literature review and meta-analysis. J Telemed Telecare. 2017;23(2):339–46.
35. Bai MY, Mobbs RJ, Walsh WR, Betteridge C. MHealth apps for enhanced management of spinal surgery patients: A review. Front Surg. 2020;7:573398.
36. Kleinpell RM. Randomized trial of a discharge planning and telehealth intervention for patients aged 65 and older after coronary artery bypass surgery. Int J Clin Cardiol. 2015;2(4).
37. World Health Organization. Adherence to long-term therapies: Evidence for action. Genève, Switzerland: World Health Organization; 2003.
38. Centers for Disease Control and Prevention. Measuring healthy days. Atlanta, GA: Centers for Disease Control and Prevention; 2000. p. 6.
39. Centers for Disease Control and Prevention. HRQOL concepts [Internet]. 2018 [cited 2022 Jul 4]. Available from: https://www.cdc.gov/hrqol/concept.htm
40. Shirley ED, Sanders JO. Patient satisfaction: Implications and predictors of success. J Bone Joint Surg Am. 2013;95(10):e69.
41. Lobo Prabhu K, Cleghorn MC, Elnahas A, Tse A, Maeda A, Quereshy FA, *et al.* Is quality important to our patients? The relationship between surgical outcomes and patient satisfaction. BMJ Qual Saf. 2018;27(1):48–52.
42. Xesfingi S, Vozikis A. Patient satisfaction with the healthcare system: Assessing the impact of socio-economic and healthcare provision factors. BMC Health Serv Res. 2016;16(1):94.

43. Asiri A, AlBishi S, AlMadani W, ElMetwally A, Househ M. The use of telemedicine in surgical care: A systematic review. Acta Inform Med. 2018;26(3):201–6.
44. Gunter RL, Chouinard S, Fernandes-Taylor S, Wiseman JT, Clarkson S, Bennett K, *et al.* Current use of telemedicine for post-discharge surgical care: A systematic review. J Am Coll Surg. 2016;222(5):915–27.
45. van der Meij E, Anema JR, Otten RHJ, Huirne JAF, Schaafsma FG. The effect of perioperative E-health interventions on the postoperative course: A systematic review of randomised and non-randomised controlled trials. PLoS One. 2016;11(7):e0158612.
46. van Egmond MA, van der Schaaf M, Vredeveld T, Vollenbroek-Hutten MMR, van Berge Henegouwen MI, Klinkenbijl JHG, *et al.* Effectiveness of physiotherapy with telerehabilitation in surgical patients: a systematic review and meta-analysis. Physiotherapy. 2018;104(3):277–98.
47. Memon A, Lec P, Lenis A, Sharma V, Wood E, Schade G, *et al.* Relationship between mobile digital sensor monitoring and perioperative outcomes: Systematic review. JMIR Perioper Med. 2021;4(1):e21571.
48. Robinson A, Husband AK, Slight RD, Slight SP. Digital technology to support lifestyle and health behaviour changes in surgical patients: systematic review. BJS Open. 2021;5(2).
49. Higgins JPT, Thomas J, Chandler J, Cumpston M, Li T, Page MJ, et al, editors. Cochrane Handbook for Systematic Reviews of Interventions. 6.3th ed. Cochrane; 2022.
50. Page MJ, McKenzie JE, Bossuyt PM, Boutron I, Hoffmann TC, Mulrow CD, *et al.* The PRISMA 2020 statement: an updated guideline for reporting systematic reviews. Syst Rev. 2021;10(1):89.
51. Hariton E, Locascio JJ. Randomised controlled trials — the gold standard for effectiveness research: Study design: randomised controlled trials. BJOG. 2018;125(13):1716.
52. Lefebvre C, Glanville J, Briscoe S, Featherstone R, Littlewood A, Marshall C, *et al.* Chapter 4: Searching for and selecting studies. In: Higgins JPT, Thomas J, Chandler J, Cumpston M, Li T, Page MJ, et al, editors. Cochrane Handbook for Systematic Reviews of Interventions. 6.3th ed. Cochrane; 2022.
53. SAGE Publications. Journal of telemedicine and telecare [Internet]. c2022 [cited 2022 Jul 4]. Available from: https://journals.sagepub.com/home/jtt
54. Mary Ann Liebert, Inc. Telemedicine and e-Health [Internet]. c2022 [cited 2022 Jul 4]. Available from: https://home.liebertpub.com/publications/telemedicine-and-e-health/54

55. McGowan J, Sampson M, Salzwedel DM, Cogo E, Foerster V, Lefebvre C. PRESS Peer Review of Electronic Search Strategies: 2015 Guideline Statement. J Clin Epidemiol. 2016;75:40–6.
56. EndNote. Product details [Internet]. 2020 [cited 2022 Jul 4]. Available from: https://endnote.com/product-details
57. Ouzzani M, Hammady H, Fedorowicz Z, Elmagarmid A. Rayyan — a web and mobile app for systematic reviews. Syst Rev. 2016;5(1).
58. Higgins JPT, Altman DG, Gøtzsche PC, Jüni P, Moher D, Oxman AD, *et al.* The Cochrane Collaboration's tool for assessing risk of bias in randomised trials. BMJ. 2011;343:d5928.
59. Higgins JPT, Savović J, Page MJ, Elbers RG, Sterne JAC. Chapter 8: Assessing risk of bias in a randomized trial. In: Higgins JPT, Thomas J, Chandler J, Cumpston M, Li T, Page MJ, et al, editors. Cochrane Handbook for Systematic Reviews of Interventions. 6.3th ed. Cochrane; 2022.
60. Boutron I, Page MJ, Higgins JPT, Altman DG, Lundh A, Hróbjartsson A. Chapter 7: Considering bias and conflicts of interest among the included studies. In: Higgins JPT, Thomas J, Chandler J, Cumpston M, Li T, Page MJ, *et al.*, editors. Cochrane Handbook for Systematic Reviews of Interventions. 6.3th ed. Cochrane; 2022.
61. Balshem H, Helfand M, Schünemann HJ, Oxman AD, Kunz R, Brozek J, *et al.* GRADE guidelines: 3. Rating the quality of evidence. J Clin Epidemiol. 2011;64(4):401–6.
62. Schünemann H, Brożek J, Guyatt G, Oxman A. GRADE handbook [Internet]. The GRADE Working Group; 2013. Available from: https://gdt.gradepro.org/app/handbook/handbook.html#h.svwngs6pm0f2
63. GradePro. [Internet]. [cited 2022 Jul 4]. Available from: https://www.gradepro.org/
64. Cochrane Training. Data extraction form intervention review — RCTs only [Internet]. [cited 2021 Dec 8].
65. Li T, Higgins JPT, Deeks JJ. Chapter 5: Collecting data. In: Higgins JPT, Thomas J, Chandler J, Cumpston M, Li T, Page MJ, et al, editors. Cochrane Handbook for Systematic Reviews of Interventions. 6.3th ed. Cochrane; 2022.
66. Cochrane. RevMan [Internet]. [cited 2022 Jul 4]. Available from: https://training.cochrane.org/online-learning/core-software-cochrane-reviews/revman
67. Deeks JJ, Higgins JPT, Altman DG. Chapter 10: Analysing data and undertaking meta-analyses. In: Higgins JPT, Thomas J, Chandler J, Cumpston M, Li T, Page MJ, *et al.*, editors. Cochrane Handbook for Systematic Reviews of Interventions. 6.3th ed. Cochrane; 2022.

68. Cohen J. Statistical power analysis for the behavioral sciences. 2nd ed. Lawrence Erlbaum Associates; 1988.
69. Sullivan GM, Feinn R. Using effect size — or why the P value is not enough. J Grad Med Educ. 2012;4(3):279–82.
70. Higgins JPT, Green S. Cochrane handbook for systematic reviews of interventions. 5.1.0th ed. Cochrane; 2011.
71. Jamovi version 1.6 [Internet]. [cited 2022 Jul 4]. Available from: https://www.jamovi.org/
72. Page MJ, Higgins JPT, Sterne JAC. Chapter 13: Assessing risk of bias due to missing results in a synthesis. In: Higgins JPT, Thomas J, Chandler J, Cumpston M, Li T, Page MJ, *et al.*, editors. Cochrane Handbook for Systematic Reviews of Interventions. 6.3th ed. Cochrane; 2022.
73. Sterne JAC, Sutton AJ, Ioannidis JPA, Terrin N, Jones DR, Lau J, *et al.* Recommendations for examining and interpreting funnel plot asymmetry in meta-analyses of randomised controlled trials. BMJ. 2011;343:d4002.
74. McKenzie JE, Brennan SE. Chapter 12: Synthesizing and presenting findings using other methods. In: Higgins JPT, Thomas J, Chandler J, Cumpston M, Li T, Page MJ, et al, editors. Cochrane Handbook for Systematic Reviews of Interventions. 6.3th ed. Cochrane; 2022.
75. Aldemir K, Gürkan A. The effect of pedometer-supported walking and telemonitoring after disc hernia surgery on pain and disability levels and quality of life. Int J Nurs Pract. 2021;27(2):e12917.
76. Applegate RL 2nd, Gildea B, Patchin R, Rook JL, Wolford B, Nyirady J, *et al.* Telemedicine pre-anesthesia evaluation: a randomized pilot trial. Telemed J E Health. 2013;19(3):211–6.
77. Bednarski BK, Nickerson TP, You YN, Messick CA, Speer B, Gottumukkala V, *et al.* Randomized clinical trial of accelerated enhanced recovery after minimally invasive colorectal cancer surgery (RecoverMI trial). Br J Surg. 2019;106(10):1311–8.
78. Bini SA, Mahajan J. Clinical outcomes of remote asynchronous telerehabilitation are equivalent to traditional therapy following total knee arthroplasty: A randomized control study. J Telemed Telecare. 2017;23(2):239–47.
79. Cassin SE, Sockalingam S, Du C, Wnuk S, Hawa R, Parikh SV. A pilot randomized controlled trial of telephone-based cognitive behavioural therapy for preoperative bariatric surgery patients. Behav Res Ther. 2016;80:17–22.
80. Chen K, Yao F, Chen X, Lin Y, Kang M. Effectiveness of telerehabilitation on short-term quality of life of patients after esophageal cancer surgery during COVID-19: a single-center, randomized, controlled study. J Gastrointest Oncol. 2021;12(4):1255–64.

81. Clari M, Frigerio S, Ricceri F, Pici A, Alvaro R, Dimonte V. Follow-up telephone calls to patients discharged after undergoing orthopaedic surgery: double-blind, randomised controlled trial of efficacy. J Clin Nurs. 2015;24(19–20):2736–44.
82. Cleeland CS, Wang XS, Shi Q, Mendoza TR, Wright SL, Berry MD, *et al.* Automated symptom alerts reduce postoperative symptom severity after cancer surgery: a randomized controlled clinical trial. J Clin Oncol. 2011;29(8):994–1000.
83. Crawford DA, Duwelius PJ, Sneller MA, Morris MJ, Hurst JM, Berend KR, *et al.* 2021 Mark Coventry Award: Use of a smartphone-based care platform after primary partial and total knee arthroplasty: a prospective randomized controlled trial. Bone Joint J. 2021a;103-B(6 Suppl A):3–12.
84. Crawford DA, Lombardi AV Jr, Berend KR, Huddleston JI 3rd, Peters CL, DeHaan A, *et al.* Early outcomes of primary total hip arthroplasty with use of a smartphone-based care platform: a prospective randomized controlled trial. Bone Joint J. 2021b;103-B(7 Suppl B):91–7.
85. Dallimore R-K, Asinas-Tan ML, Chan D, Hussain S, Willett C, Zainuldin R. A randomised, double-blinded clinical study on the efficacy of multimedia presentation using an iPad for patient education of postoperative hip surgery patients in a public hospital in Singapore. Singapore Med J. 2017;58(9):562–8.
86. DeVito Dabbs A, Song MK, Myers BA, Li R, Hawkins RP, Pilewski JM, *et al.* A randomized controlled trial of a mobile health intervention to promote self-management after lung transplantation. Am J Transplant. 2016;16(7):2172–80.
87. Doiron-Cadrin P, Kairy D, Vendittoli P-A, Lowry V, Poitras S, Desmeules F. Feasibility and preliminary effects of a tele-prehabilitation program and an in-person prehabilitation program compared to usual care for total hip or knee arthroplasty candidates: a pilot randomized controlled trial. Disabil Rehabil. 2020;42(7):989–98.
88. Downey CL, Croft J, Ainsworth G, Buckley H, Shinkins B, Randell R, *et al.* Trial of remote continuous versus intermittent NEWS monitoring after major surgery (TRaCINg): a feasibility randomised controlled trial. Pilot Feasibility Stud. 2020;6(1):183.
89. Foley NM, O'Connell EP, Lehane EA, Livingstone V, Maher B, Kaimkhani S, *et al.* PATI: Patient accessed tailored information: A pilot study to evaluate the effect on preoperative breast cancer patients of information delivered via a mobile application. Breast. 2016;30:54–8.
90. Halder GE, White AB, Brown HW, Caldwell L, Wright ML, Giles DL, *et al.* A telehealth intervention to increase patient preparedness for surgery: a randomized trial. Int Urogynecol J. 2021;33(1):85–93.

91. Harrison JD, Young JM, Solomon MJ, Butow PN, Secomb R, Masya L. Randomized pilot evaluation of the supportive care intervention "CONNECT" for people following surgery for colorectal cancer. Dis Colon Rectum. 2011;54(5):622–31.
92. He Q, Zhao J, Fan M, Wang F. Effect of continuous nursing based on wechat platform on postoperative rehabilitation of patients with lumbar disc herniation. Jpn J Nurs Sci. 2020;18(2):e12382.
93. Hou J, Yang R, Yang Y, Tang Y, Deng H, Chen Z, *et al.* The effectiveness and safety of utilizing mobile phone-based programs for rehabilitation after lumbar spinal surgery: Multicenter, prospective randomized controlled trial. JMIR MHealth UHealth. 2019;7(2):e10201.
94. Inman DM, Maxson PM, Johnson KM, Myers RP, Holland DE. The impact of follow-up educational telephone calls on patients after radical prostatectomy: Finding value in low-margin activities. Urol Nurs. 2011;31(2):83.
95. Jensen BT, Kristensen SA, Christensen SV, Borre M. Efficacy of tele-nursing consultations in rehabilitation after radical prostatectomy: a randomized controlled trial study. Int J Urol Nurs. 2011;5(3):123–30.
96. Kane LT, Thakar O, Jamgochian G, Lazarus MD, Abboud JA, Namdari S, *et al.* The role of telehealth as a platform for postoperative visits following rotator cuff repair: a prospective, randomized controlled trial. J Shoulder Elbow Surg. 2020;29(4):775–83.
97. Kassymova G, Sydsjö G, Borendal Wodlin N, Nilsson L, Kjølhede P. The effect of follow-up contact on recovery after benign hysterectomy: A randomized, single-blinded, four-arm, controlled multicenter trial. J Womens Health (Larchmt). 2021;30(6):872–81.
98. Keeping-Burke L, Purden M, Frasure-Smith N, Cossette S, McCarthy F, Amsel R. Bridging the transition from hospital to home: effects of the VITAL telehealth program on recovery for CABG surgery patients and their caregivers. Res Nurs Health. 2013;36(6):540–53.
99. Lee TC, Kaiser TE, Alloway R, Woodle ES, Edwards MJ, Shah SA. Telemedicine based remote home monitoring after liver transplantation: Results of a randomized prospective trial. Ann Surg. 2019;270(3):564–72.
100. Lee DD, Arya LA, Andy UU, Harvie HS. Video virtual clinical encounters versus office visits for postoperative care after pelvic organ prolapse surgery: A randomized clinical trial. Female Pelvic Med Reconstr Surg. 2021;27(7):432–8.
101. Lindman BR, Gillam LD, Coylewright M, Welt FGP, Elmariah S, Smith SA, *et al.* Effect of a pragmatic home-based mobile health exercise intervention

after transcatheter aortic valve replacement: a randomized pilot trial. Eur Heart J Digit Health. 2021;2(1):90–103.

102. Malmström M, Ivarsson B, Klefsgård R, Persson K, Jakobsson U, Johansson J. The effect of a nurse led telephone supportive care programme on patients' quality of life, received information and health care contacts after oesophageal cancer surgery-A six month RCT-follow-up study. Int J Nurs Stud. 2016;64:86–95.
103. Mangieri CW, Johnson RJ, Sweeney LB, Choi YU, Wood JC. Mobile health applications enhance weight loss efficacy following bariatric surgery. Obes Res Clin Pract. 2019;13(2):176–9.
104. Mata J, Pecorelli N, Kaneva P, Moldoveanu D, Gosselin-Tardiff A, Alhashemi M, *et al.* A mobile device application (app) to improve adherence to an enhanced recovery program for colorectal surgery: a randomized controlled trial. Surg Endosc. 2019;34(2):742–51.
105. McGillicuddy JW, Gregoski MJ, Weiland AK, Rock RA, Brunner-Jackson BM, Patel SK, *et al.* Mobile health medication adherence and blood pressure control in renal transplant recipients: A proof-of-concept randomized controlled trial. JMIR Res Protoc. 2013;2(2):e32.
106. Moffet H, Tousignant M, Nadeau S, Mérette C, Boissy P, Corriveau H, *et al.* Patient satisfaction with in-home telerehabilitation after total knee arthroplasty: Results from a randomized controlled trial. Telemed J E Health. 2017;23(2):80–7.
107. Moffet H, Tousignant M, Nadeau S, Mérette C, Boissy P, Corriveau H, *et al.* In-home telerehabilitation compared with face-to-face rehabilitation after total knee arthroplasty: A noninferiority randomized controlled trial. J Bone Joint Surg Am. 2015;97(14):1129–41.
108. Nelson M, Russell T, Crossley K, Bourke M, McPhail S. Cost-effectiveness of telerehabilitation versus traditional care after total hip replacement: A trial-based economic evaluation. J Telemed Telecare. 2021;27(6):359–66.
109. Nelson M, Bourke M, Crossley K, Russell T. Telerehabilitation is non-inferior to usual care following total hip replacement — a randomized controlled non-inferiority trial. Physiotherapy. 2020;107:19–27.
110. Prvu Bettger J, Green CL, Holmes DN, Chokshi A, Mather RC 3rd, Hoch BT, *et al.* Effects of virtual exercise rehabilitation in-home therapy compared with traditional care after total knee arthroplasty: VERITAS, a randomized controlled trial. J Bone Joint Surg Am. 2019;102(2):101–9.
111. Radtke S, Umeh R, Chavez M, Curiel Z, Mendez K. Utilizing telemedicine for delivery of postoperative care following minimally invasive gynecologic

surgery: A randomized controlled trial. Gynecol Minim Invasive Ther. 2021;10(3):148–53.

112. Reese PP, Bloom RD, Trofe-Clark J, Mussell A, Leidy D, Levsky S, *et al.* Automated reminders and physician notification to promote immunosuppression adherence among kidney transplant recipients: A randomized trial. Am J Kidney Dis. 2017;69(3):400–9.
113. Russell TG, Buttrum P, Wootton R, Jull GA. Internet-based outpatient telerehabilitation for patients following total knee arthroplasty: a randomized controlled trial. J Bone Joint Surg Am. 2011;93(2):113–20.
114. Schmid A, Hils S, Kramer-Zucker A, Bogatyreva L, Hauschke D, De Geest S, *et al.* Telemedically supported case management of living-donor renal transplant recipients to optimize routine evidence-based aftercare: A single-center randomized controlled trial. Am J Transplant. 2017;17(6):1594–605.
115. Tian M, Wang B, Xue Z, Dong D, Liu X, Wu R, *et al.* Telemedicine for follow-up management of patients after liver transplantation: Cohort study. JMIR Med Inform. 2021;9(5):e27175.
116. Timmers T, Janssen L, van der Weegen W, Das D, Marijnissen W-J, Hannink G, *et al.* The effect of an app for day-to-day postoperative care education on patients with Total Knee Replacement: Randomized controlled trial. JMIR MHealth UHealth. 2019;7(10):e15323.
117. Tousignant M, Moffet H, Boissy P, Corriveau H, Cabana F, Marquis F. A randomized controlled trial of home telerehabilitation for post-knee arthroplasty. J Telemed Telecare. 2011a;17(4):195–8.
118. Tousignant M, Boissy P, Moffet H, Corriveau H, Cabana F, Marquis F, *et al.* Patients' satisfaction of healthcare services and perception with in-home telerehabilitation and physiotherapists' satisfaction toward technology for post-knee arthroplasty: an embedded study in a randomized trial. Telemed J E Health. 2011b;17(5):376–82.
119. van der Linden SD, Rutten G-JM, Dirven L, Taphoorn MJB, Satoer DD, Dirven CMF, *et al.* eHealth cognitive rehabilitation for brain tumor patients: results of a randomized controlled trial. J Neurooncol. 2021;154(3):315–26.
120. van der Meij E, Anema JR, Leclercq WKG, Bongers MY, Consten ECJ, Schraffordt Koops SE, *et al.* Personalised perioperative care by e-health after intermediate-grade abdominal surgery: a multicentre, single-blind, randomised, placebo-controlled trial. Lancet. 2018;392(10141):51–9.
121. Vesterby MS, Pedersen PU, Laursen M, Mikkelsen S, Larsen J, Søballe K, *et al.* Telemedicine support shortens length of stay after fast-track hip replacement: A randomized controlled trial. Acta Orthop. 2017;88(1):41–7.

122. Vonk Noordegraaf A, Anema JR, van Mechelen W, Knol DL, van Baal WM, van Kesteren PJM, *et al.* A personalised eHealth programme reduces the duration until return to work after gynaecological surgery: results of a multicentre randomised trial. BJOG. 2014;121(9):1127–35; discussion 1136.
123. Vos JAM, Duineveld LAM, Wieldraaijer T, Wind J, Busschers WB, Sert E, *et al.* Effect of general practitioner-led versus surgeon-led colon cancer survivorship care, with or without eHealth support, on quality of life (I CARE): an interim analysis of 1-year results of a randomised, controlled trial. Lancet Oncol. 2021;22(8):1175–87.
124. Wang J, Tong Y, Jiang Y, Zhu H, Gao H, Wei R, *et al.* The effectiveness of extended care based on Internet and home care platform for orthopaedics after hip replacement surgery in China. J Clin Nurs. 2018;27(21–22):4077–88.
125. Wang T-J, Su J-H, Leung K-W, Liang S-Y, Wu S-F, Wang H-M. Effects of a mouth-opening intervention with remote support on adherence, the maximum interincisal opening, and mandibular function of postoperative oral cancer patients: A randomized clinical trial. Eur J Oncol Nurs. 2019;40:111–9.
126. Young JM, Butow PN, Walsh J, Durcinoska I, Dobbins TA, Rodwell L, *et al.* Multicenter randomized trial of centralized nurse-led telephone-based care coordination to improve outcomes after surgical resection for colorectal cancer: the CONNECT intervention. J Clin Oncol. 2013;31(28):3585–91.
127. Yu C, Liu C, Du J, Liu H, Zhang H, Zhao Y, *et al.* Smartphone-based application to improve medication adherence in patients after surgical coronary revascularization. Am Heart J. 2020;228:17–26.
128. Zhang J-E, Wong FKY, You L-M, Zheng M-C, Li Q, Zhang B-Y, *et al.* Effects of enterostomal nurse telephone follow-up on postoperative adjustment of discharged colostomy patients. Cancer Nurs. 2013;36(6):419–28.
129. Zhou K, Wang W, Zhao W, Li L, Zhang M, Guo P, *et al.* Benefits of a WeChat-based multimodal nursing program on early rehabilitation in postoperative women with breast cancer: a randomized controlled trial. J Clin Nurs. 2021;30(3–4):513–22.
130. Gupta SK. Intention-to-treat concept: A review. Perspect Clin Res. 2011; 2(3):109–12.
131. Schlomer GL, Bauman S, Card NA. Best practices for missing data management in counseling psychology. J Couns Psychol. 2010;57(1):1–10.
132. Chazapis M, Gilhooly D, Smith AF, Myles PS, Haller G, Grocott MPW, *et al.* Perioperative structure and process quality and safety indicators: a systematic review. Br J Anaesth. 2018;120(1):51–66.

133. Gilhooly D, Chazapis M, Moonesinghe SR. Prioritisation of quality indicators for elective perioperative care: a Delphi consensus. Perioper Med (Lond). 2020;9(1):8.
134. Govender R, Smith CH, Taylor SA, Barratt H, Gardner B. Swallowing interventions for the treatment of dysphagia after head and neck cancer: a systematic review of behavioural strategies used to promote patient adherence to swallowing exercises. BMC Cancer. 2017;17(1):43.
135. Tang J, James L, Howell M, Tong A, Wong G. EHealth interventions for solid organ transplant recipients: A systematic review and meta-analysis of randomized controlled trials. Transplantation. 2020.
136. Ganjali R, Ghorban Sabbagh M, Nazemiyan F, Mamdouhi F, Badiee Aval S, Taherzadeh Z, *et al.* Factors associated with adherence to immunosuppressive therapy and barriers in Asian kidney transplant recipients. ImmunoTargets Ther. 2019;8:53–62.
137. Marienne J, Laville SM, Caillard P, Batteux B, Gras-Champel V, Masmoudi K, *et al.* Evaluation of changes over time in the drug burden and medication regimen complexity in ESRD patients before and after renal transplantation. Kidney Int Rep. 2021;6(1):128–37.
138. Shinn EH, Basen-Engquist K, Baum G, Steen S, Bauman RF, Morrison W, *et al.* Adherence to preventive exercises and self-reported swallowing outcomes in post-radiation head and neck cancer patients: Oropharyngeal cancer: Swallowing exercise nonadherence. Head Neck. 2013;35(12):1707–12.
139. Marks R. Knee osteoarthritis and exercise adherence: a review. Curr Aging Sci. 2012;5(1):72–83.
140. Tripp DA, Abraham E, Lambert M, Wagg K, Bigney E, Daly E, *et al.* Biopsychosocial factors predict quality of life in thoracolumbar spine surgery. Qual Life Res. 2017;26(11):3099–110.
141. Triberti S, Savioni L, Sebri V, Pravettoni G. eHealth for improving quality of life in breast cancer patients: A systematic review. Cancer Treat Rev. 2019;74:1–14.
142. Pang L, Liu Z, Lin S, Liu Z, Liu H, Mai Z, *et al.* The effects of telemedicine on the quality of life of patients with lung cancer: a systematic review and meta-analysis. Ther Adv Chronic Dis. 2020;11.
143. Antonsson T, Wennersten A, Sörensen K, Regnér S, Ekelund M. Differences in health-related quality of life after gastric bypass surgery: A cross-sectional study. Obes Surg. 2021;31(7):3194–202.
144. Goodall RJ, Ellauzi J, Tan MKH, Onida S, Davies AH, Shalhoub J. A systematic review of the impact of foot care education on self efficacy and self care in patients with diabetes. Eur J Vasc Endovasc Surg. 2020;60(2):282–92.

145. Ponce MSH, Rosas RPE, Lorca MBF. Social capital, social participation and life satisfaction among Chilean older adults. Rev Saude Publica. 2014;48(5): 739–49.
146. Aseem R, Cribb E, Liccardo F, Daulatzai N, Smith J, Pawa N. 698 A systematic review of smartphone applications for enhanced recovery after surgery (ERAS) following colorectal surgery. Br J Surg. 2021;108(Supplement_2).
147. Chaudhry H, Nadeem S, Mundi R. How satisfied are patients and surgeons with telemedicine in orthopaedic care during the COVID-19 pandemic? A systematic review and meta-analysis. Clin Orthop Relat Res. 2021;479(1):47–56.
148. Melian C, Kieser D, Frampton C, C Wyatt M. Teleconsultation in orthopaedic surgery: A systematic review and meta-analysis of patient and physician experiences. J Telemed Telecare. 2020.
149. Nguyen C, Kortlever JTP, Gonzalez AI, Ring D, Brown LE, Somogyi JR. Attempts to limit censoring in measures of patient satisfaction. J Patient Exp. 2020;7(6):1094–100.
150. Eustache J, El-Kefraoui C, Ekmekjian T, Latimer E, Lee L. Do postoperative telemedicine interventions with a communication feature reduce emergency department visits and readmissions?-a systematic review and meta-analysis. Surg Endosc. 2021;35(11):5889–904.
151. Gandhi S, Chen S, Hong L, Sun K, Gong E, Li C, *et al.* Effect of mobile health interventions on the secondary prevention of cardiovascular disease: Systematic review and meta-analysis. Can J Cardiol. 2017;33(2):219–31.
152. Møller AM, Myles PS. What makes a good systematic review and meta-analysis? Br J Anaesth. 2016;117(4):428–30.
153. Borm GF, Fransen J, Lemmens WAJG. A simple sample size formula for analysis of covariance in randomized clinical trials. J Clin Epidemiol. 2007;60(12):1234–8.
154. Jüni P, Holenstein F, Sterne J, Bartlett C, Egger M. Direction and impact of language bias in meta-analyses of controlled trials: empirical study. Int J Epidemiol. 2002;31(1):115–23.
155. Nussbaumer-Streit B, Klerings I, Dobrescu AI, Persad E, Stevens A, Garritty C, *et al.* Excluding non-English publications from evidence-syntheses did not change conclusions: a meta-epidemiological study. J Clin Epidemiol. 2020;118:42–54.
156. Kichloo A, Albosta M, Dettloff K, Wani F, El-Amir Z, Singh J, *et al.* Telemedicine, the current COVID-19 pandemic and the future: a narrative review and perspectives moving forward in the USA. Fam Med Community Health. 2020;8(3):e000530.

157. Dobson GP. Trauma of major surgery: A global problem that is not going away. Int J Surg. 2020;81:47–54.
158. Cardozo AS, Santana RF, Rocha ICM, Cassiano KM, Mello TD, Melo UG. Phone follow-ups as a nursing intervention in the surgical recovery of prostatectomized elderly. Journal of Nursing. 2017;11(6):3005.
159. Thakar S, Rajagopal N, Mani S, Shyam M, Aryan S, Rao AS, *et al.* Comparison of telemedicine with in-person care for follow-up after elective neurosurgery: results of a cost-effectiveness analysis of 1200 patients using patient-perceived utility scores. Neurosurg Focus. 2018;44(5):E17.
160. Thornton A, Lee P. Publication bias in meta-analysis: its causes and consequences. J Clin Epidemiol. 2000;53(2):207–16.

https://doi.org/10.1142/9789819817320_0015

Chapter 15*

The Applications of Blockchain-based IoT Technology for Remote Patient Monitoring: A Scoping Review

Boyang Richard Liu, Sher Ning Felicia Tan, and Piyanee Klainin-Yobas*

Alice Lee Centre for Nursing Studies, Yong Loo Lin School of Medicine,
National University of Singapore, 10 Medical Drive, Singapore 117597, Singapore
**Corresponding author: nurpk@nus.edu.sg*

15.1 Introduction

Remote patient monitoring (RPM) is the process of monitoring the physiological status of patients remotely [1]. Internet of Things (IoT) devices, which transfer data over a network, are typically used for around-the-clock physiological monitoring of patients [2]. They work by collecting data via sensors attached or embedded within patients. The collected data are then sent to healthcare systems for patient monitoring or further analyses [1]. With that action, it is important to note that data breaches in healthcare are not uncommon. In fact, over 300 breaches were reported in 2017, and an estimate of 37 million health records were affected between 2010 and 2017 [3, 4]. Thus, this continuous collection of personal data could pose significant issues regarding its secure storage and potential misuse.

To tackle the aforementioned concerns, blockchain technology can be incorporated with IoT devices for RPM to improve the security and privacy of patient data through the following avenues. Firstly, blockchain is a decentralised, distributed ledger system maintained by a network of

*Appendices to this chapter are available for download at https://www.worldscientific.com/worldscibooks/10.1142/14420#t=suppl.

nodes [5]. Due to its decentralised nature, no single entity has control over the data on blockchain networks and it therefore tampers resistance. Furthermore, data are encrypted using hash functions and only a recipient can decrypt it. These factors ensure the security and privacy of patient data.

Secondly, blockchains can run smart contracts, which are important for data ownership and authentication of users [6]. Smart contracts are self-executing contracts that run when predetermined conditions are achieved [7]. Patients may decide who to share their data with and their decisions will be enforced by smart contracts. The ability to decide access control gives patients ownership over their own data [6]. Smart contracts also require user authentication, providing an additional layer of security. Together with access control policies, smart contracts ensure that patient data are only accessible to authorised users and shared with the appropriate parties [6].

Previous studies evaluated the applications of blockchain-based IoT technology for RPM, but there are some methodological limitations. One research [8] explored various studies on the application of blockchain-based IoT technology for RPM, but the authors employed a narrative description without statistical synthesis. In other research [9, 10], authors explored the advantages and limitations of blockchain technology in healthcare, but their findings were targeted at the wider healthcare system and, therefore, findings were not generalisable to the RPM systems. Furthermore, the application of blockchain-based IoT technology in healthcare was only discussed as subsections in past systematic reviews. However, none of those reviews addressed the IoT applications in RPM. Thus, such clear gaps in existing reviews prompted the need for this scoping review.

This scoping review aimed to highlight future research directions and the implications for practice by consolidating the best available evidence on blockchain-based IoT technology applications for RPM. To fulfil the aim, the following review questions are formulated:

1. How is blockchain-based IoT technology used for RPM among end users, including patients, healthcare professionals, and researchers?

2. What are the advantages and limitations of blockchain-based IoT technology for RPM?
3. What are the barriers and facilitators concerning the adoption of blockchain-based IoT technology for RPM?

15.2 Methods

15.2.1 *Study Design*

This scoping review was conducted based on Joanna Briggs Institution (JBI) guidelines and we used the PCC (participants, concept, context) framework to guide the eligibility criteria [11].

Types of participants. This review included studies involving healthcare professionals, patients, and/or researchers as end users of blockchain-based IoT RPM systems.

Concept. This review included studies focusing on the applications of blockchain-based IoT technology for RPM. Then, the concept was categorised into three sub-concepts: (a) the application of the technology on monitoring patients remotely, (b) advantages and limitations of the RPM system and (c) facilitators and barriers pertaining to the adoption of blockchain-based RPM systems. Articles were included if they discussed one or more sub-concepts of interest.

Context. This review included studies regardless of their country, location or setting.

Types of evidence. This review included all types of published and unpublished studies including, but not limited to, conference proceedings, journal articles, and book chapters. Theoretical, engineering, and empirical papers were all included. *Theoretical articles* describe theoretical frameworks underpinnings of a blockchain-based IoT RPM system, which have not been tested or evaluated. *Engineering articles* describe the implementation of the blockchain-based IoT RPM system and the system has been evaluated using computer simulations. *Empirical articles* describe real-world implementations or pilots of blockchain-based IoT RPM systems. Studies conducted from October 2008 onwards were included as blockchain technology only gained prominence following the publication of the Bitcoin white paper [12]. Only articles in English were included due to logistic matters.

15.2.2 *Search Strategy*

This review utilised the JBI three-step search strategy [13]. Firstly, a preliminary search using the terms "blockchain" and "remote patient monitoring" was conducted on PubMed and IEEE Xplore, followed by an analysis of text words and index terms of the articles. Keywords and terms related to blockchain, RPM, and IoT were initially identified. Secondly, both published and unpublished studies were searched using the identified keywords/index terms across 11 databases (CINAHL, Cochrane, Compendex, EMBASE, IEEE Xplore, Inspec, PsycINFO, ProQuest Dissertations and Theses Global, PubMed, Scopus, and Web of Science). Thirdly, the reference lists of the included articles were searched for additional related articles. During the search, we followed the Peer Review of Electronic Search Strategies (PRESS) guidelines to ascertain the appropriate and comprehensive of the search strategy [14]. Subsequently, the search strategy was peer-reviewed with a second reviewer, and a university medical sciences librarian was consulted to finalise the search strategy. The JBI three-step search strategy employed was pilot tested and developed iteratively.

15.2.3 *Study Selection*

The study selection process is reported using the PRISMA-ScR flow diagram [15]. All records identified from the comprehensive search were uploaded into EndNote X9 with duplicates being removed.

Two independent reviewers conducted title/abstract screening to identify potentially relevant articles, followed by full-text screening. Articles were screened against the eligibility criteria at both stages. Studies which fulfilled the eligibility criteria were included. Any disagreements that arose between the two reviewers were resolved through discussion. If consensus was not reached, a third reviewer was consulted.

15.2.4 *Data Extraction*

Data from the included studies were extracted using a modified JBI data extraction form by two independent reviewers [16]. The form captured data relevant to our concepts of interest, which then answered our review questions. The data extraction form was pilot tested by two independent reviewers on five randomly selected articles among the list of included articles [16]. It was then iteratively refined to ensure that all relevant data were accurately captured. Afterwards, data was extracted independently using the refined data extraction form from all included articles. The first reviewer contacted authors of studies with missing data. Any disagreements regarding the data extracted were resolved through discussion and/or consultations with the third reviewer.

15.2.5 *Data Analysis and Presentation*

We used a three-phase (preparation, organising, reporting) inductive content analysis [17]. This analysis was chosen because there was insufficient knowledge regarding the blockchain-based IoT technology's applications for RPM in existing literature [17]. The content analysis aims to provide a descriptive account of the applications by examining codes that were manifested and the frequency of their appearance. In the *preparation phase*, the first reviewer immersed in the extracted data from the included articles to gain a sense of the applications of blockchain-based IoT technology for RPM, followed by the identification of the units of analysis which can potentially be used to create categories. In the *organising phase*, the first reviewer conducted open coding and categories were freely generated. Categories were then grouped together to form higher-order categories through an abstraction process. In the *reporting phase*, these results were reported and presented using tables, figures and diagrams. Narrative summary was used to interpret the results in relation to the review questions. Then, two reviewers discussed and finalised the reported findings. Any disagreement was consulted with a third reviewer. As this scoping review only aims to provide a rapid overview of the literature concerning blockchain-based IoT technology for RPM, critical appraisal and risk of bias assessment of the included articles were not conducted [16].

15.3 Results

15.3.1 *Search Results*

After removing duplicates, 1,773 articles were identified in the initial search (Figure 15.1). Then, 1,607 records were excluded based on title/abstract screening, leaving 166 articles for full-text screening. Afterwards, 75 articles were excluded, leaving 91 articles. No additional articles were identified through other sources.

15.3.2 *Characteristics of Included Studies*

The 91 studies encompassed journal articles (n = 49), conference proceedings (n = 38), and serials (n = 4). Of the journal articles, *IEEE Access*, *IEEE Internet of Things Journal*, and *Sensors* featured the highest number of articles at six articles each (6/91, 6.59%). This was followed by *Sensors (Switzerland)*, which had four articles (4/91, 4.40%). The rest of the journals featured two articles or less. Of the conference proceedings, each proceeding was published in a different conference. All the included articles were in English and from 2017 onwards.

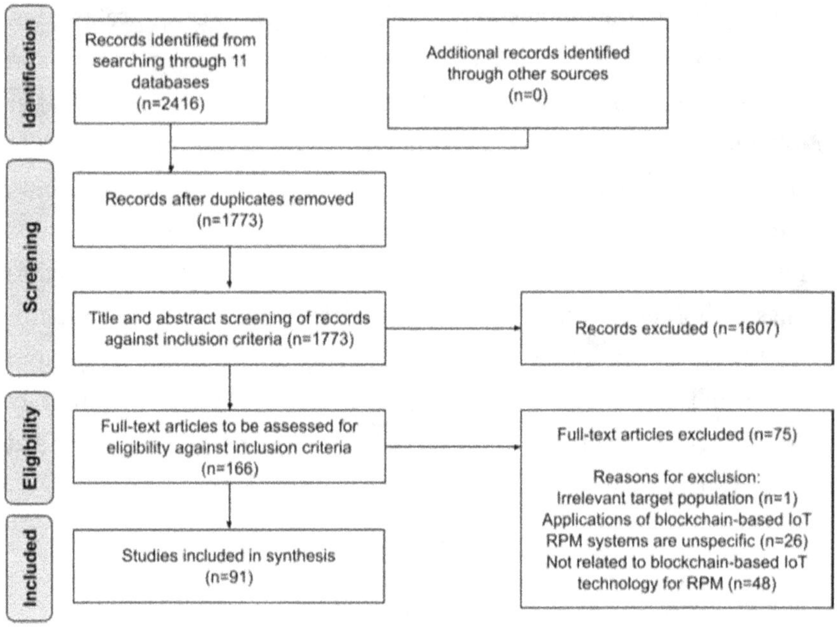

Figure 15.1 PRISMA-ScR flowchart.

The first authors of the included articles were globally represented and affiliated with 33 countries. India had the highest number of studies (19.8%, n = 18), followed by China (15.4%, n = 14), the United States of America (6.59%, n = 6), Australia (5.49%, n = 5), and South Korea (5.49%, n = 5). After grouping by World Health Organization regions, the Western Pacific had the greatest number of first authors by affiliation (29.7%, n = 27), followed by Southeast Asia (22.0%, n = 20), Eastern Mediterranean (18.7%, n = 17), Europe (15.4%, n = 14), Americas (8.79%, n = 8), and Africa (4.40%, n = 4). The affiliation of first authors by countries is summarised in Figure 15.2.

The main aims of studies were coded into ten categories. However, each article could be classified into multiple categories to better reflect its focus. The included studies addressed general applications (n = 42), improving general security (n = 30), encryption of data (n = 6),

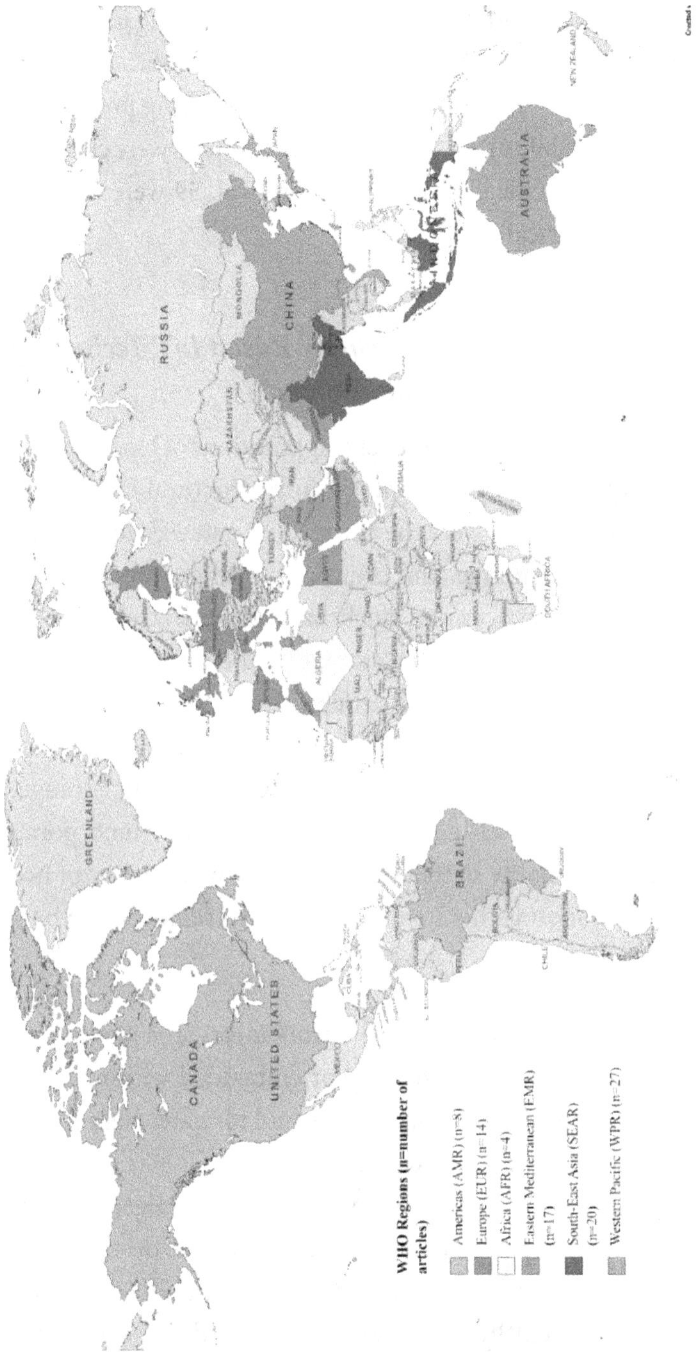
WHO Regions (n=number of articles)
Americas (AMR) (n=8)
Europe (EUR) (n=14)
Africa (AFR) (n=4)
Eastern Mediterranean (EMR) (n=17)
South-East Asia (SEAR) (n=20)
Western Pacific (WPR) (n=27)
CANADA
UNITED STATES
GREENLAND
BRAZIL
RUSSIA
MONGOLIA
CHINA
KAZAKHSTAN
AUSTRALIA

Figure 15.2 The affiliation of first authors by countries.

improving an authentication process (n = 10), improving general privacy (n = 19), managing access control of data (n = 17), data storage (n = 9), interoperability (n = 5), improving private data sharing process (n = 1), and improving scalability (n = 1). The included articles were classified into three categories. Specifically, 28 were theoretical, 59 were engineering, and four were empirical (Appendix A).

15.3.3 *The Application: Blockchain-Based IoT Technology for Remote Patient Monitoring*

Of the 42 articles focused on the general applications of blockchain-based IoT technology for RPM, we found six infrastructural layers common within them. These layers were the perception, gateway, fog computing, blockchain network, storage, and cloud computing layers. Of these six, the perception layer, gateway, and blockchain network layers were present in all articles. The fog computing, storage, and cloud computing layers were reported in 10, 35, and four articles respectively. The perception, gateway, and blockchain network ones were primary layers required for blockchain-based RPM systems. The fog computing, storage, and cloud computing ones were secondary layers that were incorporated to improve the functionality of the overall system. A summary of how the different layers work together to monitor patients remotely can be found in Figure 15.3.

Perception, Gateway and Blockchain network layers. The *perception layer* comprised sensors that were attached or embedded within the patient to collect physiological data from patients and forward them to gateway devices (such as smartphones or tablets) via WiFi, 4G/5G, Bluetooth or Zigbee [18]. Next, the *gateway layer* encompassed gateway devices that process and forward the collected data to various destinations over the blockchain network [19]. Patient data could either be sent directly to recipients like healthcare providers or could be sent to storage

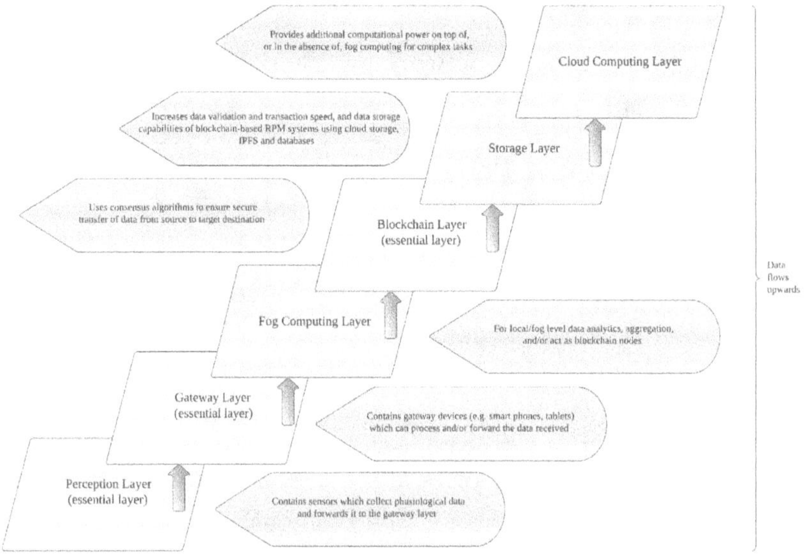

Figure 15.3 The six common infrastructural layers of blockchain-based RPM systems.

repositories. The *blockchain network layer* ensured that data were sent securely from gateway devices to target destinations through the use of consensus algorithms [20]. Consensus algorithm is a set of rules in place for all the nodes to reach an agreement regarding the legitimacy and validity of a transaction. Healthcare providers could subsequently monitor patients remotely by accessing the stored data. The blockchain network layer was also used as a platform to operate smart contracts [21].

Fog computing layer. The fog computing layer supported blockchain-based RPM systems in various areas. Two studies used fog computing for physiological data analytics and aggregation [22, 23]. Four articles used fog computing to analyse and diagnose patients with critical physiological data, followed by sending alerts to patients and healthcare providers [24–27]. Two articles used fog computing for local data processing to reduce computational time and to offload the cloud computing layer [28, 29]. Lastly, three articles utilised fog computing to support the blockchain network by functioning as participating nodes [25, 28, 30].

Storage layer. The storage layer provided data storage capabilities to increase data validation and transaction speed of blockchain-based RPM systems [31]. Six studies used cloud storage for data storage, two used IPFS for data storage [32–36], one used both cloud storage and IPFS for data storage [37], and three used unspecified third-party databases for storage [19, 30, 38].

Cloud computing layer. The *cloud computing layer* provided additional computational power on top of, or in the absence of, the fog computing layer. One study [29] incorporated cloud computing to process complex tasks that cannot be handled by fog computing. Another study [35] utilised cloud computing to store data received from gateway nodes into IPFS in the event that fog computing nodes were absent. One study [39] used cloud computing to enforce data access control set up by patients. Similarly, another study [25] used cloud computing to manage access control of patient data and utilisation through smart contracts. In addition, cloud computing also acts as nodes in a public blockchain supporting the smart contracts.

15.3.4 *Applications of Blockchain-Based IoT Technology to Domains of Care*

Monitoring patient conditions. The most commonly monitored items were vital signs, electrocardiogram, blood glucose level, and physical activity. Among the included studies, 28 monitored vital signs and others monitored electrocardiogram (n = 8), blood glucose (n = 8), and physical activity (n = 9). Furthermore, 52 studies described the use of wearable sensors to collect physiological data from patients, but did not specify which diseases or conditions were monitored.

Monitoring non-communicable diseases. Blockchain-based IoT technology was useful for monitoring non-communicable diseases including, but not limited to, diabetes mellitus, cardiovascular diseases and chronic obstructive pulmonary disease. According to the Global Burden of Disease Study [40], there were 450 million cases of diabetes mellitus, 61.7 million cases of cardiovascular diseases, and 329 million cases of chronic obstructive pulmonary disease in 2013. The high number of cases suggested the importance of managing non-communicable diseases to improve health. Through RPM, health statuses can be closely monitored to enable early intervention, improving quality of care [1].

Monitoring falls. Another frequent use case, physical activity monitoring, can be particularly helpful for detecting falls which can be quite dangerous, resulting in injuries such as acute haemorrhagic stroke or bone fracture at the hips or limbs [41, 42]. According to the Global Burden of Disease Study [40], there were 232 million cases of falls in 2013. Furthermore, as the risk of falls increases with age, an ageing population increases chances for falls to occur [43]. Thus, blockchain-based IoT technology allows for timely intervention, serving as an alert system for caregivers and hospitals.

15.3.5 *Advantages and Limitations of Blockchain-Based IoT Technology for Remote Patient Monitoring*

Advantages. The advantages of blockchain-based IoT technology for RPM largely lied in its ability to run smart contracts. Smart contracts are important in ensuring the security, privacy, and data ownership of blockchain-based RPM systems [6]. Eleven studies used smart contracts for data access control to determine access rights to the patient data [18, 44–53]. This increased data ownership among patients as they decided who to share their data with and that decision was enforced by smart contracts. Data access controls also increased the security and privacy of patients' data as only authorised data users have the rights to access the data [6]. Twelve articles used smart contracts for the authentication of patients and data users [23, 32, 46, 53–61]. Before patients and data users could utilise the RPM service, they had to first register themselves and their devices (e.g., sensors, smartphones) through smart contracts. Smart contracts captured the information and recorded it on the blockchain. The authentication process increased security as only authenticated users and devices could interact with the system [6].

Limitations. The limitations of blockchain-based IoT technology for RPM included poor scalability, high computational power requirements, transaction costs, and slow data transaction time. Ten studies raised concerns over the poor scalability of blockchain-based RPM systems [22, 27, 47, 59, 62–67]. Two mentioned requirements on high computational power [33, 65] and two addressed potentially high transaction costs [33, 53]. Lastly, two raised concerns over slow data transmission time [19, 33].

Overcoming limitations. Solutions proposed generally focused on three areas — consensus algorithm, type of blockchain network, and the use of storage repositories. Among the included articles, six used Proof of Authority (PoA) [35, 58, 68–71], four used Proof of Work (PoW) [35, 72–74], and one used Proof of Stake (PoS) [28] as their consensus algorithm. In PoA, validators staked their reputation† to validate transactions. Validators were incentivised to validate honest transactions‡, otherwise their reputation and ability to validate future transactions would be compromised [75]. In PoS, nodes were required to stake their cryptocurrency holdings to gain the right to validate transactions. PoS

† Reputation refers to the authority to validate transactions. The greater the reputation of a node in PoA, the greater its ability to validate transactions.

‡ Honest transactions refer to authentic transactions. Malicious nodes may attempt to present fraudulent transactions to tamper with data on the blockchain and thus compromise the integrity of the network.

incentivised nodes to validate honest transactions, as dishonest transactions compromise the integrity of the blockchain and decrease the value of the cryptocurrency they hold [76]. In PoW, nodes competed to generate a valid hash to a block. This process is known as mining, and only the first miner which generates a valid hash is allowed to add the block to the blockchain. This process requires great computational power and energy [77]. PoA and PoS required significantly less computational power from nodes as compared to PoW, potentially improving data transaction time and scalability of blockchain-based RPM systems [78].

Among the included articles, 33 utilised private blockchains and others used consortium (n = 13), permissioned (n = 10), public (n = 5), and hybrid blockchains (both private and public) (n = 3). These results favoured the use of permissioned networks, which included private and consortium networks, as compared to public networks. This is because permissioned blockchain networks had lower data transaction times, lower transaction costs, and higher scalability [79]. As discussed above in the infrastructure of blockchain-based RPM systems, many articles used storage repositories to store data off-chain, increasing the data transaction speed and scalability of systems [31].

15.3.5 *Facilitators and Barriers for Adoption of Blockchain-Based IoT Technology for Remote Patient Monitoring*

Facilitators. We found that financial incentives were commonly used to facilitate the adoption of blockchain-based IoT technology for RPM. In the system proposed by [80], users were rewarded with Healthcoins when they successfully validated transactions. Healthcoins were required to utilise services in the proposed system. Doctors were also rewarded with Healthcoins when their diagnosis was successfully added. Healthcoins obtained could be traded for fiat currency, or other cryptocurrencies over an exchange. In one study [35], diabetic patients were rewarded with

Glucocoins when they shared their physiological data with researchers. Glucocoins could be used to purchase insulin needles and glucometers.

Barriers. There were inadequate discussions among the included articles regarding the barriers of adoption, possibly attributed to the lack of pilot or empirical studies. Such trends show that the current focus of IoT technology has been on the development of a working system, which is necessary before pilot studies can be conducted.

15.4 Discussion

In this scoping review, we examined the applications of blockchain-based IoT technology for RPM. Existing systems were used for the monitoring of various diseases and conditions. We found that blockchain-based RPM systems were generally composed of six layers: perception, gateway, fog computing, blockchain network, storage, and cloud computing layers. Their advantages and limitations were also reported.

This review suggested that blockchain-based RPM systems played an important role in non-communicable disease management and falls monitoring. The systems were simple and straightforward solutions to mitigate the detrimental effects of uncontrolled non-communicable diseases and falls. The high proportion of studies devoted to the development of blockchain-based RPM systems for the monitoring of these physiological data has demonstrated strong interest in this area. However, there is a lack of discussion pertaining to the use of blockchain-based RPM systems for these domains of care. In previous reviews [8, 9, 81], the use of blockchain technology for RPM were only briefly discussed. There was no focus on the application of blockchain-based RPM systems for specific domains of care. Instead, these reviews merely described existing systems and their intended functions in RPM. However, the lack of discussion for the specific domains of care are likely attributed to the nature of those reviews and the novelty of the subject. In those reviews, the focus was on providing a review on the wider applications of blockchain in healthcare. As blockchain RPM systems is an emerging topic, specific focus on the domains of care were not adequately explored. Nevertheless, the findings in this review show that blockchain-based RPM systems hold great potential for non-communicable disease and falls management.

Unfortunately, the application of blockchain-based IoT technology is still in an infantile stage. This is attributed to two key reasons. Firstly, the technology must provide a satisfactory solution for the scalability issue before it can be widely adopted. The volume of patient data collected is likely to overload the existing blockchain-based RPM systems [10]. While solutions were proposed to overcome scalability concerns through consensus algorithms, these solutions still have drawbacks. Specifically, PoA is a consensus algorithm but it reduces properties of decentralisation [82]. PoS, another consensus algorithm, still faces several security issues such as bribe attacks or grinding attacks [83].

Secondly, the lack of widespread adoption is also attributed to the absence of a unified standard for blockchain-based RPM systems. A standard on security, privacy, scalability, and interoperability needs to be set to ensure the efficacy of blockchain-based RPM systems. This notion is also reflected in an existing systematic review [81], which suggested that the standards are essential to give stakeholders the confidence to adopt the RPM systems. Hence, a future research direction is to develop a unified standard for blockchain-based RPM systems.

The two issues mentioned must be addressed before blockchain-based RPM systems can be industrialised. Currently, the only notable advantage they have over traditional IoT-based RPM systems is the increased security and privacy of patient data [84]. Traditional RPM systems entail similar performance in monitoring the same diseases or conditions with a higher scalability [84]. Thus, blockchain-based RPM systems need to operate at the same efficiency as the traditional RPM systems before they can be considered as viable replacements.

Looking forward, there must be facilitators for the adoption of these systems at a user level. Our findings suggested that financial incentives can be used to encourage the adoption amongst individuals. This is not surprising because financial incentives are effective motivators for behavioural changes [85, 86]. However, the use of financial incentives may be divisive to different societal groups [87]. Using the system conceptualised by one research [45] as an example, patients sell their data to researchers using smart contracts. Patients of lower socioeconomic status may feel obliged to earn the incentives. As a result, incentives may be framed as a form of punishment instead [87]. Therefore, system developers need to tread carefully around the plausible implications regarding the use of financial incentives to promote adoption.

On the other hand, the barriers for adoption of the technology amongst individuals were not adequately discussed. This is expected given that many blockchain-based RPM systems are still novel without many real-world tests and experimentations, making it difficult to identify concrete barriers. A previous study [9] highlighted the lack of interest in new technology, especially among the elderly, being a major stumbling block. This is expected as blockchain is a novel and complicated concept. This coincides with the Theory of Diffusion of Innovation [88], which explains that elderly individuals are less likely to adopt new technologies unless they see clear benefits. Hence, future designs of blockchain-based RPM systems need to be simple and user friendly, with clear tangible benefits.

15.4.1 *Implications for Future Practice and Research Direction*

From our findings, blockchain-based IoT technology is useful for remote monitoring of non-communicable diseases and falls. It is known that the risk of multiple non-communicable diseases and falls increases with age. Coupled with the fact that many communities are ageing, the ability to monitor health remotely and provide healthcare would appear to be a pressing concern [43, 89]. Therefore, societies with an ageing population can consider adopting blockchain-based IoT technology to monitor their health remotely. However, blockchain-based IoT RPM systems are mostly in their conceptual stages. Until large-scale pilot studies have been conducted to evaluate the feasibility and effectiveness of such systems, stakeholders should adopt a wait-and-see approach. Finally, scalability issues and the lack of a unified standard need to be addressed since they remain as key barriers holding back industry-wide implementations [84].

15.4.2 *Strengths and Limitations of this Review*

The strength of our review lies in the comprehensiveness of our search. We conducted our search on 11 databases to capture all relevant literature. We included articles as long as they were related to the applications of blockchain-based IoT technology for RPM, even if the focus was only on a part of the broader system. The broad inclusion criteria allowed us to gain a valuable overview of all current accomplishments in this field.

However, we admit there might be several limitations with our scoping review. Firstly, given that scoping is not required to perform critical quality appraisal or risk of bias assessment [16], results and implications need to be interpreted with due diligence. Secondly, due to the reviewers' limited language flexibility, only articles written in English were included for review. Potential important articles in other languages might be excluded [90].

15.5 Conclusion

In all, the advancement in modern technology enables healthcare professionals to monitor patients remotely using IoT devices [1]. Blockchain-based RPM systems have potential uses in non-communicable disease and falls monitoring. This allows healthcare professionals to develop treatment for early prevention, or to provide timely intervention during acute events. Yet, the volumes of personal information collected raise red flags regarding the secure storage and handling of these data. Despite blockchain-based RPM systems offering an innovative solution for data security and privacy [6, 91], they are mostly conceptual without any real-world implementations. Scalability considerations and the lack of unified standards remain as major stumbling blocks, preventing widespread adoption [91]. Future research should focus on addressing these barriers.

References

1. Farias FA, Dagostini CM, Bicca Y, de, Falavigna VF, Falavigna A. Remote patient monitoring: A systematic review. Telemed J E Health. 2020;26(5):576–583.
2. Ratta P, Kaur A, Sharma S, Shabaz M, Dhiman G. Application of blockchain and internet of things in healthcare and medical sector: Applications, challenges, and future perspectives. J Food Qual. 2021;2021:1–20.
3. McCoy TH, Perlis RH. Temporal trends and characteristics of reportable health data breaches, 2010–2017. JAMA. 2018;320(12):1282–1284.
4. Talesh SA. Data breach, privacy, and cyber insurance: How insurance companies act as "compliance managers" for businesses. Law Soc Inquiry. 2018;43(2):417–440.
5. Abou Jaoude J, George Saade R. Blockchain applications — usage in different domains. IEEE Access. 2019;7:45360–45381.
6. Zheng Z, Xie S, Dai HN, Chen W, Chen X, Weng J, Imran M. An overview on smart contracts: Challenges, advances and platforms. Future Gener Comput Syst. 2020;105:475–491.
7. Christidis K, Devetsikiotis M. Blockchains and smart contracts for the internet of things. IEEE Access. 2016;4:2292–2303.
8. Tandon A, Dhir A, Islam AKMN, Mäntymäki M. Blockchain in healthcare: A systematic literature review, synthesizing framework and future research agenda. Comput Ind. 2020;122:1–21.
9. Agbo C, Mahmoud Q, Eklund J. Blockchain technology in healthcare: A systematic review. Healthcare. 2019;7(56):1–30.
10. Durneva P, Cousins K, Chen M. The current state of research, challenges, and future research directions of blockchain technology in patient care: Systematic review. J Med Internet Res. 2020;22(7):e18619.

11. Peters M, Godfrey C, McInerney P, Munn Z, Tricco A, Khalil H. Chapter 11: Scoping reviews. JBI Manual for Evidence Synthesis. https://doi.org/10.46658/jbimes-20-12
12. Nakamoto S. Bitcoin: A peer-to-peer electronic cash system. Retrieved March 3, 2022, from https://bitcoin.org/bitcoin.pdf
13. Aromataris E, Riitano D. Constructing a search strategy and searching for evidence. Am J Nurs. 2014;114(5):49–56.
14. McGowan J, Sampson M, Salzwedel DM, Cogo E, Foerster V, Lefebvre C. PRESS peer review of electronic search strategies: 2015 guideline statement. J Clin Epidemiol. 2016;75:40–46.
15. Tricco AC, Lillie E, Zarin W, O'Brien KK, Colquhoun H, Levac D, *et al.* PRISMA extension for scoping reviews (PRISMA-SCR): Checklist and explanation. Ann Intern Med. 2018;169(7):467–473.
16. Peters MDJ, Marnie C, Tricco AC, Pollock D, Munn Z, Alexander L, *et al.* Updated methodological guidance for the conduct of scoping reviews. 2021;19(1):3–10.
17. Elo S, Kyngäs H. The qualitative content analysis process. J Adv Nurs. 2008;62(1):107–115.
18. Saravanan M, Shubha R, Marks AM, Iyer V. Smead: A secured mobile enabled assisting device for diabetics monitoring. 2017 IEEE International Conference on Advanced Networks and Telecommunications Systems (ANTS). https://doi.org/10.1109/ants.2017.8384099
19. Griggs KN, Ossipova O, Kohlios CP, Baccarini AN, Howson EA, Hayajneh T. Healthcare blockchain system using smart contracts for secure automated remote patient monitoring. J Med Syst. 2018;42(7):130.
20. Shyamala Devi M, Swathi P, Nitesh Kumar Sah M, Jahangir A, Upadhyay SS. Edge technology enabled IoT blockchain-based health monitoring for chronically sick patients. Lect Notes Netw Syst. https://doi.org/10.1007/978-981-16-0666-3_44
21. Kazmi HS, Nazeer F, Mubarak S, Hameed S, Basharat A, Javaid N. Trusted remote patient monitoring using blockchain-based smart contracts. Lect Notes Netw Syst. https://doi.org/10.1007/978-3-030-33506-9_70
22. Dai HN, Wu Y, Wang H, Imran M, Haider N. Blockchain-empowered edge intelligence for internet of medical things against COVID-19. IEEE Internet Things Mag. 2021;4(2):34–39.
23. Kembo SH, Mpofu P, Mukorera BT, Jacques S. Blockchain-secured health wearables in smart homes utilising raspberry pi web of things gateways. 2nd African Int Conf Ind Eng Oper Manag (IEOM). 2020:2269–2280.

24. Aujla GS, Jindal A. A decoupled blockchain approach for edge-envisioned IoT-based healthcare monitoring. IEEE J Sel Areas Commun. 2021;39(2):491–499.
25. Egala BS, Priyanka S, Pradhan AK. SHPI: Smart healthcare system for patients in ICU using IoT. 2019 IEEE Int Conf Adv Netw Telecommun Syst (ANTS). https://doi.org/10.1109/ants47819.2019.9118084
26. Islam A, Shin SY. BHMUS: Blockchain based secure outdoor health monitoring scheme using UAV in smart city. 2019 7th Int Conf Inf Commun Technol (ICoICT). https://doi.org/10.1109/icoict.2019.8835373
27. Saha R, Kumar G, Kumar N, Kim TH, Devgun T, Thomas R, *et al.* Internet of things framework for oxygen saturation monitoring in COVID-19 environment. IEEE Internet Things J. 2022;9(5):3631–3641.
28. Uddin MA, Stranieri A, Gondal I, Balasubramanian V. A decentralized patient agent controlled blockchain for remote patient monitoring. 2019 Int Conf Wireless Mobile Comput, Netw Commun (WiMob). https://doi.org/10.1109/wimob.2019.8923209
29. Uddin MA, Stranieri A, Gondal I, Balasubramanian V. Blockchain leveraged decentralized IoT eHealth framework. Internet Things. 2020;9:100159.
30. Rahman MA, Rashid M, Barnes S, Hossain MS, Hassanain E, Guizani M. An IoT and blockchain-based multi-sensory in-home quality of life framework for cancer patients. 2019 15th Int Wirel Commun Mob Comput Conf (IWCMC). https://doi.org/10.1109/iwcmc.2019.8766496
31. Xie J, Yu FR, Huang T, Xie R, Liu J, Liu Y. A survey on the scalability of blockchain systems. IEEE Netw. 2019;33(5):166–173.
32. Azbeg K, Ouchetto O, Andaloussi SJ, Fetjah L, Sekkaki A. Blockchain and IoT for security and privacy: A platform for diabetes self-management. 2018 4th Int Conf Cloud Comput Technol Appl (Cloudtech). https://doi.org/10.1109/cloudtech.2018.8713343
33. Dey T, Jaiswal S, Sunderkrishnan S, Katre N. HealthSense: A medical use case of internet of things and blockchain. 2017 Int Conf Intell Sustain Syst (ICISS). https://doi.org/10.1109/iss1.2017.8389459
34. Ersotelos N, Bottarelli M, Al-Khateeb H, Epiphaniou G, Alhaboby Z, Pillai P, Aggoun A. Blockchain and IoMT against physical abuse: Bullying in schools as a case study. J Sensor Actuator Netw. 2020;10(1):1–20.
35. Fernández-Caramés TM, Froiz-Míguez I, Blanco-Novoa O, Fraga-Lamas P. Enabling the internet of mobile crowdsourcing health things: A mobile fog computing, blockchain and IoT based continuous glucose monitoring system for diabetes mellitus research and care. Sensors. 2019;19(15):1–24.

36. Rahman MA, Rashid MM, Le Kernec J, Philippe B, Barnes SJ, Fioranelli F, *et al.* A secure occupational therapy framework for monitoring cancer patients' quality of life. Sensors. 2019;19(23):1–30.
37. Siddiqui A, Qaddour J, Ullah S. Securing healthcare IoT (HIoT) monitoring system using blockchain. 2021 Twelfth Int Conf Ubiquitous Future Netw (ICUFN). https://doi.org/10.1109/icufn49451.2021.9528625
38. Jeong SH, Shen JH, Ahn B. A study on smart healthcare monitoring using IoT based on blockchain. Wirel Commun Mob Comput. 2021;2021:1–9.
39. Indumathi J, Shankar A, Ghalib MR, Gitanjali J, Hua Q, Wen Z, Qi X. Blockchain based internet of medical things for uninterrupted, ubiquitous, user-friendly, unflappable, unblemished, unlimited health care services (BC IoMT U6 HCS). IEEE Access. 2020;8:216856–216872.
40. Global Burden of Disease Study 2013 Collaborators. Global, regional, and national incidence, prevalence, and years lived with disability for 301 acute and chronic diseases and injuries in 188 countries, 1990–2013: A systematic analysis for the Global Burden of Disease Study 2013. Lancet. 2015;386(9995):743–800.
41. Ambrose AF, Cruz L, Paul G. Falls and fractures: A systematic approach to screening and prevention. Maturitas. 2015;82(1):85–93.
42. Langlois JA, Rutland-Brown W, Thomas KE. Traumatic brain injury in the United States: Emergency department visits, hospitalizations, and deaths. PsycEXTRA Dataset. https://doi.org/10.1037/e721222007-001
43. Ambrose AF, Paul G, Hausdorff JM. Risk factors for falls among older adults: A review of the literature. Maturitas. 2013;75(1):51–61.
44. Alamri B, Javed IT, Margaria T. Preserving patients' privacy in medical IoT using blockchain. In: Int Conf Edge Comput. 2020:103–110. https://doi.org/10.1007/978-3-030-76066-3_5
45. Colman A, Chowdhury MJ, Chhetri MB. Sharing wearable health data using user-defined blockchain policies. Lecture Notes Inst Comput Sci Soc Inform Telecommun Eng. https://doi.org/10.1007/978-3-030-76066-3_5
46. Gao Y, Lin H, Chen Y, Liu Y. Blockchain and SGX-enabled edge-computing-empowered secure IoMT data analysis. IEEE Internet Things J. 2021;8(21):15785–15795.
47. Hewa T, Braeken A, Ylianttila M, Liyanage M. Multi-access edge computing and blockchain-based secure telehealth system connected with 5G and IoT. GLOBECOM 2020 — IEEE Global Commun Conf. https://doi.org/10.1109/globecom42002.2020.9348125

48. Jain P, Anand A, Saria M, Kumari R, Bothra P, Sultana M. A prototype proposal for AI based smart integrated platform for doctors and patients. 2020 8th Int Conf Reliab Infocom Technol Optim (ICRITO). https://doi.org/10.1109/icrito48877.2020.9197871
49. Li P, Xu C, Jin H, Hu C, Luo Y, Cao Y, *et al.* ChainSDI: A software-defined infrastructure for regulation-compliant home-based healthcare services secured by blockchains. IEEE Syst J. 2020;14(2):2042–2053.
50. Patil RM, Kulkarni R. Universal storage and analytical framework of health records using blockchain data from wearable data devices. 2020 2nd Int Conf Innov Mechanisms Ind Appl (ICIMIA). https://doi.org/10.1109/icimia48430.2020.9074909
51. Rahman MZ, Surekha S, Satamraju KP, Mirza SS, Lay-Ekuakille A. A collateral sensor data sharing framework for Decentralized Healthcare Systems. IEEE Sensors J. 2021;21(24):27848–27857.
52. Reffad H, Djenaoui A, Alti A. Distributed Secure Services Based on IoT and Blockchain for e-Health Remote Care. ICCSA 2021: The 2nd International Conference on Computer Science's Complex and their Application, May 25–26, 2021, Algeria. http://ceur-ws.org/Vol-2904/11.pdf
53. Younis M, Lalouani W, Lasla N, Emokpae L, Abdallah M. Blockchain-enabled and data-driven smart healthcare solution for secure and privacy-preserving data access. IEEE Syst J. 2021:1–12.
54. ElRahman SA, Alluhaidan AS. Blockchain technology and IoT-edge framework for sharing healthcare services. Soft Comput. 2021;25(21):13753–13777.
55. Iqbal J, Umar AI, Amin N, Waheed A. Efficient and secure attribute-based heterogeneous online/offline signcryption for body sensor networks based on Blockchain. Int J Distrib Sens Netw. 2019;15(9):1–23.
56. Kumar R, Tripathi R. Towards design and implementation of security and privacy framework for internet of medical things (IoMT) by leveraging blockchain and IPFS technology. J Supercomput. 2021;77(8):7916–7955.
57. Pham H, Tran TH, Nakashima Y. A secure remote healthcare system for hospital using blockchain smart contract. 2018 IEEE Globecom Workshops (GC Wkshps). https://doi.org/10.1109/glocomw.2018.8644164
58. Sharmila AH, Jaisankar N. Edge intelligent agent assisted hybrid hierarchical blockchain for continuous healthcare monitoring & recommendation system in 5G WBAN-IoT. Comput Netw. 2021;200:108508.
59. Shukla S, Thakur S, Hussain S, Breslin JG, Jameel SM. Identification and authentication in Healthcare Internet-of-Things using integrated fog computing based blockchain model. Internet Things. 2021;15:100422.

60. Tomaz AE, Nascimento JC, Hafid AS, De Souza JN. Preserving privacy in mobile health systems using non-interactive zero-knowledge proof and blockchain. IEEE Access. 2020;8:204441–204458.
61. Wang W, Qiu C, Yin Z, Srivastava G, Gadekallu TR, Alsolami F, Su C. Blockchain and PUF-based lightweight authentication protocol for wireless medical sensor networks. IEEE Int Things J. 2021;9(11):1.
62. Awad Abdellatif A, Samara L, Mohamed A, Erbad A, Chiasserini CF, Guizani M, O'Connor MD, Laughton J. Medge-Chain: Leveraging edge computing and blockchain for efficient medical data exchange. IEEE Int Things J. 2021;8(21):15762–15775.
63. Cernian A, Tiganoaia B, Sacala I, Pavel A, Iftemi A. PatientDataChain: A blockchain-based approach to integrate personal health records. Sensors. 2020;20(22):6538.
64. Jita H, Pieterse V. A framework to apply the internet of things for medical care in a home environment. Proc 2018 Int Conf Cloud Comput Internet Things (CCIOT); 2018. https://doi.org/10.1145/3291064.3291065
65. Sneha S, Panjwani A, Lade B, Randolph J, Vickery M. Alleviating challenges related to FDA-approved medical wearables using blockchain technology. IT Prof. 2021;23(4):21–27.
66. Uddin MA, Stranieri A, Gondal I, Balasubramanian V. Blockchain leveraged task migration in Body Area Sensor Networks. 2019 25th Asia-Pacific Conf Commun (APCC). https://doi.org/10.1109/apcc47188.2019.9026409
67. Wang J, Fan S, Alexandridis A, Han K, Jeon G, Zilic Z, Pang Y. A multistage blockchain-based secure and trustworthy smart healthcare system using ECG characteristic. IEEE Int Things Mag. 2021;4(3):48–58.
68. Ali MS, Vecchio M, Putra GD, Kanhere SS, Antonelli F. A decentralized peer-to-peer remote health monitoring system. Sensors. 2020;20(6):1656.
69. Elsayeh M, Ezzat KA, El-Nashar H, Omran LN. Cybersecurity architecture for the internet of medical things and connected devices using blockchain. Biomed Eng Appl Basis Commun. 2021;33(02):2150013.
70. Mohammed R, Alubady R, Sherbaz A. Utilizing blockchain technology for IoT-based healthcare systems. J Phys Conf Ser. 2021;1818(1):012111.
71. Muofhe M, Dlodlo N, Terzoli A. An internet of things-based system integrated with blockchain to manage patient data in the healthcare sector. 2019 Open Innovations (OI). https://doi.org/10.1109/oi.2019.8908221
72. Barka E, Dahmane S, Kerrache CA, Khayat M, Sallabi F. STHM: A secured and trusted healthcare monitoring architecture using SDN and blockchain. Electronics. 2021;10(15):1–15.

73. Deng H, Meng X, Guo J, Xi E, Zhao H. A framework of blockchain-based security for WBANS. 2020 3rd Int Conf Smart BlockChain (SmartBlock). https://doi.org/10.1109/smartblock52591.2020.00021
74. Makka S, Arora G, Mopuru B. IoT based health monitoring and record management using distributed ledger. J Phys Conf Ser. 2021;2089(1):012030.
75. Hasan O, Brunie L, Bertino E. Privacy-preserving reputation systems based on blockchain and other cryptographic building blocks: A survey. ACM Comput Surv. 2022;55(2):1–37.
76. King S, Nadal S. PPcoin: Peer-to-peer crypto-currency with proof-of-stake. https://decred.org/research/king2012.pdf
77. O'Dwyer KJ, Malone D. Bitcoin mining and its energy footprint. Proc 25th IET Irish Signals & Systems Conf 2014 & China-Ireland Int Conf Info Commun Technol (ISSC/CIICT); 2014. https://doi.org/10.1049/cp.2014.0699
78. Bach LM, Mihaljevic B, Zagar M. Comparative analysis of blockchain consensus algorithms. Proc 2018 41st Int Conv Inf Commun Technol, Electron Microelectron (MIPRO). https://doi.org/10.23919/mipro.2018.8400278
79. Solat S, Calvez P, Naït-Abdesselam F. Permissioned vs permissionless blockchain: How and why there is only one right choice. J Softw. 2021;16(3):95–106.
80. Xu J, Xue K, Li S, Tian H, Hong J, Hong P, Yu N. Healthchain: A blockchain-based privacy preserving scheme for large-scale health data. IEEE Int Things J. 2019;6(5):8770–8781.
81. Azbeg K, Ouchetto O, Andaloussi SJ, Fetjah L. A taxonomic review of the use of IoT and blockchain in healthcare applications. IRBM. 2021.
82. Oliveira MT, Reis LHA, Medeiros DSV, Carrano RC, Olabarriaga SD, Mattos DMF. Blockchain reputation-based consensus: A scalable and resilient mechanism for distributed mistrusting applications. Comp Netw. 2020;179:107367.
83. Nguyen CT, Hoang DT, Nguyen DN, Niyato D, Nguyen HT, Dutkiewicz E. Proof-of-stake consensus mechanisms for future blockchain networks: Fundamentals, applications and opportunities. IEEE Access. 2019;7:85727–85745.
84. Ahmad RW, Salah K, Jayaraman R, Yaqoob I, Ellahham S, Omar M. The role of blockchain technology in telehealth and telemedicine. Int J Med Inform. 2021;148:104399.
85. Giles EL, Robalino S, McColl E, Sniehotta FF, Adams J. The effectiveness of financial incentives for health behaviour change: Systematic review and meta-analysis. PLoS One. 2014;9(3):e90347.

86. Haff N, Patel MS, Lim R, Zhu J, Troxel AB, Asch DA, Volpp KG. The role of behavioral economic incentive design and demographic characteristics in financial incentive-based approaches to changing health behaviors: A meta-analysis. Am J Health Promot. 2015;29(5):314–323.
87. Hoskins K, Ulrich CM, Shinnick J, Buttenheim AM. Acceptability of financial incentives for health-related behavior change: An updated systematic review. Prev Med. 2019;126:105762.
88. Rogers EM. Diffusion of innovations. Simon & Schuster; 2010.
89. Hung WW, Ross JS, Boockvar KS, Siu AL. Recent trends in chronic disease, impairment and disability among older adults in the United States. BMC Geriatr. 2011;11(1):47.
90. Smith J, Noble H. Bias in research. Evid Based Nurs. 2014;17(4):100–101.
91. Hölbl M, Kompara M, Kamišalić A, Nemec Zlatolas L. A systematic review of the use of blockchain in healthcare. Symmetry. 2018;10(10):470.
92. Ali Süzen A, Duman B. Protecting the privacy of IoT-based health records using blockchain technology. In: Int Med Things. 2021:35–54.
93. Attia O, Khoufi I, Laouiti A, Adjih C. An IoT-blockchain architecture based on Hyperledger framework for healthcare monitoring application. 2019 10th IFIP Int Conf on New Technol, Mobility Security (NTMS). https://doi.org/10.1109/ntms.2019.8763849
94. Bera B, Mitra A, Das AK, Puthal D, Park Y. Private blockchain-based AI-envisioned home monitoring framework in IoMT-enabled COVID-19 environment. IEEE Consum Electron Mag. 2021:1–1.
95. Bhawiyuga A, Wardhana A, Amron K, Kirana AP. Platform for integrating internet of things based smart healthcare system and blockchain network. 2019 6th NAFOSTED Conf on Info Comput Sci (NICS). https://doi.org/10.1109/nics48868.2019.9023797
96. Buzachis A, Celesti A, Fazio M, Villari M. On the design of a blockchain-as-a-service-based health information exchange (BaaS-HIE) system for patient monitoring. 2019 IEEE Symp on Computers and Commun (ISCC). https://doi.org/10.1109/iscc47284.2019.8969718
97. Cheng JC, Lee NY, Chi C, Chen YH. Blockchain and smart contract for digital certificate. 2018 IEEE Int Conf on Applied System Invention (ICASI). https://doi.org/10.1109/icasi.2018.8394455
98. Christy A, Anto Praveena MD, Suji Helen L, Vaithyasubramanian S. A framework for monitoring patient's vital signs with internet of things and blockchain technology. Comp Netw Big Data IoT. 2021:697–708.
99. Dwivedi A, Srivastava G, Dhar S, Singh R. A decentralized privacy-preserving healthcare blockchain for IoT. Sensors. 2019;19(2):332.

100. Ejaz M, Kumar T, Kovacevic I, Ylianttila M, Harjula E. Health-blockedge: Blockchain-edge framework for reliable low-latency digital healthcare applications. Sensors. 2021;21(7):2502.
101. Guo R, Zhuang C, Shi H, Zhang Y, Zheng D. A lightweight verifiable outsourced decryption of attribute-based encryption scheme for blockchain-enabled wireless body area network in fog computing. Int J Distrib Sens Netw. 2020;16(2):155014772090679.
102. Hameed K, Bajwa IS, Sarwar N, Anwar W, Mushtaq Z, Rashid T. Integration of 5G and block-chain technologies in smart telemedicine using IoT. J Healthc Eng. 2021;2021:1–18.
103. Hu N, Su S, Tang C, Wang L. Wearable-sensors based activity recognition for smart human healthcare using internet of things. 2020 Int Wireless Commun Mobile Comput (IWCMC). https://doi.org/10.1109/iwcmc48107.2020.9148197
104. Ismail S, Almadasaf R, Chehab S, Alghamdi S, Almutairi A, Alasmari B, Altherwy R. Edge IoT-cloud framework based on blockchain. 2020 2nd Int Conf Comput Inform Sci (ICCIS). https://doi.org/10.1109/iccis49240.2020.9257647
105. Jamil F, Ahmad S, Iqbal N, Kim DH. Towards a remote monitoring of patient vital signs based on IoT-based blockchain integrity management platforms in smart hospitals. Sensors. 2020;20(8):2195.
106. Juyal S, Sharma S, Harbola A, Shukla AS. Privacy and security of IoT based skin monitoring system using blockchain approach. 2020 IEEE Int Conf Electron Comput Commun Technol (CONECCT). https://doi.org/10.1109/conecct50063.2020.9198409
107. Kumar A, Kumar Sharma D, Nayyar A, Singh S, Yoon B. Lightweight proof of Game (LPoG): A proof of work's extended lightweight consensus algorithm for wearable kidneys. Sensors. 2020;20(10):2868.
108. Li CT, Shih DH, Wang CC, Chen CL, Lee CC. A blockchain based data aggregation and group authentication scheme for electronic medical system. IEEE Access. 2020;8:173904–173917.
109. Liang X, Shetty S, Tosh D, Bowden D, Njilla L, Kamhoua C. Towards blockchain empowered trusted and accountable data sharing and collaboration in mobile healthcare applications. EAI Endorsed Trans Pervasive Health Technol. 2018;4(15):159338.
110. Liang X, Zhao J, Shetty S, Liu J, Li D. Integrating blockchain for data sharing and collaboration in mobile healthcare applications. 2017 IEEE 28th Annu Int Symp Personal Indoor Mobile Radio Commun (PIMRC). https://doi.org/10.1109/pimrc.2017.8292361

111. Mehbodniya A, Neware R, Vyas S, Kumar MR, Ngulube P, Ray S. Blockchain and IPFS integrated framework in bilevel Fog-Cloud network for security and privacy of IoMT devices. Comput Math Methods Med. 2021;2021:1–9.
112. Monte GD, Pennino D, Pizzonia M. Scaling blockchains without giving up decentralization and security. Proc 3rd Workshop Cryptocurrencies Blockchains Distrib Syst. 2020. https://doi.org/10.1145/3410699.3413800
113. Mubarakali A. Healthcare services monitoring in cloud using secure and robust healthcare-based blockchain (SRHB) approach. Mob Netw Appl. 2020;25(4):1330–1337.
114. Oikonomou FP, Mantas G, Cox P, Bashashi F, Gil-Castineira F, Gonzalez J. A blockchain-based architecture for secure IoT-based health monitoring systems. 2021 IEEE 26th Int Workshop Comput Aided Model Design Commun Links Netw (CAMAD). https://doi.org/10.1109/camad52502.2021.9617803
115. Oikonomou FP, Ribeiro J, Mantas G, Bastos JM, Rodriguez J. A hyperledger fabric-based blockchain architecture to secure IoT-based health monitoring systems. 2021 IEEE Int Mediterranean Conf Commun Netw (MeditCom). https://doi.org/10.1109/meditcom49071.2021.9647521
116. Pradhan NR, Rout SS, Singh AP. Blockchain based smart healthcare system for chronic-illness patient monitoring. 2020 3rd Int Conf Energy Power Environ: Towards Clean Energy Technol. https://doi.org/10.1109/icepe50861.2021.9404496
117. Przytarski D, Stach C, Gritti C, Mitschang B. A blueprint for a trustworthy health data platform encompassing IoT and blockchain technologies. EPiC Ser Comput. 2021;76:57–65.
118. Puri V, Kataria A, Sharma V. Artificial intelligence–powered decentralized framework for internet of things in healthcare 4.0. Trans Emerg Telecommun Technol. 2021;e4245.
119. Ray PP, Chowhan B, Kumar N, Almogren A. BIoTHR: Electronic health record servicing scheme in IoT-Blockchain ecosystem. IEEE Int Things J. 2021;8(13):10857–10872.
120. Ren Y, Leng Y, Zhu F, Wang J, Kim HJ. Data storage mechanism based on blockchain with privacy protection in wireless body area network. Sensors. 2019;19(10):2395.
121. Sassi M, Abid M. Security and privacy protection in the e-health system: Remote monitoring of COVID-19 patients as a use case. Netw Intell Syst Security. 2021:829–843.
122. Shahbazi Z, Byun YC. Towards a secure thermal-energy aware routing protocol in wireless body area network based on blockchain technology. Sensors. 2020;20(12):3604.

123. Son S, Lee J, Kim M, Yu S, Das AK, Park Y. Design of secure authentication protocol for cloud-assisted telecare medical information system using blockchain. IEEE Access. 2020;8:192177–192191.
124. Srivastava G, Parizi RM, Dehghantanha A, Choo KKR. Data sharing and privacy for patient IoT devices using blockchain. Commun Comput Inform Sci. 2019;334–348.
125. Uddin MA, Stranieri A, Gondal I, Balasubramanian V. Continuous patient monitoring with a patient centric agent: A block architecture. IEEE Access. 2018;6:32700–32726.
126. Wadud MA, Amir-Ul-Haque Bhuiyan TM, Uddin MA, Rahman MM. A patient centric agent assisted private blockchain on hyperledger fabric for managing remote patient monitoring. 2020 11th Int Conf Electr Comput Eng (ICECE). https://doi.org/10.1109/icece51571.2020.9393124
127. Wang J, Han K, Alexandridis A, Chen Z, Zilic Z, Pang Y, Jeon G, Piccialli F. A blockchain-based eHealthcare system interoperating with WBANS. Future Gener Comput Syst. 2020;110:675–685.
128. Xiao L, Han D, Meng X, Liang W, Li KC. A secure framework for data sharing in private blockchain-based WBANS. IEEE Access. 2020;8:153956–153968.
129. Xu J, Meng X, Liang W, Peng L, Xu Z, Li KC. A hybrid mutual authentication scheme based on blockchain technology for WBANS. Commun Comput Inform Sci. 2019;350–362.
130. Xu J, Meng X, Liang W, Zhou H, Li KC. A secure mutual authentication scheme of blockchain-based WBANS. China Commun. 2020;17(9):34–49.
131. Zaabar B, Cheikhrouhou O, Ammi M, Awad AI, Abid M. Secure and privacy-aware blockchain-based remote patient monitoring system for internet of healthcare things. 2021 17th Int Conf Wireless Mobile Comput Netw Commun (WiMob). https://doi.org/10.1109/wimob52687.2021.9606362

https://doi.org/10.1142/9789819817320_0016

Chapter 16*

Perceptions of Tobacco Endgame Strategies Among Youths and Adults Globally: A Qualitative Systematic Review

Annabelle Lim,[1], Koong Heng Nung[2], and Piyanee Klainin-Yobas[3,*]

[1]*5 Lower Kent Ridge Rd, Singapore 119074*

[2]*Koong & Ho Surgery Centre, 38 Irrawady Road, Mt Elizabeth Novena Specialist Centre Singapore*

[3]*Alice Lee Centre for Nursing Studies, Yong Loo Lin School of Medicine, National University of Singapore, Centre for Translational Medicine, Block MD6, 14 Medical Drive, Singapore 117599*

**Corresponding author: nurpk@nus.edu.sg*

16.1 Introduction

The World Health Organization regards tobacco smoking as an "epidemic", contributing to eight million deaths annually. Smoking is the leading cause of preventable deaths in the United States [1], and the number of deaths attributed to smoking is the second highest globally [2]. In 2019, an estimated 155 million individuals aged 15–24 years were tobacco smokers. About 82% of current smokers initiated between age 14 and 25 years, and 18.5% of smokers began smoking regularly by age 15 [3].

To combat the tobacco epidemic, the World Health Organization launched the Framework Convention on Tobacco Control (FCTC) in 2003. This is an evidence-based treaty, currently ratified by 180 signatory countries, enacted to reduce tobacco use. The FCTC aims to place: (a) a comprehensive ban on tobacco advertising, sponsorship and promotion;

* Appendices to this chapter are available for download at https://www.worldscientific.com/worldscibooks/10.1142/14420#t=suppl.

(b) strong health warnings on tobacco packaging; (c) protection from second-hand smoke in indoor workplaces, public places and public transportation; and (d) recently, measures to reduce the smuggling of tobacco products [4].

However, there is contention over the effectiveness of the FCTC in addressing tobacco supply-side issues and reducing cigarette consumption. An interrupted time-series study and in-sample forecast event modelling [5] reported no significant changes in global population-weighted cigarette consumption per adult between pre- and post-FCTC trends. Therefore, the FCTC has been encouraged as a single strategy.

Despite its many criticisms, countries like Australia, the United Kingdom, Ireland and France have placed efforts to implement the FCTC, imposing plain packaging regulations with large graphic health warnings on cigarette packages [6]. Following this, the tobacco industry took legal action against Australia based on intellectual property violations. Australia eventually won the case; however, other countries were not successful in their acts against big tobacco companies and their legal tactics to continuously promote cigarette use.

Endgame strategies were developed to target demand and supply of tobacco, and to counteract tobacco industry exploitation tactics. The strategies aim to permanently and rapidly reduce the prevalence of smoking [7], putting an end to tobacco use in a defined geographic area. Some Endgame strategies are summarised below:

(a) A "regulated market model" that removes incentives from selling tobacco products and creates incentives for promotion of less harmful products, while striving to maintain the inherent free market competition [8];
(b) Reduction of nicotine to non-addictive levels, preventing addiction when young people begin smoking, avoiding harmful long-term effects, and hastening the cessation process [9];

(c) Imposing a "sinking lid" on the industry to address supply side of tobacco, gradually reducing sales and production quotas [10];
(d) Establishing tobacco-free generations — prohibiting possession of tobacco by all persons born after a specified birth year; and with the support of the mass public, imposition of abolition of tobacco manufacture and sale [11].

Evaluation of public perception and support for Endgame policies are crucial to inform policymakers and policy adjustments to best suit target populations [12]. Furthermore, Endgame policies are medium to long-term strategies [13], affecting young adults whose opinions influence policy as they reach the voting age. The Endgame goal risks losing momentum without the active support of young adults. Therefore, both adults' and young adults' perceptions and opinions on Endgame goals are crucial to informing policy priorities and advocacy strategies.

16.1.1 *Gaps in Existing Reviews*

A qualitative review [14] was previously conducted, which gathered information on the implementation, benefits, challenges and public support for Endgame strategies. However, it did not synthesise and utilise experiences of the public to inform policy adjustments. This meta-synthesis will minimise the gaps by synthesising evidence regarding the implementations of Endgame methods in different countries. The review question is "What are perceptions of the implementation of Tobacco Endgame strategies among youths and adults globally?"

16.2 Method

This systematic review was conducted in accordance with the Joanna Briggs Institute (JBI) approach for qualitative synthesis [15], meta-synthesis framework [16, 17] and Preferred Reporting Items for Systematic

Reviews and Meta Analyses (PRISMA) statement [18]. Data selection, critical appraisal and data extraction were carried out by two independent reviewers. Any disagreements arising during the process were resolved through discussions and/or recommendations from a third reviewer.

16.2.1 *Eligibility Criteria*

The participant (P), phenomena of interest (I), context (Co) framework was used to settle the eligibility criteria. This review considered studies that: (a) involved young adults and adults regardless of smoking status (P), (b) discussed the implementation of Endgame strategies and their impacts on populations (I), and (c) were implemented in any country worldwide (Co). Furthermore, this review considers all types of qualitative design reported in English, without any restriction in publication years.

16.2.2 *Information Resources*

A comprehensive search was conducted across seven electronic databases. Published studies were identified through PubMed, CINAHL, Scopus, EMBASE and Cochrane Central. Grey literature was searched using ProQuest and MedNar. Rigorous measures were undertaken to ensure all relevant studies were retrieved. Furthermore, hand search was performed on two main journals (*Tobacco Control, Nicotine & Tobacco Research* and *BMJ*), and reference lists of all included studies and existing systematic reviews.

16.2.3 *Search Strategy*

A three-phase search strategy was utilised, according to JBI's recommendations [15]. The Peer Review of Electronic Search Strategies (PRESS) Evidence-Based Checklist was used to guide the search strategy [18]. An initial limited search of PubMed was conducted to identify possible keywords. Subsequently, a comprehensive search strategy was developed (including various index terms, MeSH terms, and other control vocabulary), combining with Boolean operators (AND or OR). An experienced librarian was consulted to ensure the comprehensiveness of search strategy.

16.2.4 *Critical Appraisal and Data Extraction*

All included studies were appraised using the Critical Appraisal Skills Programme (CASP) tool [15]. The two reviewers rated each study. Inter-rater agreement was 98% among the two reviewers. Information from included studies was extracted using the JBI QARI Data Extraction Tool for Qualitative Research [15], including specific details about the population, study methods, and outcomes of significance to the review question. Findings and illustrations were assigned a level of credibility.

16.2.5 *Data Synthesis*

Data was synthesised using inductive thematic analysis to examine underlying ideas and conceptualisations. There are six steps: (a) getting familiar with the qualitative data, (b) generating initial codes from the data, (c) searching for possible themes among initial codes, (d) reviewing and revising the created themes, (e) defining and naming the themes, and (f) writing up findings [15]. The reviewers read and re-read data from all included studies, generated new codes, and collated the new codes into potential themes. Each theme was reviewed and defined to achieve new and organised understanding of the experiences of the Endgame strategies.

16.3 Results

A comprehensive search yielded 329 records after removal of duplicates. 17 studies reported between 2011 and 2022 were included, involving 556 participants (Figure 16.1). Studies were conducted mostly in New Zealand (n = 10), followed by North America (n = 3), Finland (n = 1), India (n = 1), and Belgium (n = 1). Characteristics of included studies are reported in Figure 16.1.

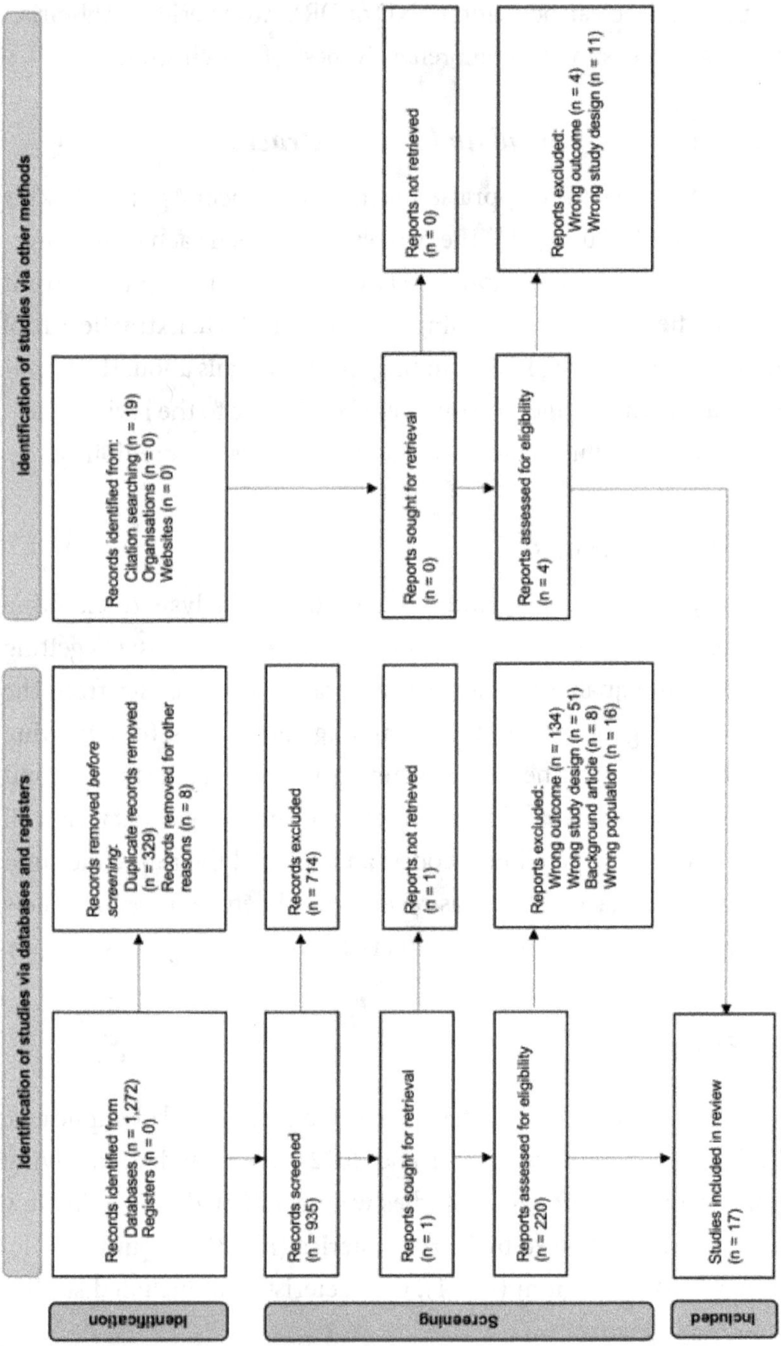

Figure 16.1 The PRISMA diagram of the search selection.

Table 16.1 Synthesised themes and subthemes.

	Synthesised Themes	**Synthesised Subthemes**
1	Perceptions of Tobacco Endgame goals	Not applicable
2	Perspectives on Tobacco Endgame strategies	2.1 Diminishing tobacco accessibility and purchase 2.2 Imposing ban on tobacco sale 2.3 Creating a tobacco-free generation
3	Smokers' intention to quit	Not applicable
4	Barriers to achieving the Endgame	4.1 Intending to use alternative sources 4.2 Identifying relevant psychosocial factors
5	Overcoming barriers and achieving Endgame goals	5.1 Rendering legislations and regulations 5.2 Reaching out and engaging the community through education

49 original themes were reported across 17 studies. Afterwards, we synthesised the original findings and identified five new themes: (a) perceptions of Tobacco Endgame goals, (b) perspectives on Tobacco Endgame strategies, (c) smokers' intention to quit, (d) barriers to achieving Endgame goal, and (e) Endgame solutions (Table 16.1).

16.3.1 *Theme 1: Perception of Tobacco Endgame Goals*

The Endgame had clear goals in permanent and rapid reduction of tobacco use. There were mixed responses to such goals as displayed in Table 16.2. While some people expressed support for the Endgame goal, others had reservations about how they could be achieved, and others felt that they would not be possible. Some smokers believed that the Endgame goal would push them to stop smoking. However, they might feel frustrated with the initial implementation. On the contrary, some smokers felt that the goals are not achievable while others stated that the Endgame goal would negatively affect tourism.

Table 16.2 Perception of Tobacco Endgame goals.

Theme 1	Original Quotations
Perception of Tobacco Endgame goals	"I think that'll be great for smokers. I reckon that that'll really push us to stop... I can say confidently that I reckon about 70% of smokers deep down would be keen for that, and they'll look at it as another way of sort of — that that's a good push for them to stop." [19] "I mean I like smoking but I don't like smoking...I don't think anyone should start...I'll be really pissed off when they make it smoke-free and I can't buy cigarettes anymore...but in the long run, I think smoking's something our country could do without." [19] "That's fine if they want to do it. How they are going to do it is a different story." [19] "In your *** dreams. I think that, sorry, try to make New Zealand smoke-free, just try it. It's not going to happen." [19] "Until there is the political will to put the tobacco industry really in its place, then… this is just another pie in the sky." [20] "I also think too, we . . . have a responsibility to pass the message on to our families." [21] "In theory this looks very good. But I think ah, New Zealand can't be like that. One main reason, our biggest income is from tourism and they are chain smokers. You can't say that 'ok you coming here, you can't smoke'. They say 'oh, I am not going there.'" [22]

16.3.2 *Theme 2: Perspectives on Endgame Strategies*

16.3.2.1 *Subtheme 2.1 Diminishing Tobacco Accessibility and Purchase*

One of the Endgame strategies is to reduce tobacco sales and production quotas [10]. Many participants expressed their agreement with the strategy (Table 16.3). They felt that making **the tobacco purchase**

Table 16.3 Perspectives on Endgame strategies (Theme 2).

Subtheme 2.1	**Original Quotations**
Diminishing tobacco accessibility and purchase	"...you can't have that kind of goal when they're selling them in the shops...It's too readily available." [19] "Just [have] only certain place or places where they're selling cigarettes. Some people don't want to travel far and they'll just say 'I'm not going to smoke.'" [19] "You're going after the person who's selling the products versus the person who's addicted." [20] "If you...come to buy three items, say one of them is smokes... you wanted to buy bread, milk and some groceries — but I don't stock smokes — they don't stop here — they'll go somewhere else." [29] I think that [raising the legal age of purchase] points much more strongly towards the severity of smoking and it says that as a nation and a government we realise how dangerous this product is… That's a clear marker for young people." [30] "It's weird how they sell it with...food and stuff... it's just wrong for me. They should have...a R18 shop for them or something." [19] "At least that stops it being something that's easily acquirable for young people...it takes it out of their sort of price range." [19] "In the last five years the only thing that's messaged has been the price. The only thing that's ever caught my eye is, 'oh, man, I remember when I started smoking — they were only $10.'" [23] "We used to buy packets of 30s but now we only ever buy 20s." [23] "Sometimes I give up on smoking tobacco to smoke illegal substances cos it's cheaper. It's way cheaper." [23] "I'll buy smokes regardless. If they're $100 this week I'd still buy them...but then I'd have to go without something else." [25]

(*Continued*)

Table 16.3 (*Continued*)

Subtheme 2.1	Original Quotations
	"I know it wouldn't be a popular opinion but to reduce the price to help people, sort of, not become stressed in their own life...it would help them to have more money in their pocket, and then they may begin to like it, and then want to step away from smoking too." [25]
	"Tobacco sales have gone down...It's a good thing and a bad thing. A good thing because people are smoking less." [24]
	"Such a package that has no colour at all, that would not appeal to me to buy it. I don't know why, but... probably because it simply looks bad. That's why I would never buy such a white package." [31]
	"Yes, the message 'smoking kills' and then on the back the picture... The message catches the attention much more on the white package...I mean, you would more likely believe the message on the white package." [31]
	"People…don't just go into the shop and buy like oh, any old crap, you know. You go in there and you know what you want." [21]
	"It will take a bit more time...Maybe half a minute, a minute or something like that...Yes, definitely not good because in the busy time, we've got three or four customers at a time and if we take longer time, customer don't like, you know?" [29]
	"It would make it so much easier to quit. I wouldn't have, yeah... I know they've got the cabinets behind them now and you can't see what's in them. But you know what's in there... And you walk into a shop and they're always right behind the counter. Like they're right there as soon as you walk in the door... It's like, 'Oh, f***. I need a pack of smokes.'" [28]
	"[It would mean] the idea of smoking isn't in [young people's] face all the time." [30]
	"The more difficult you make it for young people to obtain the cigarette, the harder it [uptake] would be; I think that's perfect." [27]

inconvenient and involving travel efforts would reduce smoking or would encourage smoking cessation. Policymakers asserted that the inconvenient strategy would be politically viable because of its focus on sellers, not on smokers' and people's rights. However, most retailers expressed concern that their business would be affected. Specifically, smokers would only purchase groceries and items at shops where tobaccos are accessible.

Raising a legal age of tobacco purchase was perceived to be important. Policymakers in New Zealand stated that such a strategy would send a clear message, especially to young adults, regarding the government's stance on smoking and its dangers. Furthermore, **increasing tobacco price** was believed to reduce tobacco consumption and to trigger smoke cessation. However, some smokers would switch to use other substances to cut costs or would forgo other basic needs to purchase tobacco. One participant suggested the tobacco price be decreased to lower people's financial burden, thereby reducing the need to smoke as a stress-relieving strategy. Retailers were hesitant to support the price increase strategy, which might lower their profits from "holding money on the shelf" [24].

Plain packages of tobacco aimed to "make smoking less glamorous…without encroaching on people's civil liberties" [19]. Many youth smokers selected their choice of tobacco with brand, claiming they would not purchase tobacco with plain white packaging. Health warnings printed on the plain packages were perceived as prominent and convincing, prompting them to quit. Therefore, it might be useful in preventing the initiation of smoking and inducing cessation rates among young smokers. Nevertheless, some adult smokers stated that the plain packaging would not change their smoking and purchasing habits. On the retailers' perspectives, they believed the strategy would affect their business as the packaging products would delay the purchase.

16.3.2.2 *Subtheme 2.2: Imposing Ban On Tobacco Sale*

Policymakers in USA supported a complete sale ban because "people could rally around…banning the industry" [20], which could change the tobacco landscape. Some smokers supported the ban, as it would send a clear message aligning with the Endgame, and the ban would discourage them to smoke. However, some respondents felt that the ban would only eliminate the tobacco access, but it will not eradicate the root cause of the issue. Other respondents believed that people might not respond well to the prohibition law (Table 16.4).

In India, public responses to the tobacco were not all positive. Many youths observed that black markets emerged and tobacco prices rose following the sale ban. Some respondents initially supported the ban, but they later realised that the ban would exacerbate financial pressure on lower-income families. Other youths noticed the discrepancy between the government's ban policy and "corrected state police" who continued to smoke in public. Nonetheless, the ban could be effective, as some participants witnessed their friends quit smoking.

Additionally, policymakers in Finland perceived that the implementation of a display ban since 2010 had been an "effective means" [26] to curb tobacco purchase and consumption. Participants believed that the display ban would encourage the intention to quit and would reduce the reminder and need to smoke. Nonetheless, one retailer did not notice any decrease in tobacco sales following a display ban, suggesting that implementing this policy alone might not be effective.

16.3.2.3 *Subtheme 2.3 Creating a Tobacco-Free Generation*

Policymakers in USA described a tobacco-free generation (TFG) approach as "*palatable*", "*marketable*" and "*doable*" [20]. The TFG approach "*focuses on young people who have not started yet and will never know the difference*" [20], thus preventing the need for future changes in behaviour (Table 16.4). In New Zealand, policymakers commented that creating a TFG was not only a regulation but also "a strong political and social movement" and "powerful story" to achieve the Endgame goals. Some people in New Zealand supported the implementation of smoke-free

Table 16.4 Perspectives on Endgame strategies (Theme 2).

Subtheme	Original Quotations
2.2 Imposing ban on tobacco sale	"It's really trying to eliminate access to tobacco...And that...is not going to address the issue." [20] "Banning sales is...a prohibition approach, which I just don't think is effective." [20] "...if we're going to do this, let's do this...[banning smoking] makes more sense...this [reducing smoking to five percent or below] isn't going to help people stop smoking. This is just, 'Oh, we're going to try.'" [25] "If they [cigarettes] weren't on the shelves...I probably wouldn't feel as compelled." [25] "...the ban on tobacco products introduced by the government of Manipur is not effective enough. It has led to the rise of price almost to double from the actual price, smuggling, and black marketing... As a result, instead of quitting tobacco it has greatly affected the economy of the poor addicted users, which directly or indirectly has affected the livelihood of the entire family members." [32] "If the government... is actually serious...they would have properly followed up on the ban. They would have appointed a separated police force instead of the corrupt state police who they themselves are smoking and chewing." [32] "...some of [their] friends quitting, because they could no longer afford to buy due to the rise of price." [32] "The easiest way to change behaviour is to not to have to." [20]
Subtheme 2.3 Creating a tobacco-free generation	"I think there shouldn't also be smoking in CBD [central business district] areas...just to socially change people's mentality of having the right to smoke." [19] "If I'm shopping, I have a smoke out the street. Whereas if you can't then you hold off that extra hour...the little things like that all lead up to... giving up." [25] "If you've got an addiction to smoking...you'll go back to your car, you'll go around the corner, you'll find somewhere." [25] "I think initially there'd be an outcry about it, but given that we've been able to implement having smoke-free inside, I don't see any problem with us also having smoke-free outside." [30]

(*Continued*)

Table 16.4 (*Continued*)

Subtheme	Original Quotations
	"It would make it so much easier to quit. I wouldn't have, yeah... I know they've got the cabinets behind them now and you can't see what's in them. But you know what's in there... And you walk into a shop and they're always right behind the counter. Like they're right there as soon as you walk in the door... It's like, 'Oh, f***. I need a pack of smokes.'" [28]
	"You're not selling a regulation...you're really selling an idea of a smoke-free generation...I think it's something you could get a really strong political and social movement around. I think it's a very powerful story there." [30]
	"...it would just change the world in a few years. Like, if you stop... the young, the next generation will stop. Then when they're the leaders of their generation, or generations below them...it just will get better and better and better, the younger they go." [28]
	"not many people know the disadvantages so it'll take them a really long time...to find out for themselves. So I think definitely stopping them is a big option just because it takes [so] long to realise the disadvantages of it." [28]
	"I feel like banning smoking has many more benefits, rather than saying, "Oh, it's freedom, so we should have it, we should keep it." [28]
	"...It's better for everyone in the long run on...the wider scale and for the future...people should be. . .open to thinking about those... wider implications." [28]
	"I understand why they're doing it. Yeah, to stop the youth getting into it but what I'm saying is don't bring it in on the current people who are already there. If it's a new business, ok." [22]

areas, and de-normalisation of smoking as a social norm. Therefore, children would see less and less tobacco in their day-to-day lives [25].

Many young adults supported the TFG approach, one of which stated that this approach will "change the world in a few years" [28]. Specifically, the TFG will lead the next generations towards smoke-free societies. Furthermore, smoking prohibition had more benefits over the "freedom" to smoke [28]. The TFG should be created now, instead of waiting until youths suffer the consequences of smoking and quit it on their free will. Other respondents asserted that the TFG approach would be "*solely about protection*" [28], and it will be beneficial in the long run, "the wider scale and for the future" [28]. Additionally, some retailers supported the TFG approach, because it would not affect the current market of adult smokers, while helping reduce youth smoking [22].

16.3.3 *Theme 3: Facilitating Smokers' Intention to Quit*

Across the included studies, many smokers expressed their intention to quit smoking (Table 16.5). They thought that reduced tobacco availability

Table 16.5 Facilitating smokers' intention to quit.

Theme 3	Original Quotations
Facilitating smokers' intention to quit	"I don't want to smoke forever, and obviously that would probably be the best motivator." [28] "...'cause it would make me stop... If it wasn't available...I wouldn't be doing it. Pretty much." [28] "Some people say they are going to quit, and I say that is good." [24] "...If it was less than 5%, you'd just feel like such...a weirdo smoking, really, being such a small group of the population and you were still doing it, (laughs) and you know?... The less and less it gets the worse and worse you feel..." [28] "I don't think it would impact my smoking at all... I'm quite happy to be part of that 5%, if need be... I mean, you'd still feel a little bit shitty about yourself. But I, I don't view myself under those stereotypes, so I still don't think it would touch me really." [28] "People respond better to positive affirmation and positive feedback...I just think it needs to be handled really carefully so that people who are smokers aren't made to feel bad or lesser than." [25]

would encourage them to quit. One smoker had the intention to quit smoking. However, she expressed the fear of quitting to "losing…the best friend" [25] and losing the dependability on tobacco. Furthermore, retailers across studies shared their experience with smokers who "*quit because they were forced to*" [24], and those who expressed intention to quit due to tobacco regulation.

In New Zealand, a smoke-free goal is defined as the prevalence of smoking less than 5% [28]. Such a goal triggered various public responses, and one smoker believed that it will be "the best motivator" [28]. Some smokers shared that the goal would make them feel like "a weirdo smoking" where they become the minority of their society. The smaller the prevalence, the worse they would feel. Furthermore, they suggested the utilisation of "positive affirmation and positive feedback" to handle the fragile and sensitive situation. It would be important not make smokers feel inferior [25]. Nevertheless, other smokers did not think that "the 5% prevalence" would impact their smoking behaviours and they were happy to be part of the minority.

16.3.4 *Theme 4: Barriers to Achieving Endgame Goals*

16.3.4.1 *Subtheme 4.1 Intending to Use Alternative Sources*

Different Endgame strategies have been implemented in many countries and reducing tobacco advertisement might lead to different reactions (Table 16.6). Some smokers stated that they might grow their own tobacco while others did not think that would be worth the effort. Some smokers mentioned re-rolling tobacco into a smaller size to cut costs whereas other smokers would find alternative sources outside the country. Across the included studies, respondents were convinced that the prohibition law would encourage higher tobacco in black markets. This scenario took place in India, where black markets and illegal sources emerged following a complete sale ban. In line with this, a young smoker believed that shopkeepers would continue to make money, and she would purchase tobacco from "shops who sold secretly".

Table 16.6 Barriers to achieving Endgame goals (Theme 4).

Subtheme	Original Quotations
4.1 Intending to use alternative sources	"If they stop tobacco...being imported into the country, I'm sure smokers will find a way in growing their own tobacco." [19]
	"If they get rid of smoking, then people will still find a way to grow tobacco, smoke, whatever..." [28]
	"It won't worry me, cos at the end of the day, if they stopped it, and banned it, I'd just start growing my [expletive] own." [21]
	"I wouldn't mind if New Zealand was smoke-free because then I'd just have to stop. I'm not going to grow my own tobacco plants and fork out like $60 a week for tobacco from some old man that lives in the whops [remote country area], like I wouldn't do that." [19]
	"We'd buy a $21 packet of tailies, break them all up, which would give us 40 grams of tobacco...then we'd re-roll them into smaller cigarettes which would make them stretch..." [23]
	"Say they took smokes out entirely, people are gonna start growing a black market... It's not gonna erase smoking. And you'll end up getting people buying it from overseas." [22]
	"It has opened up a road to price rise, black marketing, etc., of various tobacco products. Making the poor users hard to afford at the same time they can't quit taking tobacco." [32]
	"An illegal drug. Then they'll start having to traffic it and bring it from other countries." [20]
	"Yeah it won't make any major difference if you...import the tobacco from ah, other countries." [29]
	"...banning of sales of tobacco has led to making more profit to the shopkeepers, because I myself would not quit even after the products are banned. I kept going to the shops who sell secretly." [32]
4.2 Identifying relevant psychosocial factors	"Some kids...still smoking because...people in their household smoked." [20]
	"Cause there's still so many of them smoking, and still parents letting, you know, 12-year-olds smoke. I think that if that was addressed a little bit more…" [19]

(*Continued*)

Table 16.6 (*Continued*)

Subtheme	Original Quotations
	"...parents teach you not to smoke when you grow up. But then...you go and watch them smoking. So, you're like, 'I want to be like Mum...or Dad'...I feel bad for my sister 'cause...I know she smokes 'cause we all smoke in the house." [28]
	"Because of my mother, she also always smokes BRAND X and those were the first cigarettes that I tried and I became attached to them, more as a habit." [31]
	"The other reasons they might be smoking [such as stress brought on by economic hardship or racial discrimination] are not going to be mitigated by the policies that we are pushing...And I think the more that we ignore that, the more people are going to push back and fight the policies." [33]
	"Every young person I know who smokes...they either don't give up because of stress or they don't want to give up because it's their one opportunity to get outside, to...do something that brings them some stress relief." [30]
	"We're not going to get to zero unless we're actually really addressing...the reasons why they're still smoking." [20]
	"Just because people have to drive an extra 2 km to get their tobacco...they will still buy it...if you're a smoker and you want a cigarette, you're gonna walk that distance, aren't you?" [22]
4.3 Balancing between people's freedom and public interests	"How are you going to sell it politically in a climate where 'nanny-state' is poison?" [34]
	"It's a choice that we make for ourselves. It's not a choice that the government should be making for us." [25]
	"...this is not freedom. This is giving them a product that damages their health... It's not something good to do." [28]
	"It is kind of taking their choice away from them, but it is for a good cause, it is a good reason to do it." [28]
	"A choice, yes, totally agree, but I don't think people are informed enough to actually make that choice when it comes to tobacco..." [27]

Table 16.6 (*Continued*)

Subtheme	Original Quotations
	"[It's] a phrase coined by the tobacco industry as a way of... getting out of any responsibility for any tobacco sales or addiction made by people under 18. It's their scapegoat phrase." [27] "Cause all that does is just hurt predominantly poor people who are already struggling to pay their bills." [19] "Those communities that are hardest hit, most concentrated with tobacco permits...have the most advertising." [20] "What's really important, is to really begin to engage other folks that are impacted by commercial tobacco...and those include communities of colour. It includes LGBT communities. It includes other priority populations." [20]

16.3.4.2 *Subtheme 4.2 Identifying Relevant Psychosocial Factors*

Psychosocial factors that might hamper people to quit smoking encompassed: smoking in household, stress, addition, and perceived lack of freedom (Table 16.6). In many households, **parents regularly smoked**, and they allowed their children to smoke at young ages. Subsequently, the children developed the smoking behaviour. Similarly, several smokers testified that they began to smoke because they observed and mimicked their parents' smoking behaviour (Table 16.6).

Across the included studies, many participants identified "**addiction**" as a strong driving force for continued smoking despite tobacco regulations. Smokers admitted that "people will always find a way" [25]. Retailers regarded addiction as a main reason for the failure of tobacco legislation. According to retailers, smokers would be willing to travel long distances to obtain tobacco. Furthermore, some policymakers highlighted the need to identify underlying causes of smoking such as addiction, **stress** and day-to-day hardships. They felt that any legislation would not be successful without addressing underlying causes.

16.3.4.3 *Subtheme 4.3 Balancing Between People's Freedom and Public Interests*

Across the included studies, the issue of "nanny state" was raised in relation to smoke legislations (Table 16.6). Some smokers argued that their choices should not be made by the government. Other respondents viewed that the tobacco legislations would predominantly hurt low-income people who had been struggling to pay their bills. In this regard, policymakers argued that such communities were the main targets of commercial tobacco and, therefore, the legislations would be suitable. From policymakers' perspective, people's freedoms should not be violated. Nevertheless, the freedom should not be given to harmful matters, and many people have not been sufficiently informed about tobacco.

16.3.5 *Theme 5: Overcoming Barriers and Achieving Endgame Goals*

16.3.5.1 *Subtheme 5.1 Rendering Legislations and Regulations*

People anticipated government actions in terms of looking after their people, keeping them safe, preventing harm, minimising bureaucracy, and taking quick actions to serve taxpayers (Table 16.7). Furthermore, national policies should send clear statements, without mixed messages, especially to young adults. To achieve this, the intended messages should be complemented by appropriate legislation to clearly indicate the government's stance on tobacco. In addition to reducing demands, there is a need to decrease the supply, and relevant parties should think about "stronger supply-side management." Specifically, stronger actions are required to manage the powerful tobacco industries, which would fight very hard for their profits.

16.3.5.2 *Subtheme 5.2 Reaching Out and Engaging the Community Through Education*

To accomplish the Endgame strategies, there is a need to reach out and understand people in the communities. Smokers expressed various

Table 16.7 Overcoming barriers and achieving Endgame goals.

Subtheme	Original Quotations
5.1 Rendering legislations and regulations	"The government essentially is supposed to keep you safe, and they're not supposed to...make things readily available that are gonna actively harm you." [28] "Yes — I think the Government has [the] right to look after the people." [29] "Just, you know, keep your bureaucracy down to a minimum. Don't make it another body that swallows our taxes." [21] "It's sort of a contradiction. That it's bad for you, don't do it, yet it's sold everywhere and it's like a normal product." [27] "We can't be giving our young people messages around health and how it's not good for you when we actually allow it to be sold in our communities everywhere... Those two things don't sit together well." [30] "We have looked at demand...but we need to look at supply-side and [the]...regulation of that, or management of that in a better way. ....got to get politicians or the community to think about...stronger supply-side management." [34] "[it]...seems to more effectively reduce their [tobacco companies'] power base within the country." [34] "...there's tobacco companies. They've got so much power, so much money, they're going to fight it tooth [and nail]...every step of the way." [21]
5.2 Reaching out and Engaging the community through education	"If you talk to someone like face to face and give them advice that will be more effective. You just have like booths where you can meet people and talk with them and have a face-to-face conversation. They must be like, especially like ex-smokers: 'I just quit smoking. Come and talk to me, and I have like that experience and I can give you way better advice rather than because I don't smoke.'" [19] "People tend to look at you like in disgust if you are smoking. But a lot of them, they, they don't understand what it's actually like to be a smoker, and it's not as easy as just throwing them away and never smoking again." [25]

(*Continued*)

Table 16.7 (*Continued*)

Subtheme	Original Quotations
	"I'd felt a little bit embarrassed by them trying to give me support...cause I just didn't want to admit to myself that I was a smoker at the time...I didn't want to have that label on me." [25] "People don't necessarily reach out a hand to help someone that says, 'Ah, I don't wanna smoke,' you know? Like you can go and say, 'Hey, I've got a drug problem,' and you get...you know what I mean? But if you go to someone and say, 'Hey, I have...a smoking addiction,' people don't look at you like, 'Oh hey, I'll help you.' That's more of a, 'Oh, give up.' You know?" [25] "Beef up cessation services in a comprehensive way so that it is relevant to the communities that are most affected." [33] "The populations that have the least resources to come up to hours-long city council meetings." [33] "I think...that knowledge is better, having — putting the rules and regulation in place I think might have an adverse effect to what we're trying to get." [27] "Making that access [to risk information] um, readily available and constantly available...the proximity of that information to their daily lives is important." [27] "If smoking is off their radar screen in their everyday lives, it...is harder to engage them in the idea that they need to do more about it." [34] "...We want to actually — we want to find young people who are going to lead the country and the world, and you have to give them the tools to be able to do that. So it's, yeah, it's giving our young ones more tools." [30] "People get really upset when they feel they've been duped, especially young people." [30] "We are in a time of young people starting to kind of question the status quo around the power of big companies, and if there's a sense they're being used just to achieve profit for a large company, then there's potentially a useful message in there." [30]

concerns such as being afraid to admit the problem and to be labelled as "smoker"; feeling "embarrassed" to seek support concerning their smoking behaviour; being afraid of people's negative reactions; and feeling the lack of intentional support from people in communities. They requested for face-to-face meetings with people that could help them (such as ex-smokers) to help them overcome the smoking problem. Furthermore, they asked for "comprehensive services" in communities.

Policymakers valued strengthening smoke cessation services that tailored to minority groups. Engaging communities through education would be promising for vulnerable populations and regulations without community support might falter. Equipping people with knowledge would empower them to make better decisions and to follow regulations. Raising the awareness of smoking might create the urgency to take action against the tobacco issue in communities. Furthermore, policymakers perceived the potential to further the education to nurture young leaders to lead the Endgame and impact future generations.

16.3.6 *Quality of Evidence*

The strength of findings was assessed using GRADE-CERQual (Appendix A). Public perception of the Endgame goal, perspectives on Endgame strategies, barriers to achieving the Endgame and Endgame solutions were met with moderate confidence. Smokers' intention to quit were met with low confidence due to some concerns over methodology and adequacy; however, it was coherent and provided detailed and relevant data, therefore is suitable for use in this synthesis.

16.4 Discussion

This review aimed to explore people's perceptions towards the implementation of Tobacco Endgame strategies in different countries. 17 studies from five countries were included. Results from meta-synthesis derived five themes and seven subthemes. Most study participants (smokers, non-smokers and policymakers) supported the Tobacco Endgame goals, due to feelings of responsibility for future generations and public health.

The first two themes of this review concerned "Perception of Endgame Goal" and "Perspectives on Endgame Strategies". Diminishing tobacco accessibility, imposing complete tobacco ban, and establishing TFG were part of the Endgame strategies. The Incentive Salience Theory of Addiction postulated that day-to-day reward cues can trigger reward-seeking motivation, the "want" for tobacco [36]. While strategies to limit tobacco access help reduce tobacco reward cues, a complete tobacco ban and TFG methods remove reward cues completely. Overall, the TFG approach was envisioned as the most politically favourable because it did not penalise current smokers, and would only prevent the occurrence of future smokers.

Facilitating smokers' intention to quit became an emerging new theme in this review. Some people expressed their willingness to quit due to reduced access to tobacco, government legislation, among others. However, other smokers declined to quit given the government policy. The Psychological Reactance theory [38] can be used to explain the variations in smokers' behaviours. Specifically, the theory postulated that individuals react differently to unpleasant motivational stimuli that might affect their autonomy, freedom and self-determination. Smokers with high levels of psychological reactance would resist rigorous measures (such as the smoke-free goal) and they were more likely to continue to smoke.

Our finding highlights "Barriers to achieving the Endgame goals," including alternative sources of tobacco, psychological factors (parents' smoke behaviour, stress and addiction) and individual's perceived freedom. According to the Thorndike's Stimulus-Response Learning theory, [39] smoking is a learned behaviour and it can be developed into a habit. This highlights the urgency for effective legislations to send clear messages and to restrict tobacco use, breaking the cycle of the learned smoking habit in youths. Furthermore, stress might exacerbate tobacco use, perpetuating a negative reinforcement cycle [40] in smokers. Tobacco would provide temporary relief from stressors, and smokers return to smoking when they return to their previous aversive mental states caused by stressors [40].

Additionally, "Overcoming barriers and achieving Endgame goals" addressed strategies that could help mitigate barriers. Findings reveal that the public expects the government to protect its citizens, therefore pertinent messaging and policy strategies could be the watershed moment for public support and efficacy of legislation [41]. Eliminating existing mixed messaging is therefore crucial for Endgame success, reducing demand and hence crippling the tobacco industry, and complemented with education, engagement and support that are widely known to positively correlate with changes in smoking behaviour [42]. Integration of education, support and engagement with legislation is pivotal in ensuring its effectiveness and sustainability [43]. Strengthening engagement and social support may alleviate disparate effects of tobacco legislation due to existing social inequalities and address sociopolitical concerns, hence boosting public support for Endgame strategies. Appropriate education strategies equip the public with knowledge to make better decisions, further reducing the power of tobacco industries to manipulate the public for its continued profit [44].

16.4.1 *Strengths and Limitations*

This systematic review conducted a comprehensive search, entailing published, grey literature and other sources. Hence, it is less likely to face the issue of publication bias. Nevertheless, there are some methodological limitations. Specifically, most of the included studies were carried out in New Zealand, due to the novel nature of the topic. Findings may thus be skewed to suit the sociopolitical climate of New Zealand. However, findings from our review would enhance the understanding of the implementation of Tobacco Endgame strategies. Synthesised themes and subthemes may inform policymakers in other countries.

16.4.2 *Implications*

Our review suggested that only regulations or engagement alone was not sufficient to accomplish the Tobacco Endgame goals. The regulations targeting smokers might be perceived as threats, whilst the engagement strategies did not strictly enforce the tobacco law. Accordingly, we recommend that a combination of both strategies be implemented. Firstly, we recommend the increase of social support structures for youths, and to decrease any support for existing smokers. These strategies will prevent smoking in young adults. They will also break the negative reinforcement cycle among existing smokers and will create constructive ways to deal with daily stressors. Developing support groups in community settings may help vulnerable people to feel a sense of belonging, which may remove the need to smoke under social pressure.

Secondly, the TFG movement has garnered favourable feedback among leaders in New Zealand. Accordingly, we recommend other countries to consider implementing the TFG with an intensive public education campaign as a long-term Tobacco Endgame solution. This will minimise pressure on existing smokers to change their habits within the timeframe. Thirdly, more transparency between governments and their people is crucial to address underlying inequalities, allowing the government to exercise their right and responsibility to care for its people. Our findings suggested people might show greater willingness to support Tobacco Endgame policies given less bureaucracy, improved transparency, and more aid to vulnerable populations affected by Endgame policies. Fewer 'nanny state' arguments may arise, and policies may see more success.

16.4.3 *Recommendations for Future Research*

Future research may further investigate the effectiveness of Tobacco Endgame policy on various political climates, to further inform policy-makers for more countries. More research may delve into the effects of supply-side policies on the public, their perception before or after the

Endgame strategy implementation in conjunction with demand-side policies. Furthermore, more research may investigate underlying inequalities and equity issues hindering Endgame success, and how to best address them, to resolve systemic issues preventing elimination of tobacco use.

16.5 Conclusion

This systematic review highlights the perceptions of youths and adults on the Tobacco Endgame strategies, which received support from some participants. However, governments faced challenges of balancing regulation with engagement, and addressing underlying inequalities to ensure benefit to all demographics. More support should be provided to address underlying causes for continuing or initiating smoking, implementation of a politically feasible solution like TFG, with education and increased transparency between governments and its people, to protect public health and future generations.

References

1. Lariscy JT. Smoking-attributable mortality by cause of death in the United States: An indirect approach. SSM Popul Health. 2019;7:100349.
2. Murray CJL, Aravkin AY, Zheng P, *et al.* Global burden of 87 risk factors in 204 countries and territories, 1990–2019: A systematic analysis for the Global Burden of Disease Study 2019. Lancet. 2020;17:1223–49.
3. The global burden of tobacco [Internet]. The Lancet Public Health; 2021 [cited 2024 Sep 24]. Available from: https://www.thelancet.com/infographics-do/tobacco
4. World Health Organization. The WHO Framework Convention on Tobacco Control: A decade of saving lives [Internet]. 2015 [cited 2024 Sep 9]. Available from: https://www.who.int/hongkongchina/news/detail/25-02-2015-the-who-framework-convention-on-tobacco-control-a-decade-of-saving-lives
5. Hoffman SJ, Poirier MJP, Katwyk SRV, *et al.* Impact of the WHO Framework Convention on Tobacco Control on global cigarette consumption: Quasi-experimental evaluations using interrupted time series analysis and in-sample forecast event modelling. BMJ. 2019;19:l2287.

6. Moodie C, Angus K, Bauld L, *et al.* Plain tobacco packaging: A systematic review [Internet]. London: Public Health Research Consortium; 2012 [cited 2024 Sep 9]. Available from: http://eppi.ioe.ac.uk/cms/Default.aspx?tabid=3327
7. Puljević C, Morphett K, Hefler M, *et al.* Closing the gaps in tobacco endgame evidence: A scoping review. Tob Control. 2022;31:365–75.
8. Borland R. A strategy for controlling the marketing of tobacco products: A regulated market model. Tob Control. 2003;12:374–82.
9. Benowitz NL, Henningfield JE. Reducing the nicotine content to make cigarettes less addictive. Tob Control. 2013;15(Suppl 1):s14–s17.
10. Wilson N, Thomson GW, Edwards R, *et al.* Potential advantages and disadvantages of an endgame strategy: A "sinking lid" on tobacco supply. Tob Control. 2013;22(Suppl 1):s18–s21.
11. Berrick AJ. The tobacco-free generation proposal. Tob Control. 2013;22(Suppl 1):s22–s26.
12. Burstein P. The impact of public opinion on public policy. In: Princeton University Press eBooks. 2021. p. 325–45.
13. Jaine R, Healey B, Edwards R, *et al.* How adolescents view the tobacco endgame and tobacco control measures: Trends and associations in support among 14–15 year olds. Tob Control. 2014;24:449–54.
14. McDaniel PA, Smith EA, Malone RE. The tobacco endgame: A qualitative review and synthesis. Tob Control. 2015;25:594–604.
15. Munn Z. The JBI Approach to qualitative synthesis [Internet]. 2022 [cited 2024 Sep 9]. Available from: https://jbi-global-wiki.refined.site/space/MANUAL/4688131/2.4+The+JBI+Approach+to+qualitative+synthesis
16. Greenhalgh T, Robert G, Macfarlane F, *et al.* Storylines of research in diffusion of innovation: A meta-narrative approach to systematic review. Soc Sci Med. 2005;61:417–30.
17. Lachal J, Revah-Levy A, Orri M, *et al.* Metasynthesis: An original method to synthesize qualitative literature in psychiatry. Front Psychiatry. 2017;8:269.
18. McGowan J, Sampson M, Salzwedel DM, *et al.* PRESS peer review of electronic search strategies: 2015 guideline statement. J Clin Epidemiol. 2016;75:40–6.
19. Maubach N, Hoek JA, Edwards R, *et al.* "The times are changing": New Zealand smokers' perceptions of the tobacco endgame. Tob Control. 2012;22:395–400.
20. Smith EA, McDaniel PA, Malone RE. Leadership perceptions of endgame strategies for tobacco control in California. J Public Health Manag Pract. 2019;25:554–61.
21. Edwards R, Peace J, Russell M, *et al.* Qualitative exploration of public and smoker understanding of, and reactions to, an endgame solution to the tobacco epidemic. BMC Public Health. 2012;12:782.

22. Robertson L, Marsh L, Hoek J, *et al.* Regulating the sale of tobacco in New Zealand: A qualitative analysis of retailers' views and implications for advocacy. Int J Drug Policy. 2015;26:1222–30.
23. Gifford H, Waa A, Cvitanovic L, *et al.* Exploring Indigenous perspectives on tobacco tax: How some Māori families are responding in Aotearoa New Zealand. Tob Control. 2021;30:e144–9.
24. Chavez G, Minkler M, McDaniel PA, *et al.* Retailers' perspectives on selling tobacco in a low-income San Francisco neighbourhood after California's $2 tobacco tax increase. Tob Control. 2018;28:657–62.
25. Barbalich I, Gartner C, Edwards R, *et al.* New Zealand smokers' perceptions of tobacco endgame measures: A qualitative analysis. Nicotine Tob Res. 2021;24:93–9.
26. Timberlake DS, Laitinen U, Kinnunen JM, *et al.* Strategies and barriers to achieving the goal of Finland's tobacco endgame. Tob Control. 2020;29:398–404.
27. Hoek J, Ball J, Gray R, *et al.* Smoking as an "informed choice": Implications for endgame strategies. Tob Control. 2016;26:669–73.
28. Hoek J, Lee E, Teddy L, *et al.* How do New Zealand youth perceive the smoke-free generation policy? A qualitative analysis. Tob Control. 2022;33:346–52.
29. Guthrie J, Hoek J, Darroch E, *et al.* A qualitative analysis of New Zealand retailers' responses to standardised packaging legislation and tobacco industry opposition. BMJ Open. 2015;5:e009521.
30. Ball J, Hoek J, Tautolo ES, *et al.* New Zealand policy experts' appraisal of interventions to reduce smoking in young adults: A qualitative investigation. BMJ Open. 2017;7:e017837.
31. Van Hal G, Van Roosbroeck S, Vriesacker B, *et al.* Flemish adolescents' perceptions of cigarette plain packaging: A qualitative study with focus group discussions. BMJ Open. 2012;2:e001424.
32. Shimray RA. The effects of complete ban of smokeless tobacco products in the State of Manipur: A qualitative study. IOSR J Humanit Soc Sci. 2016;21: 10–20.
33. Smith EA, McDaniel PA, Malone RE. California advocates' perspectives on challenges and risks of advancing the tobacco endgame. J Public Health Policy. 2020;41:321–33.
34. Edwards R, Russell M, Thomson G, *et al.* Daring to dream: Reactions to tobacco endgame ideas among policy-makers, media and public health practitioners. BMC Public Health. 2011;11:580.
35. Perry J. Trust in public institutions: Trends and implications for economic security [Internet]. United Nations; 2021 [cited 2024 Sep 9]. Available from: https://www.un.org/development/desa/dspd/2021/07/trust-public-institutions/

36. Olney JJ, Warlow SM, Naffziger EE, *et al.* Current perspectives on incentive salience and applications to clinical disorders. Curr Opin Behav Sci. 2018;22: 59–69.
37. Steindl C, Jonas E, Sittenthaler S, *et al.* Understanding psychological reactance. Z Psychol. 2015;223:205–14.
38. Muncan B, Walters SM, Ezell J, *et al.* "They look at us like junkies": Influences of drug use stigma on the healthcare engagement of people who inject drugs in New York City. Harm Reduct J. 2020;17:53.
39. Nevin JA. Analyzing Thorndike's law of effect: The question of stimulus-response bonds. J Exp Anal Behav. 1999;72:447–50.
40. May AC, Aupperle RL, Stewart JL. Dark times: The role of negative reinforcement in methamphetamine addiction. Front Psychiatry. 2020;11:144.
41. Wood BH, Gardner J, Leask J, *et al.* Toward effective government communication strategies in the era of COVID-19. Humanit Soc Sci Commun. 2021;8:1–11.
42. Burns RJ, Rothman AJ, Fu SS, *et al.* The relation between social support and smoking cessation: Revisiting an established measure to improve prediction. Ann Behav Med. 2014;47:369–75.
43. UNESCO. Strengthening the rule of law through education: A guide for policymakers [Internet]. 2019 [cited 2024 Sep 9]. Available from: https://unesdoc.unesco.org/ark:/48223/pf0000366771
44. World Health Organization. Tobacco industry interference: A global brief [Internet]. 2012 [cited 2024 Sep 9]. Available from: https://paho.org/hq/dmdocuments/2012/WNTD-brochure.pdf

https://doi.org/10.1142/9789819817320_bmatter

Index